2023 Harvard Health Annual

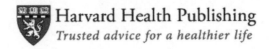

Harvard Health Publishing
Trusted advice for a healthier life

Harvard Health Annual 2023

Consulting Editor: Howard LeWine, M.D., Chief Medical Editor, Harvard Health Publishing,
and Editor in Chief, *Harvard Men's Health Watch*
Book Editor: Rebecca Shannonhouse

Faculty Editors:
Deepak L. Bhatt, M.D., M.P.H., Editor in Chief, *Harvard Heart Letter*
Toni Golen, M.D., Editor in Chief, *Harvard Women's Health Watch*
Anthony L. Komaroff, M.D., Editor in Chief, *Harvard Health Letter*

Contributing Editors:
Julie Corliss, Executive Editor, *Harvard Heart Letter*
Heidi Godman, Executive Editor, *Harvard Health Letter*
Maureen Salamon, Executive Editor, *Harvard Women's Health Watch*
Matthew Solan, Executive Editor, *Harvard Men's Health Watch*

ISBN 978-1-61401-305-1
10 9 8 7 6 5 4 3 2 1

This publication is intended to provide readers with accurate and timely medical news and information. It is not intended to give personal medical advice, which should be obtained directly from a licensed health care provider. We regret that we cannot respond to individual inquiries about personal health matters. Websites listed in this book are accurate at the time of publication.

Table of Contents

1   **Foreword**

3   **Chapter 1:** Inflammation

21   **Chapter 2:** Mind, Memory, and Mood

47   **Chapter 3:** Blood Pressure and Cholesterol

67   **Chapter 4:** Cardiovascular Health

95   **Chapter 5:** Smart Eating

125   **Chapter 6:** Pain Management for Arthritis and More

153   **Chapter 7:** Cancer Prevention and Early Detection

177   **Chapter 8:** Fit and Active

210   **Chapter 9:** Women's Health

239   **Chapter 10:** Men's Health

267   **Chapter 11:** Healthy Habits

282   **Chapter 12:** Health and Wellness Technology

299   **Chapter 13:** Savvy Patient

Foreword

If you've fallen behind on health screenings and the lifestyle habits that will give you the best odds of achieving and maintaining good health, you're not alone. Like many others, you might have been so busy just trying to adapt to the changing landscape of the pandemic that you may have missed out on recent research findings that can help optimize your health. Maybe you've also had a difficult time keeping up with all your routine medical care and now realize that you've lost ground on your long-term health goals. The good news is that it's not too late to reset your priorities. This year's annual will help bring you up to date on actionable health information that will get you back on course.

For example, a growing body of evidence demonstrates that inflammation, a normal physiological process that's long been recognized for its role in healing, can have dire health consequences when it simmers within the body in a chronic state. Research has found that many less-than-desirable daily habits, such as an unhealthy diet, sedentary lifestyle, and persistent stress, promote chronic inflammation. This, in turn, is linked to the development of some of our most challenging diseases, including heart disease, dementia, and diabetes.

To give you insights into the health risks of chronic inflammation and the steps you can take to protect yourself, this year's annual includes an entire chapter devoted to the topic. Here, you'll learn important facts, including:

- The effect that chronic inflammation has on your heart, brain, and joints
- The foods you can eat to help dampen the negative effects of chronic inflammation
- The factors you should consider when deciding whether to get a blood test that measures a biomarker of chronic inflammation.

Because our health is so profoundly affected by our daily habits, we've also included a chapter covering healthy habits that are designed to keep our bodies and minds functioning at their highest levels. For example, how often do you forget to get enough fluids throughout the day? Do you go to bed each night at the optimal time for your heart health? How often do you use one of the most effective methods for helping combat stress? You'll find answers to all these questions—and more—in the healthy habits chapter.

In addition, this year's annual includes a chapter on noteworthy advancements in health and wellness technology. Here, you'll learn about the ways in which virtual reality is now being used to effectively treat chronic pain, the various easy-to-use gadgets that can help you cope when your memory is fuzzy, the precautions you should take if you rely on a wearable device to detect atrial fibrillation, and other updates on technology that can offer new solutions for your health needs.

As part of our dedication to exceptionally high standards for health information, we also seek to include in this book the scientific research that may not have attracted the level of attention it deserves. In this year's annual, you'll read about many topics that have slipped beneath the public's radar, such as recent findings on the effect of loneliness on one's risk for dementia and why it's so important to be screened for prediabetes.

Along with this, you'll read about the ways in which medical professionals are refining the traditional warnings on body fat and looking beyond numerical blood pressure targets to create a more individualized risk profile for heart disease. To clear up widespread misconceptions about the use of low-dose aspirin to help reduce heart attack and stroke risk, you'll get a clear-eyed, evidence-based description of the people who can benefit most from aspirin therapy and those for whom the increased risk for serious side effects outweighs aspirin's potential benefit. You'll also learn about promising research on new drug treatments for heart failure, the leading cause of hospitalization for adults over age 65.

We all know, however, that staying healthy requires more than simply taking a pill. Exercise is one of the most effective—yet under-utilized—"prescriptions" for good health. I'm not an athlete, but I exercise almost daily. That's because it not only makes me feel good, but I also recognize the powerful, wide-ranging benefits exercise provides—especially for my heart and brain. Whether you exercise regularly or don't even own a pair of walking shoes, you'll find information in these pages that will help take you to the next level of physical fitness. If you're looking to ramp up your daily activity, there's excellent advice in these pages on creating achievable, yet meaningful fitness goals. If you already exercise, you'll learn about the smartest ways to avoid injuries and often-overlooked activities that will help keep your workouts fun and engaging.

Of course, we'd be remiss if we didn't also include fresh new approaches to nutrition. The food choices you make every day have a powerful impact on your strength and vitality but also your body's ability to withstand various diseases. Maintaining a healthy diet doesn't have to be a chore. In fact, you'll find various approaches to make your meals and snacks not only nutritious but also downright delicious.

This is just a sampling of all the information included in this year's *Harvard Health Annual*. We hope that you will take full advantage of the potentially life-changing recommendations you'll find in these pages. While the book is designed to be read in its entirety, the table of contents and index make it easy to return to the chapters that are most applicable to you and your family.

We encourage you to use the annual to help formulate questions for your own doctors and deepen your partnership with your medical professionals. There's the saying that "it takes a village to raise a child." It could also be said that it takes a "village" to live your healthiest and best life. We are proud to share our wisdom with you—and to be a part of the team that not only helps keep you informed but also cheers you on toward greater health and well-being!

Howard E. LeWine MD

Howard LeWine, M.D.
Harvard Medical School

Chapter 1
Inflammation

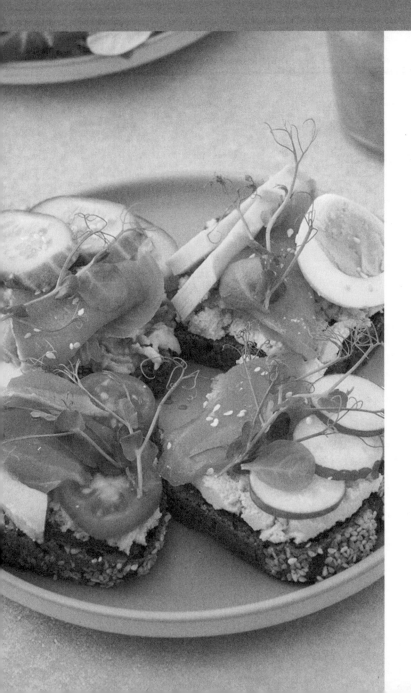

Take Action!
5 Things You Can Do Now

1 **Avoid processed foods.** They are pro-inflammatory and can contribute to joint pain and swelling. (page 5)

2 **Eat a Mediterranean-style diet.** High intake of fruits, vegetables, and healthy fats helps dampen chronic inflammation. (page 8)

3 **Beware of home CRP kits.** Self-testing for this inflammation marker may lead to misinterpretation. (page 11)

4 **Take steps to reduce stress.** Curbing stress and adopting a healthy lifestyle can lower the inflammation response. (page 13)

5 **Schedule dedicated exercise times on your calendar.** Regular exercise turns down the heat of chronic inflammation. (page 18)

A brief history of inflammation

Inflammation is hardly a new discovery. In the first century, Roman physician Aulus Cornelius Celsus first described the four hallmark signs or "pillars" of inflammation: rubor (redness), tumor (swelling), calor (heat), and dolor (pain). This simplistic definition was based on symptoms, rather than an understanding of the deeper physiological processes. Two centuries later, Galen, the physician to Roman emperor Marcus Aurelius, recognized that inflammation was the body's response to injury.

Until the beginning of the 19th century, much of the thinking around inflammation was based on speculation and reasoning, rather than on true science. It wasn't until technological advances enabled scientists to peer through microscopes and witness the actual cellular activities at work during inflammatory reactions that the scientific underpinnings of the process began to emerge. Scientists watched in wonder as white blood cells migrated to the site of the injury or infection, where some started gobbling up germs, while others swept up cellular debris. Biologists postulated that inflammation wasn't a single event, as had been previously assumed, but rather a series of steps that started with an injury to the tissues and ended with their repair.

In 1871, Rudolf Virchow, the German scientist known as the "father of modern pathology," added a fifth sign to Celsus's four: loss of function in the affected area. He described the process of inflammation as a manifestation of disease arising from the release of nutrients from damaged blood vessels, which caused a rush of cells to the site. Virchow was also the first to surmise that, while short-term (acute) inflammation promoted healing, long-term (chronic) inflammation could have damaging implications, including the development of cancer.

While pathologists studied the ways in which the human body responds to disease and injury, and immunologists investigated how the immune system reacts to foreign invaders, the fledgling pharmaceutical industry of the 19th century began searching for ways to dampen inflammation. Although aspirin had been discovered in the late 1890s and used for joint inflammation, a highlight of drug discovery came in 1962, when Merck researchers identified a rodent model on which they could test potential anti-inflammatory medications. This model dramatically sped up the drug development process and led to the introduction a year later of the nonsteroidal

Diseases linked to chronic inflammation

When you have chronic inflammation, your body is in a constant state of high alert. The release of inflammatory chemicals can affect many different systems in your body and be a cause or consequence of multiple diseases.

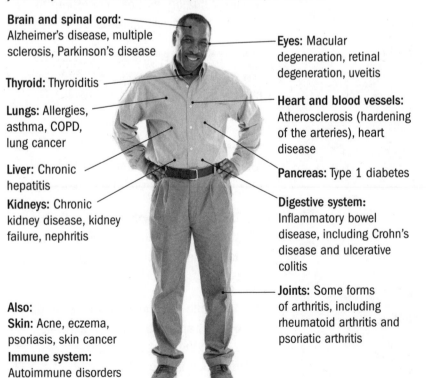

Brain and spinal cord: Alzheimer's disease, multiple sclerosis, Parkinson's disease

Thyroid: Thyroiditis

Lungs: Allergies, asthma, COPD, lung cancer

Liver: Chronic hepatitis

Kidneys: Chronic kidney disease, kidney failure, nephritis

Also:
Skin: Acne, eczema, psoriasis, skin cancer
Immune system: Autoimmune disorders such as lupus

Eyes: Macular degeneration, retinal degeneration, uveitis

Heart and blood vessels: Atherosclerosis (hardening of the arteries), heart disease

Pancreas: Type 1 diabetes

Digestive system: Inflammatory bowel disease, including Crohn's disease and ulcerative colitis

Joints: Some forms of arthritis, including rheumatoid arthritis and psoriatic arthritis

anti-inflammatory drug (NSAID) indomethacin (Indocin), which is still used to treat gout and other inflammatory conditions today. However, the mechanism behind the effects of indomethacin and aspirin remained elusive until the 1970s, when pharmacologist John Vane discovered that these drugs work by blocking the production of pain-promoting hormones called prostaglandins. His finding led to the development of ibuprofen (Advil, Motrin), naproxen (Aleve), and the more than 20 other NSAIDs we now have available to reduce inflammation.

In our time, scientists have also elucidated the role genetics plays in the inflammatory process and the benefits of lifestyle choices like diet and exercise in controlling it. Today, we realize that inflammation encompasses a complex interplay of many different events, by which tissue damage activates signals that launch and perpetuate the immune response to both eliminate the threat and repair damaged tissues. We have tools at our disposal that no other generation has had for understanding and dealing with inflammation.

Chronic inflammation and your joints

Why the immune system is sometimes the culprit in joint pain.

When you suffer a joint injury—maybe a banged-up knee or a twisted ankle—a little inflammation is part of the healing process. Puffy, red, tender joints may indicate that your immune system is working to remove damage and promote the growth of new tissue, a healthy kind of inflammation. But sometimes the immune system launches unhealthy, chronic inflammation in the joints, for no apparent reason. This leads to pain, stiffness, and joint damage known as inflammatory arthritis.

The attack on joints

It's often unknown what triggers the immune system to unleash an assault on the joints, but we do know what the cells are up to once they're in action.

"In a common type of inflammatory arthritis like rheumatoid arthritis, a variety of immune cells can be found in the lining and fluid of the joint. These cells attract other immune cells and together lead to thickening of the joint lining, new blood vessel formation, and—ultimately—joint damage," says rheumatologist Dr. Robert Shmerling, medical editor of the Harvard Special Health Report *Fighting Inflammation* (www.health.harvard.edu/ui).

Chronic inflammation in the joints can damage cartilage, bones, tendons (which attach muscle to bones), or ligaments (which hold joints together);

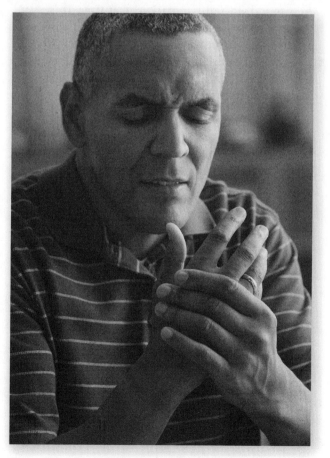

Rheumatoid arthritis often causes hand and wrist pain.

irritate nerves; and produce a long list of symptoms, including pain, swelling, and stiffness. The joint damage may be progressive and irreversible.

Types

There are many types of inflammatory arthritis. Common ones include these:

Rheumatoid arthritis (RA). RA occurs when the immune system attacks the lining of the joints, especially in the hands, wrists, and feet. RA may also affect the heart, lungs, and eyes.

Gout. Gout is characterized by a buildup of uric acid, which can form crystals in the joints—especially in the big toe, and sometimes in the hands, wrists, or knees. The crystals activate a temporary inflammatory response that can become chronic.

Calcium pyrophosphate deposition disease (CPPD, or pseudogout). In CPPD, calcium crystals settle in the joints, especially the knee, wrist, shoulder, ankle, or elbow. Like the uric acid crystals in gout, the calcium crystals in CPPD prompt the body to respond with inflammation; over time, this may become chronic.

Psoriatic arthritis. About 30% of people with psoriasis (an autoimmune condition that causes raised patches of scaly skin) develop psoriatic arthritis, which can affect the knees, ankles, wrists, or fingers.

What about osteoarthritis?

Osteoarthritis, a wearing away of the smooth cartilage lining joints, has long been considered a noninflammatory form of arthritis. "But we now recognize that some inflammatory cells are present in osteoarthritis, although the inflammation is usually much less dramatic than in rheumatoid arthritis or other types of inflammatory arthritis," Dr. Shmerling says.

The finding of mild chronic inflammation in osteoarthritis has been significant enough for researchers to begin investigating whether the condition can be treated with some of the same types of medications used to treat inflammatory arthritis.

Treatment

Many types of drugs are used to treat inflammatory arthritis. They include

- nonsteroidal anti-inflammatory drugs (NSAIDs), such as ibuprofen (Advil, Motrin), which reduce levels of prostaglandins—chemicals that promote inflammation
- oral or injected steroids, which reduce inflammation and suppress the immune system
- injections or intravenous infusions of nonbiologic disease-modifying antirheumatic drugs (DMARDs), such as methotrexate (Rheumatrex, Trexall), which suppress the immune system
- injections or infusions of biologic DMARDs, antibodies such as adalimumab (Humira) that suppress the immune system in a more targeted way than nonbiologic DMARDs
- Janus kinase (JAK) inhibitors, such as tofacitinib (Xeljanz), which interrupt inflammatory signals
- drugs that lower uric acid levels (for gout).

Results with drug treatment are often good. "Medications to lower uric acid can essentially eliminate gout. And the development of newer drugs for rheumatoid arthritis, including biologics and Janus kinase inhibitors, makes it possible for far more people than in the past to experience remission and protection from ongoing joint damage," Dr. Shmerling says.

Other ways to live with arthritis

Other ways to help reduce pain and inflammation include exercising, avoiding processed foods (which promote inflammation), reducing stress, not smoking, and getting enough sleep. Wearing a splint or brace on affected joints and seeking physical therapy may also ease your pain and keep you mobile and active.

An anti-inflammatory diet may be good for your joints

Changing your diet can't cure conditions like arthritis, but it may help prevent or manage them.

Foods that reduce inflammation inside the body are all the rage these days—and for good reason. Eating these foods over time has been linked to a lower risk of numerous health conditions, including heart and blood vessel problems and chronic diseases such as diabetes.

But can a diet rich in anti-inflammatory foods also help your joints?

"Research seems to show a benefit when it comes to prevention," says Natalie McCormick, a research fellow in medicine at Harvard Medical School. "Studies, such as the Nurses' Health Study, have found that not only can an anti-inflammatory diet help to prevent arthritis, but it may also prevent conditions like heart disease and diabetes that people with arthritis are more likely to develop."

Eat a healthy diet over the years, and you may be less prone to conditions such as gout or other types of arthritis. The benefit is less clear if you've got joint problems already, says McCormick. But it may still help.

"Diet can be part of disease management," she says. "But it's not necessarily a cure-all for joint pain on its own."

Understanding inflammation

Inflammation inside the body occurs when your immune system leaps into action to heal an infection or injury by sending in an army of white blood cells. If you have a cut, the area around it may turn red or swell as this healing process occurs. But once the problem is under control, inflammation recedes, and your body returns to normal.

Chronic inflammation is not so helpful to your

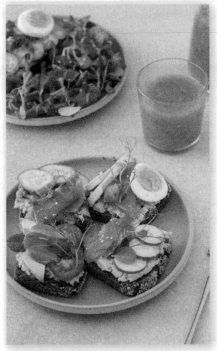

What you eat might affect the health of your joints.

body. If you are under chronic stress, are obese, or have an autoimmune disorder, inflammation doesn't go away. It persists, damaging the body and potentially leading to problems such as arthritis, heart disease, or cancer.

Eating the right diet may help to switch off this inflammatory process, protecting your body from harm. There are still many unknowns about how the food you eat relates to the levels of inflammation in your body. But evidence of a potential benefit is growing.

"When researchers first started looking at diets that produced anti-inflammatory effects, they were interested in whether they could reduce heart disease and cancer. But over the years, other benefits have emerged," says McCormick. This includes the protection that these diets may afford the joints.

Some painful joint conditions are potentially triggered or exacerbated by inflammation in the body. For example, gout, which is caused by a buildup of a substance called uric acid, occurs when tiny crystals form in the joints. These crystals irritate the tissues in the joint and can trigger chronic inflammation. Even osteoarthritis, which was once thought of as just wear and tear on joints, is now known to be associated with chronic inflammation, albeit less than what is seen in other types of arthritis.

Choosing the right diet

There are two main dietary patterns that are thought to produce anti-inflammatory benefits, says McCormick. These are the Mediterranean diet and the

DASH diet. The Alternative Healthy Eating Index, which measures diet quality, can also be used to work toward a similar healthy eating pattern that has been shown to improve health—lots of fruits and vegetables; healthy fats, such as olive oil; whole grains; and lean meats, fish, and legumes. These diets don't include many of the foods in a Western-style diet, such as highly processed and sugary foods and drinks and red and processed meats.

Researchers have noted a reduction in various measures of inflammation inside the body, such as a substance called C-reactive protein, in people who regularly opt for an anti-inflammatory dietary pattern. People who eat a Western-style diet have seen the opposite effect. Over time, a healthy dietary pattern may reduce your risk of developing a painful joint condition. An anti-inflammatory eating pattern over the years may cut your risk of gout by as much as 60%, says McCormick.

A steady diet of anti-inflammatory foods may also help to reduce joint pain for people living with osteoarthritis and potentially slow the progression of damage. To get the most benefit, you've got to eat a variety of anti-inflammatory foods, ideally over a number of years, she says. While questions still need to be answered about the role of food in fighting inflammation, what is known is that the foods that appear to reduce inflammation also tend to be good for you for other reasons. So, there is really no drawback to adding more of these foods into your daily meal plan.

You don't necessarily have to pick one anti-inflammatory diet over another, says McCormick. Rather, you can mix and match elements to suit your personal lifestyle and tastes. Red meats and sugary beverages are associated with increased risk of gout, says McCormick. So, you should eliminate those if possible. Choosing a healthy eating pattern may have broad health benefits protecting against a variety of conditions.

"You don't have to choose one type of food to prevent one condition and something else for another," she says.

Foods that fight inflammation

Load your meals with healthy foods that offer maximum inflammation-fighting potential.

In the fight against chronic inflammation—a state of persistent activation of the immune system—your diet is a powerful weapon. Eating healthy foods helps quiet chronic inflammation, and it benefits your health in other ways (like lowering cholesterol levels). Chronic inflammation often is seen with, and may contribute to, chronic diseases such as diabetes, cardiovascular disease, and cognitive decline.

Where do you find inflammation-fighting foods? They're all part of a Mediterranean-style diet, which consists of fruits, vegetables, legumes, whole grains, nuts, seeds, lean proteins, and small amounts of dairy foods and olive oil.

"Plant-based foods provide us with vitamins, minerals, fiber, and phytochemicals—plant chemicals that appear to fight free radicals [molecules that damage cells] and may protect our cells against inflammation, cancer growth, and viruses," says

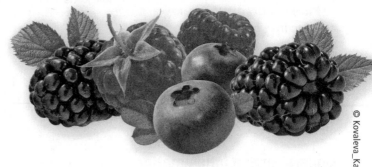

Berries contain anthocyanins, which have anti-inflammatory effects.

Kathy McManus, director of the Department of Nutrition at Harvard-affiliated Brigham and Women's Hospital. "Fish, nuts, and plant oils contain healthy unsaturated fats, which are good for your blood vessels, heart, and brain."

Here are some foods that support the quest to keep inflammation in check.

Berries

Strawberries, raspberries, blueberries, and blackberries may just seem like sweet treats. But berries are also hard-working inflammation fighters. Berries contain phytochemicals called anthocyanins, which give the fruits their red and purple hues. Anthocyanins have an anti-inflammatory effect on cells and are associated with lower risks of heart disease, cognitive decline, and diabetes.

Fatty fish

Fatty fish—such as salmon, tuna, and sardines—are abundant sources of omega-3 fatty acids, which have been shown to reduce cardiovascular disease risk. That benefit might be due to reduced inflammation in the body, especially in the blood vessels (protecting them against the buildup of plaque).

Some evidence has found that eating fatty fish is associated with lower levels of C-reactive protein, an inflammatory marker in the blood.

Leafy greens

Green leafy vegetables—such as arugula, chard, kale, and spinach—are loaded with vitamins A, B, C, E, and K, as well as important minerals (iron, magnesium, and potassium) and phytochemicals. Spinach is associated with a reduction in inflammation levels over time, slowed cognitive decline, and reduced risks for coronary artery disease and stroke.

Nuts and seeds

Tiny but mighty, nuts and seeds (such as pistachios, almonds, sunflower seeds, and pumpkin seeds) are rich in fiber and other nutrients that help keep your gut bacteria healthy and in turn may help tamp down brain inflammation. Certain nuts and seeds—such as walnuts, flaxseeds, chia seeds, and hemp seeds—are also good sources of omega-3 fatty acids.

What to eat

To get enough foods that fight inflammation, eat at least two servings of fatty fish per week and at least five servings of fruits and vegetables per day (two fruits, three vegetables). It's okay to enjoy a handful of nuts or seeds each day. And you'll want to bulk up on fiber sources, such as legumes like beans and lentils (women older than 50 need 21 grams of fiber per day; men need 30 grams per day).

"For the most impact, get the widest variety of plant-based foods possible in each meal. For example, make a big green salad with several kinds of greens and colorful vegetables, seeds, berries, and a simple dressing of a little olive oil and vinegar," McManus suggests. "Or cook whole grains such as quinoa or brown rice, and stir in the greens of your choice, beans, and colorful vegetables like carrots, squash, and tomatoes."

It's easiest to toss extra plant foods into a meal when you have them on hand. "If produce seems to spoil faster than you can use it, keep it in your freezer, divided into small amounts. That way, you can reach for fruits and vegetables when you need them," says McManus.

And as much as possible, avoid eating processed foods. They typically contain high amounts of calories, added sugars, unhealthy saturated fats, and salt, and are associated with chronic inflammation.

Autoimmune conditions and heart disease

Threats to the heart may be under-treated in people with conditions that boost inflammation.

When the body's immune system goes awry and mistakenly attacks its own tissues, it triggers an outpouring of white blood cells and other substances. Known as inflammation, this largely invisible, insidious process is the hallmark of autoimmune systemic inflammatory diseases (see "Mysterious immune system misfires" on the next page).

Inflammation is also at the heart of cardiovascular disease. When fatty plaque builds up inside arteries, the body perceives it as foreign and enlists a similar arsenal of white blood cells. These further ignite an inflammatory response, creating conditions that encourage the blood clots that are responsible for most heart attacks and strokes.

So it's perhaps not surprising that people with autoimmune inflammatory diseases are more likely to have heart attacks and to die of cardiovascular disease than people in the general population. Growing recognition of this problem—and the related treatment challenges for affected patients—has spurred a new specialty known as cardio-rheumatology, says Dr. Katherine Liao, codirector of the Cardiovascular Rheumatology Clinic at Harvard-affiliated Brigham and Women's Hospital.

"For many years, there weren't good therapies for rheumatoid arthritis and related inflammatory diseases," she says. But that changed about two decades ago, with the development of targeted drugs known as biologics that modify the body's response to inflammation. With these improved therapies, people started living longer. Soon, cardiovascular disease emerged as a leading cause of death for people with these conditions.

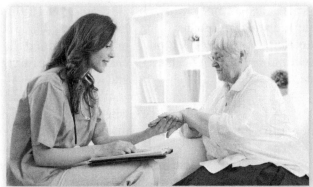

Autoimmune conditions such as psoriasis and rheumatoid arthritis may worsen heart disease.

© vgajic | Getty Images

More deadly heart attacks

Heart attacks are twice as likely to be fatal in younger adults with systemic inflammatory conditions, according to a study co-authored by Dr. Liao in the March 30, 2021, *European Journal of Preventive Cardiology*. People with inflammatory conditions were more likely to have higher blood pressure, but they had similar rates of high cholesterol and diabetes compared with people without inflammatory disease.

Just like diabetes, systemic inflammatory conditions such as psoriasis, lupus, and rheumatoid arthritis should be considered "risk enhancers" when it comes to estimating a person's odds of heart problems. Still, the heart risks from these less-common conditions may be underappreciated. In the recent study, people with inflammatory diseases were less likely to be prescribed aspirin and statins, although both can help lower the risk of a repeat heart attack.

Treatment options

Currently, there aren't clear guidelines about how to best prevent and manage cardiovascular disease in people with systemic inflammatory diseases beyond what is recommended for the general population.

Mysterious immune system misfires

Your immune system normally protects your body against viruses, bacteria, and other invaders. But sometimes immune cells launch an inappropriate attack against the body's own tissues. The resulting conditions, known as autoimmune systemic inflammatory diseases, include these:

Psoriasis. The inflammation in psoriasis affects the skin, causing a pink or dull-red, scaly skin rash that occurs in patches, usually on the back of the elbow, in skin folds, and on the scalp. About one in three people with psoriasis also has a type of inflammatory arthritis known as psoriatic arthritis, which causes joint inflammation (especially in the fingers, toes, or knees) and morning stiffness in addition to the characteristic rash.

Rheumatoid arthritis. The immune system attack targets tissue lining the joints, creating inflammation marked by swelling, pain, and stiffness. It typically strikes multiple joints at once, especially in the hands and feet. Other symptoms include morning stiffness that lasts more than an hour and fatigue.

Systemic lupus erythematosus. The inflammatory process in lupus can affect almost any organ in the body, triggering a wide array of symptoms. Common early symptoms include fever and joint pain similar to rheumatoid arthritis. One distinct symptom is a rash across the bridge of the nose and cheeks, called a "butterfly rash." The immune system attack can also damage the heart, lungs, kidneys, and blood vessels.

Some medications used to treat rheumatoid arthritis and related conditions may lower the risk for dying from heart disease, including methotrexate (Rheumatrex, Trexall) and biologic drugs known as TNF-alfa inhibitors. These include infliximab (Remicade), adalimumab (Humira), and etanercept (Enbrel).

Nonsteroidal anti-inflammatory drugs (NSAIDs), which include ibuprofen (Advil, Motrin), naproxen (Aleve, Naprosyn), and celecoxib (Celexa), may be prescribed to control pain and swelling. But these drugs can raise blood pressure and are linked to a higher risk of a heart attack. At Dr. Liao's clinic, cardiologists and rheumatologists work closely together to provide the best possible care for people with both conditions.

Should you monitor this chronic inflammation marker?

Think twice before getting a C-reactive protein test on your own.

Chronic inflammation is the common denominator in many diseases, and you might be tempted to get a blood test to gauge your risk. It's easy enough: in many states, certain labs will test you for an inflammation marker called C-reactive protein (CRP) without an order from your doctor. Just be careful. Self-ordered CRP tests come with some real pitfalls.

What is CRP testing?

CRP is a protein your liver makes when it senses injury, infection, or inflammation in the body. The protein helps the immune system heal the injury or fight the infection.

CRP levels can increase substantially in response to everything from a cold or a bad cut to autoimmune disease, cancer, heart disease, or obesity.

Doctors order a test measuring CRP—sometimes called a high-sensitivity C-reactive protein (hsCRP) test—to monitor many different health conditions. For example, CRP may be measured (among other blood markers) to assess how active rheumatoid arthritis is, or to see how well medications that

---

IN THE JOURNALS

Beyond blood pressure: Added benefits from the DASH diet

The Dietary Approaches to Stop Hypertension (DASH) eating pattern doesn't just lower blood pressure. It also reduces inflammation, heart injury, and heart strain, according to a study published in the June 1, 2021, *Journal of the American College of Cardiology.*

Long considered one of the healthiest diets for the heart, the DASH diet features whole grains, fruits, vegetables, and low-fat dairy products as well as fish, poultry, beans, nuts, and healthy oils. For the study, researchers measured three cardiovascular biomarkers (substances known to reflect heart health) in stored blood samples from the original DASH study in the late 1990s. Participants followed either a DASH diet or a typical American diet, and within those two groups, each was assigned to one of three sodium levels (low, medium, or high) for four weeks.

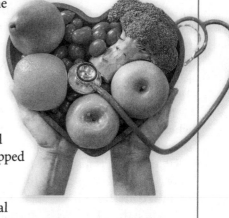

Among people on the DASH diet, biomarkers linked to heart injury and inflammation dropped by 18% and 13%, respectively, compared with a typical diet. Biomarkers for heart injury and heart strain went down 20% to 23% among those following the low-sodium DASH diet.

reduce inflammation are working. CRP is also used as a predictor of cardiovascular disease, heart attack, or stroke. For someone with an intermediate risk for cardiovascular disease, the CRP test can help a doctor decide whether to prescribe medicine to help reduce the risk.

Self-ordered tests

Increasingly, CRP tests are marketed to health-conscious consumers as a way of determining whether they have chronic inflammation. There are two ways to get one of these self-ordered tests.

One way is at certain "anytime" walk-in labs. A customer simply makes an appointment to have blood drawn, then pays for the test out of pocket (cost: about $40 to $80).

Another is from an online lab that will send a collection kit (cost: $40 to $60). When the collection kit arrives, the customer uses a finger-prick method to obtain a small blood sample, then mails the sample to the lab.

To get results, the customer logs on to the lab's website, or the lab might call or send a letter.

Potential problems

Getting a self-ordered CRP test comes with downsides. One is cost: many health insurers will not cover self-ordered tests, and you need to pay up front when you order one. Here are other potential problems.

Home kits may lead to errors. "Collecting a blood sample at home with a finger stick can introduce errors that affect the final results. For example, if you have to 'milk' your finger to obtain more blood, you might dilute the blood with other fluids, which would mean your sample may have a falsely decreased amount of important blood markers," says Dr. Nader Rifai, a professor of pathology at Harvard Medical School and a pioneer in CRP testing.

It's not the whole story. While a lab will tell you what your CRP level is, it won't explain what that snapshot of inflammation means for your health. A CRP test result is just one piece of evidence, and it may conflict with other evidence, especially in certain conditions.

"While the CRP level is one marker of how active rheumatoid arthritis is, the CRP level is sometimes normal even when rheumatoid arthritis is active, and high even when other evidence shows that the arthritis is inactive," notes rheumatologist Dr. Robert Shmerling, associate professor of medicine at Harvard Medical School and medical editor of the Harvard Special Health Report *Fighting Inflammation* (www.health.harvard.edu/ui).

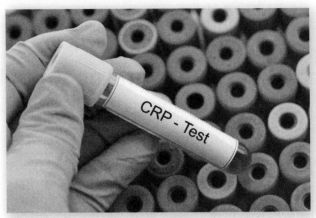

C-reactive protein, a marker of inflammation, can be measured with a simple blood test.

Results may cause anxiety. Seeing a lab result that indicates a high CRP level, without talking to your doctor about it, may provoke unnecessary feelings of distress.

Results could create a false sense of security. For example: "If the test result comes back in the lower cardiovascular disease risk range, it's not a guarantee that you're out of the woods and can forget about preventive measures," says Dr. Peter Libby, a cardiologist at Harvard-affiliated Brigham and Women's Hospital, whose research has helped explain the role of inflammation in cardiovascular disease.

It might lead to unnecessary treatment. "If people get a CRP test on their own and it's a little high, I'm concerned they may go buy supplements with unproven value that contain hidden unhealthy ingredients," Dr. Libby says. "Or maybe they'll get an unnecessary imaging test that doesn't need their doctor's order, which exposes them to radiation."

What you should do

If you're interested in measuring your CRP for any reason, talk to your doctor about it first. Perhaps the doctor will agree the test would be useful, and can order a test at a trusted lab that's covered by your insurance or is less expensive than tests from walk-in or online labs.

What if you're healthy and just curious about your CRP level? It might be better to keep your curiosity from getting the best of you. "It's not at all clear that looking for evidence of low-grade inflammation in a person without a suspicion of inflammatory disease is a good idea," Dr. Shmerling says.

"It would frustrate me if people plunk down their dollars on tests that may lead to aggravation and anxiety, but they don't do the simple things to fight chronic inflammation," Dr. Libby says. "I'd rather that they exercise regularly, eat a healthy diet, get sufficient sleep, don't smoke, limit alcohol intake, and take their prescribed medications."

Can medication tame chronic inflammation?

The answer isn't "yes" for everyone. Here's what you need to know about it.

Many diseases are marked by chronic inflammation—the persistent activation of the immune system.

Although we have lots of medications to quiet acute (short-term) inflammation—like an attack of gout—they're not often effective in preventing chronic inflammation. And some people don't realize that. "I've had patients come in and say, 'I keep reading that inflammation is a killer. Can you give me something for it?' There's a lot of misconception about it," notes Dr. Robert Shmerling, a rheumatologist and medical editor of the Harvard Special Health Report *Fighting Inflammation* (www.health.harvard.edu/ui).

Medications

There are many medications to manage inflammatory disease. Here are some of the most common.

Nonsteroidal anti-inflammatory drugs (NSAIDs). NSAIDs, such as ibuprofen (Advil, Motrin), inhibit compounds called prostaglandins that promote inflammation. "You might need ibuprofen to treat rheumatoid arthritis, especially if you're waiting for other medications to work better or deciding which medications to take," Dr. Shmerling says. NSAID risks, especially when taken long-term, include stomach ulcers, bleeding, and heart attacks.

Corticosteroids. These very powerful anti-inflammatory drugs, such as prednisone, suppress the immune system's ability to cause inflammation. They may be taken orally or by injection to treat inflammation that occurs anywhere—including the heart, lungs, feet (such as with gout), or gastrointestinal tract (for inflammatory bowel disease symptoms). You can also get joint injections of steroids to tame arthritis flare-ups. Steroids can have significant side effects like

weight gain, bone thinning, and mood swings. For that reason, they are safest when used temporarily.

Immunosuppressants. These drugs, such as

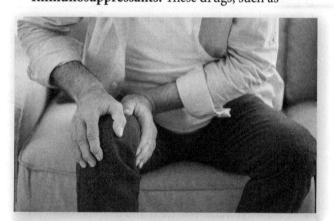

Understanding inflammation

When the immune system is alerted to damage or danger in the body—such as infection or injury—it sends cells that fight invading microbes, clean up debris, and begin the healing process. The response is called acute inflammation, and it's temporary. But sometimes the immune response continues over a long period, injuring a specific part of the body. This chronic inflammation can be triggered by any number of inflammatory diseases, such as rheumatoid arthritis (which attacks the lining of the joints) or inflammatory bowel disease (which attacks the digestive tract lining). Chronic inflammation can also result from an unhealthy lifestyle—being sedentary, smoking, eating an unhealthy diet, not getting enough sleep, drinking too much alcohol, or being stressed all the time. Those habits promote inflammation throughout the body, and play a role in the development of Alzheimer's disease, heart disease, and diabetes.

methotrexate (Rheumatrex, Trexall) or tofacitinib (Xeljanz), are chemical compounds that suppress the immune response by inhibiting the production of inflammatory substances. This can slow or even halt damage to the body from many kinds of disease, including rheumatoid arthritis, inflammatory bowel disease, lupus, or psoriasis. The drugs also reduce the body's ability to fight infection, so anyone using them must be monitored very carefully.

Biologics. Biologics—such as adalimumab (Humira), infliximab (Remicade), and etanercept (Enbrel)—are given as injections or infusions, and they suppress the immune system in a much more targeted way than most immunosuppressants. Biologics are derived from living cells, and they are engineered to target and block specific proteins or cells involved in inflammation. Since they are more selective than immunosuppressants, biologics are often more effective. But they, too, increase the risk for infection, and you must be monitored closely for infection if you take them.

Other approaches

Treating the underlying reason that triggers inflammation can be important. For example, taking pills to reduce levels of uric acid in your blood leads to fewer crystals getting into joints, thereby reducing attacks of gout.

To dampen chronic inflammation, make healthy lifestyle choices. "It's not a pill, but it's the best prevention measure we have to help people avoid chronic inflammation and its complications," Dr. Shmerling says. "It's inexpensive and has few side effects. And even making small improvements, like cutting out processed foods and taking a 10-minute walk each day, can make a difference."

Chronic gut inflammation: Coping with inflammatory bowel disease

An unhealthy lifestyle and genetics may collide to trigger IBD.

Like any area of the body, the gastrointestinal tract can suffer the effects of chronic inflammation. The same persistent activation of the immune system that can occur in your joints (causing inflammatory arthritis) or arteries (provoking plaque buildup) can also take place in the gastrointestinal tract, inflaming or damaging the lining of the intestines and other parts of the digestive system. This gut inflammation may be caused by a variety of diseases (such as celiac disease), or it may be due to inflammatory bowel disease (IBD).

IBD usually appears in one's teens or 20s, but it can also occur in older age. "People over age 60 make up about 15% of new cases of IBD. It's a second peak in incidence that we don't yet understand," says gastroenterologist Dr. Lawrence S. Friedman, professor of medicine at Harvard Medical School and the Anton

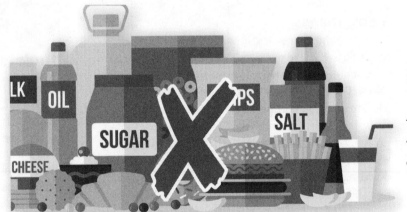

Avoid processed foods; they contain food additives, and some may be tied to IBD flares.

R. Fried, M.D., Chair of the Department of Medicine at Newton-Wellesley Hospital.

IBD types and symptoms

There are two main types of inflammatory bowel disease.

Crohn's disease. Crohn's is characterized by inflammation anywhere along the entire digestive tract, from the mouth to the anus (most commonly in the end of the small intestine and beginning of the large intestine, or colon). "Bowel involvement may be patchy, with some segments affected and others normal. The inflammation typically involves the entire thickness of the bowel wall, from the lining on the inside, through the muscle layer, to the surrounding tissue," Dr. Friedman says.

Ulcerative colitis. This disease occurs in the rectum and often extends up into the colon, sometimes involving the entire length of the colon. Unlike Crohn's disease, ulcerative colitis inflammation is limited to the lining of the rectum and colon, and doesn't invade deeper tissue. No matter which type of IBD you have, you may experience flare-ups of diarrhea, abdominal cramps, fatigue, gas, bloating, bloody stools, loss of appetite, or weight loss. In some cases, inflammation develops in other organs, such as the skin, eyes, joints, liver, heart, or lungs. Unrelenting inflammation of the bowel also increases the risk of future bowel cancer.

IBD causes

It's unclear what causes IBD. Doctors suspect it's a combination of the following.

Lifestyle factors. IBD risk goes up with a diet high in saturated fat, red meat, or processed foods. Smoking raises the risk for Crohn's disease.

Medications. Nonsteroidal anti-inflammatory drugs, antibiotics, and birth control pills are among the drugs that may increase IBD risk.

Altered gut bacteria. The gut is home to 100 trillion microbes. Most are "good," helping us digest food and fight harmful bacteria. "But if the composition of gut bacteria is altered, some bacteria may trigger an inflammatory response," Dr. Friedman says.

A leaky gut. The inner lining of the intestines is a tight barrier made of millions of cells. If this barrier leaks, gut bacteria or their toxins may get into the bowel wall, bloodstream, or lymph nodes, triggering an immune response and inflammation.

Genetics. "We've identified many genetic variants [mutations] that may predispose you to getting inflammatory bowel disease. And some gene mutations may lead to altered immune function. For example, one gene variant appears to weaken the gut

barrier," says Dr. Ramnik Xavier, director of the Center for the Study of Inflammatory Bowel Disease at Harvard-affiliated Massachusetts General Hospital and Kurt Isselbacher Professor of Medicine, Harvard Medical School.

Managing disease

The goal of IBD treatment is remission: suppressed symptoms, lower blood levels of inflammatory markers, and normal-looking bowel and tissue biopsies. The following approaches can help you achieve remission and prevent flare-ups.

Medications. Crohn's and ulcerative colitis are often treated with the same types of drugs, including anti-inflammatory medications (such as corticosteroids), immune system suppressors, or biologics (which target proteins involved in inflammation). "But you must be treated by someone who knows the range of therapeutic options and how to manage their side effects," Dr. Friedman advises.

Surgery. If medications don't work, you may need to have the diseased part of the bowel removed.

A healthy lifestyle. Eating a healthy diet, avoiding processed foods (which contain additives, some of which may be associated with IBD flares), exercising, maintaining a healthy weight, not smoking, and getting enough sleep are all keys to staying healthy with IBD.

Is it possible to live well with IBD? "Yes—it's not the debilitating disease it used to be. We have very good medications and surgery as a backup. Older people respond as well as younger people," Dr. Friedman says, "and we can keep most people feeling well and active and living a normal lifestyle."

Good germs, bad germs

The immune system has a vested interest in rooting out harmful microbes such as bacteria, viruses, fungi, and parasites, which is why it quickly deploys white blood cells to surround and consume these hostile organisms. There is a good reason for the attack. The diseases they cause can range from something minor like the common cold to a potentially fatal disease such as meningitis.

However, not every germ is bad for you and deserving of destruction. In fact, you have an entire world of microbes living harmoniously with you—on your skin, and inside your digestive system, nose, and other areas of your body. These trillions of beneficial bacteria, known collectively as the microbiome, act a lot like your own cells, breaking down nutrients and synthesizing the vitamins you need to stay healthy, as well as protecting you from more harmful germs. Some of these microorganisms—like *Bifidobacterium*—actually help to harness damaging inflammation by stimulating the growth of immune cells that control the inflammatory response. The immune system is trained to distinguish these friendly bacteria from harmful ones so that it does not attack the microorganisms that are good for your health.

Researchers have also discovered that a little bit of exposure to both healthful and harmful germs early in life might be a good thing, priming our immune system to respond more effectively to pathogens in the future. In effect, this exposure "teaches" your immune system how to respond to threats, so that it can regulate the inflammatory response and prevent the type of overreaction that can lead to allergies and asthma.

The role of the microbiome in inflammatory diseases

The human body is more than simply a collection of cells, tissues, and organs. An entire microscopic world, teeming with more than 100 trillion bacteria, fungi, viruses, and protozoa, inhabits your gut and other parts of your body. These microorganisms outnumber your own cells by a factor of 10 to one.

While some members of your microbiome can make you sick, most live harmoniously and even helpfully within you. Beneficial bacteria help your body digest food, produce vitamins, protect you against the harmful bacteria, and inhibit inflammation.

Although the makeup of your microbiome remains fairly stable, certain environmental factors—including a high-calorie, high-fat diet and drugs like antibiotics—can change its composition. Some of these changes can damage the barrier that keeps these bacteria out of the bloodstream. Once the barrier is damaged, bacteria may cause inflammation in the digestive

tract and throughout the body (although just how this happens is uncertain). Research has found that an imbalance in the microbiome, called dysbiosis, may contribute to the development of autoimmune diseases like inflammatory bowel disease, rheumatoid arthritis and other inflammatory types of arthritis, type 1 diabetes, multiple sclerosis, and lupus.

Studies are currently investigating whether probiotics (foods and supplements that contain live beneficial bacteria) and prebiotics (foods and supplements that feed and encourage the growth of beneficial bacteria) might help to treat people with autoimmune diseases. So far, this research has been inconclusive. Another promising therapy under investigation is fecal transplantation, which transfers a sample of the microbiome from a healthy donor to a person with autoimmune disease. And still other research is focused on how certain diets—such as the Mediterranean diet—might alter the gut microenvironment in a way that dampens inflammation in autoimmune diseases.

How diet can transform the microbiome

You can see the effects of a healthy diet pretty easily in the forms of weight loss and energy gain. When you eat anti-inflammatory foods, a lot happens under the surface, too. Not only do markers of inflammation in your blood drop, but your gut also undergoes a real and dramatic population shift.

The gut microbiota (the bacteria and other microorganisms that inhabit your digestive tract) include both beneficial bacteria that aid in processes like digestion and nutrient absorption, and harmful bacteria that contribute to inflammation, illness, and metabolic dysfunction. When it comes to these tiny residents, diversity is an asset. People with a more diverse population of bacteria in their digestive tract tend to have less chronic, low-grade inflammation than those with less diversity.

Certain styles of eating—such as a low-sugar, low-fat, high-fiber diet—promote a wider variety of microorganisms in your gut. Probiotics, consumed either as foods (sauerkraut, kimchi, kefir, miso) or supplements, contain beneficial bacteria themselves. Other foods, called prebiotics (which contain fermentable fibers that bacteria like to feed on), are found in foods like onions, bananas, leeks, garlic, oats, and soybeans.

A look at psoriasis

Medications and other standard therapies can help you manage this common skin condition.

Psoriasis is among the most common skin diseases, and once it shows up, it never entirely goes away. "Unfortunately, there is no cure for psoriasis," says Dr. Flavia Fedeles, a dermatologist with Harvard-affiliated Massachusetts General Hospital. "But you can take steps to reduce flare-ups and manage their severity when they do appear."

Causes and appearance

Psoriasis appears as reddish patches of skin covered with silvery scales. It can cause intense itchiness and pain. You might feel like you're being poked with needles or on fire. Breakouts can appear almost anywhere on the body, depending on which version of the condition you have (see "Know your psoriasis" on the next page).

Psoriasis develops when the immune system prompts certain areas of your skin to produce new cells more rapidly than usual, which leads to thickening and scaling. It's not clear what makes this happen. The condition tends to go through cycles. Flare-ups can last weeks or even months, followed by remission for several months or even a year or longer. While psoriasis strikes more men than women, genetics are a more significant factor in who gets it. Most people with psoriasis have inherited one or more genes that affect the immune system in a way to make them prone to it.

Various types of stimuli can make the immune system go haywire and trigger flare-ups. The most common is stress, which causes the body to release chemicals that boost inflammation. Weight gain also contributes to outbreaks. Flare-ups can be a response to certain medications, like beta blockers used to control high blood pressure or heart rate, or lithium used to treat bipolar disorder. (If you think your flare-ups are related to your medication use, check with your doctor about changing drugs or adjusting dosage.)

Current treatments

There are many psoriasis treatments available, which may be used alone or in combination. "Several factors go into the decision of which to use, including the body surface area affected, whether a person has psoriatic arthritis or other medical problems, and the potential risk of side effects," says Dr. Fedeles.

The goal of treatment is to reduce your psoriasis to no more than 1% of your body surface area (about equal to the top of your hand) within three months, according to the National Psoriasis Foundation.

"If you don't reach the 1% goal during this time frame, your doctor may have you continue treatment for an additional three months," says Dr. Fedeles. You and your doctor may choose to accept a less aggressive goal, such as 3% (or less) of your skin surface. If you still don't meet the target after six months, your doctor may explore other options, like increasing

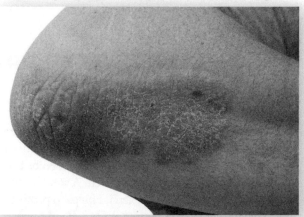

While psoriasis can appear almost anywhere on the body, the elbow is a frequent spot.

medication dosage or switching to another one.

Here are some of the common treatments your doctor may recommend:

Topical medications. These prescription and over-the-counter creams, ointments, and lotions are applied directly to the skin. People also should maintain a daily skin care regimen using lubricants like unscented moisturizers.

Phototherapy. Also called light therapy, this treats extensive or widespread psoriasis. Here, artificial ultraviolet B rays penetrate the skin to slow the growth of affected skin cells. The light intensity, duration of exposure, and number of treatments vary. It's common for psoriasis to initially worsen with this treatment before it improves.

Oral vitamin A derivatives. These medications treat moderate to severe psoriasis involving large areas of skin. They sometimes cause severe side effects, like hair loss; thin nails; dry mouth, eyes, and skin; bleeding gums; nosebleeds; headache; and joint or muscle pain.

Biologic therapy. These drugs suppress the immune system. They come in pill or injection form and treat moderate to severe psoriasis or when a person has joint involvement (psoriatic arthritis). There are many FDA-approved drugs available and more in the pipeline.

Healthy habits. This includes maintaining a healthy weight, following a healthy diet, exercising regularly, and reducing stress. You should also give up smoking and limit alcohol consumption, as both can worsen psoriasis.

Know your psoriasis

Psoriasis comes in four main patterns:

Plaque psoriasis, the most common type, is marked by patches on the trunk and limbs, especially the elbows and knees, and on the scalp. Fingernails and toenails may become thick and pitted and separate from their nail beds.

Inverse psoriasis, a plaque type of psoriasis, tends to affect skin creases, such as those under the arm and around the groin and buttocks. The red patches may be moist rather than scaly.

Pustular psoriasis is characterized by small pustules (bulging patches of skin filled with fluid) spread over the body.

Guttate psoriasis causes many teardrop-sized patches that are more prominent on the body than the face.

Regular exercise can turn down the heat of chronic inflammation

The government and most major health organizations urge us all to get at least 150 minutes (two-and-a-half hours) of aerobic activity plus two or three strength training sessions every week. A solid body of research shows that regular exercise helps to protect the heart and brain, strengthen the bones, and prevent diseases like dementia, type 2 diabetes, heart disease, and depression. It may even lengthen your life.

Exercise causes many changes in the body that produce these positive effects. But one important factor that is often underappreciated is that it helps fight low-grade chronic inflammation—the same type of inflammation that underlies so many chronic diseases.

The research into exercise and inflammation is still young, but it has already yielded fascinating insights. For example, regular exercise seems to control inflammation in multiple ways. By helping to prevent excess weight gain, it indirectly heads off the proliferation of inflammation-promoting macrophages in fat tissue.

Exercise can also have more direct effects on levels of pro-inflammatory cytokines. For example, in a study by researchers at the University of California San Diego, just 20 minutes of moderate aerobic exercise lowered production of TNF. The authors noted that the anti-inflammatory effect may come from catecholamines, hormones the adrenal glands release during exercise.

The caveat is that if you overdo it—say, by exercising at too high an intensity or for too long—an exercise session can damage muscles and connective tissue and *provoke* an inflammatory response. Before starting or ramping up an exercise program, you should speak with your doctor, especially if you have heart disease or musculoskeletal problems. If you work out on a regular basis and know your limits, however, the effects should be overwhelmingly beneficial.

Exercise of all types is good. The point is that you need to do it regularly and observe basic precautions to avoid injury.

Gum disease and heart health: Probing the link

Bacteria and inflammation may underlie the long-observed connection between oral health and cardiovascular disease.

About two-thirds of people over 65 have gum disease—more formally known as periodontal disease. It starts when plaque, a sticky film of bacteria and food, builds up around the teeth. In the earliest stage of gingivitis, irritated gums can bleed easily. Left untreated, periodontal disease can worsen and, in its most severe form, cause the teeth to loosen and fall out.

Compared with people who have healthy gums, people with periodontal disease are about twice as likely to have a heart attack. Shared risk factors—including smoking, an unhealthy diet, or lack of access to health and dental care—may explain some of this association. However, some bacterial and viral infections also appear to increase the risk of heart attack and stroke. And growing evidence suggests that bacteria and inflammation may underlie the link between the mouth and the heart.

"Your mouth is a gateway to the rest of your body, so it's not surprising that your oral health can affect your overall health and vice versa," says Dr. Tien Jiang, a prosthodontist in the Department of Oral Health Policy and Epidemiology at the Harvard School of Dental Medicine.

Hundreds of different types of bacteria occur naturally in the mouth. Some, fed by sugars, release acids that break down the outer layer of your teeth, causing cavities. Other types of bacteria form plaque that—if not removed by regular brushing and flossing—hardens into tartar, Dr. Jiang explains. Only a professional dental cleaning can remove these hard, calcified deposits.

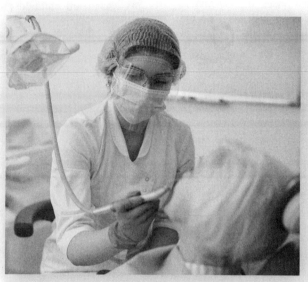

Have your teeth professionally cleaned regularly for optimal health.

Bacteria on the move?

The bacteria responsible for periodontal disease can travel to blood vessels throughout the body. In fact, periodontal bacteria have been found in the fatty debris (atherosclerosis) that clogs arteries located far from the mouth—and in blood clots from people who have experienced heart attacks.

"In both gum disease and heart disease, we find bacteria in places where they're not supposed to be," says Dr. Jiang. The body's immune response to these misplaced bacteria triggers an outpouring of white blood cells. The resulting inflammation may lead to tiny clots and cause a heart attack or stroke.

In addition, many factors linked to a higher risk of heart disease—diabetes, high blood pressure, high cholesterol, and obesity—are all more common in people with periodontal disease, according to a 2021 review article about oral health and cardiovascular disease in the *American Journal of Preventive Cardiology.*

One way to treat periodontal disease is for dentists and hygienists to use manual scalers or ultrasound devices to scrape away tartar above and below the gum line. Known as scaling and root planing, this deep cleaning is more extensive than the twice-yearly cleanings people typically get at the dentist. But while treating periodontal disease may help bring down levels of inflammatory markers in the bloodstream, there's limited evidence it can reduce heart attacks or other cardiovascular problems.

Preventing periodontal disease

To prevent gum disease, daily brushing and flossing are essential—and can even reverse gingivitis before it worsens. If you've slacked off on your flossing, you may notice a little bleeding when you start up again, says Dr. Jiang. When that happens, some people get nervous and stop flossing. But don't worry; just get back into the habit and chances are the bleeding will improve within a few days, she advises. If it doesn't, and you notice other signs of gum disease (see box), schedule an appointment with your dentist.

A healthy diet can also help, says Dr. Jiang. Most people know that hard or chewy candy and other sticky sweets promote cavities. But sugary drinks like sodas (especially if you sip them throughout the day) also feed the bacteria that cause cavities and gum disease. "That's also true for refined carbohydrates that stick to your teeth, like crackers and breads made with white flour," says Dr. Jiang. What's more, a sugary diet is itself associated with higher heart disease risk.

Signs of gum disease

If you experience any of these signs, you may have periodontal disease:

▶ swollen, red, or tender gums

▶ gums that bleed easily

▶ pus between the teeth and gums

▶ bad breath

▶ buildup of hard yellow or brown deposits along the gum line

▶ teeth that are moving apart or loose

▶ dental appliances no longer fit well.

Chapter 2

Mind, Memory, and Mood

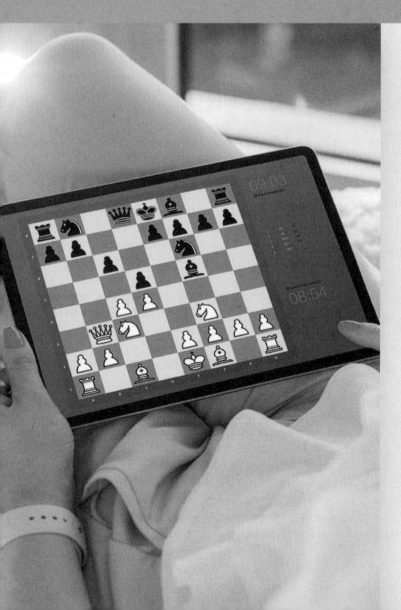

Take Action!
5 Things You Can Do Now

1 **Take the stairs.** Activity may reduce dementia risk. (page 25)

2 **Wake up early.** It may reduce your risk for depression. (page 32)

3 **Schedule a dental check-up.** New research links tooth loss with cognitive decline. (page 33)

4 **Include both coffee and tea in your diet.** The combo is tied to dementia risk reduction. (page 45)

5 **Track how long you sleep each night.** Less than six hours and more than nine may hurt your memory. (page 46)

Thoughts on optimism

Research says people with a positive outlook live longer. But what if you're not inherently optimistic? Can you change your outlook on life?

You know the type: some people manage to remain upbeat even during the most trying times. You probably think "How do they do it?" But a better question to ask is "Can I do it, too?"

Science continues to find that people with an optimistic outlook enjoy healthier and longer lives. A study recently published in the journal *PNAS* involving more than 70,000 people found that those who rated themselves as having high optimism were more likely to live to age 85 or older compared with less optimistic individuals.

The power of optimism is not just having a sunny disposition, but applying this mindset to make positive change, according to Laura Kubzansky, co-director of the Kum Sheung Center for Health and Happiness at the Harvard T.H. Chan School of Public Health. "Optimism is more goal-oriented," she says. "Optimistic people generally have the perspective that with the right approach and right action they can solve problems and improve the situation."

Different mindset

It's not clear exactly how optimism affects health. Investigators have considered both biological and behavioral mechanisms. For example, optimistic people tend to have lower levels of inflammation and healthier cholesterol levels compared with less optimistic people. But they also are more likely to engage in healthy behaviors like staying active, eating right, not smoking, and not abusing alcohol.

"We still are not sure if this mindset directly impacts biological functioning toward healthier profiles, or if it primarily makes people embrace healthy habits, or if it's a combination of both," says Kubzansky. But this brings up the central question about

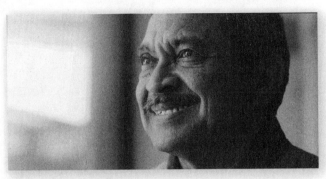

Some people are naturally optimistic, but for others it's possible to learn to change their mindset.

health and optimism: can you become more optimistic?

Factors at play

Kubzansky says that optimism is approximately 25% to 30% heritable. "But this means there is room for other factors to influence optimism quite substantially." Researchers have found that certain factors can influence one's optimism, such as income, education, geography, and social status. "So changing people's environments and social structural factors may be one way to change optimism levels," says Kubzansky.

Still, she believes people can learn to be more optimistic without such changes. "It's not always easy, and it takes dedication, but it's possible for people to change their mindset." Here are four practices she suggests that could help you build more optimism.

Look for opportunities. When difficult events happen, turn your focus toward a more positive alternative. For example, if you are stuck waiting for an appointment, use this unexpected free time to call a friend or read a book. If an injury or sickness has derailed your usual workouts, focus on what you can do, like gentle stretching or using resistance bands. "These substitute activities can make you feel more positive and remind you that difficult circumstances will not necessarily continue, and you can overcome barriers to get there," says Kubzansky.

Focus on your strengths. Here is an exercise from the Greater Good Science Center at the University of California, Berkeley. Reflect on your personal strengths, like creativity, perseverance, kindness, curiosity. Choose one and plan how to use it today. For example, for perseverance, make a list of tasks you have found challenging recently, then try to tackle each one. If you choose curiosity, attempt an activity you've never tried before. Repeat this process every day for a week. You may use the same personal strength across multiple days or try using a different one each day. Another way to assess your character strengths is to take the free Values in Action (VIA) Survey at www.viacharacter.org/survey/account/register.

Practice gratitude. Optimists often are thankful for what they have and share it with others. Keep a gratitude journal where you list the many gifts and blessings for which you are thankful, like your current health, a kind gesture you received, a great meal you enjoyed.

Create a mental image of your best possible self. Where do you see yourself in five or 10 years? This exercise helps you address three essential questions:

- What are you doing now?
- What is important to you?
- What do you care about and why?

The answers can help you focus on new goals and areas of improvement you've always wanted to pursue, but couldn't because of other life obligations, like work and raising kids. "This can help turn your attention toward something stimulating and exciting, which can increase your sense of great possibilities and a more positive future," says Kubzansky.

ASK THE DOCTOR

by ANTHONY L. KOMAROFF, M.D.

What's the connection between the gut and brain health?

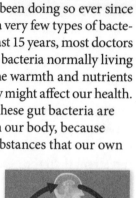

Q *I've heard that the bacteria and other germs that live in our intestines can affect our brain, including whether we get some brain diseases. Can that be true? If so, how does that happen?*

A It very likely is true. More than a century ago, we discovered that bacteria live in our intestines, in our mouth and nose, and on our skin. Indeed, they've been doing so ever since the very first humans walked the earth. We knew that a very few types of bacteria could cause diseases of the gut. However, until the past 15 years, most doctors (myself included) assumed that the vast majority of the bacteria normally living in our gut were just freeloaders, taking advantage of the warmth and nutrients in our body to remain alive. We didn't imagine that they might affect our health.

Over the past 15 years, though, we've learned that these gut bacteria are capable of producing substances that affect the cells in our body, because some of those substances are similar or identical to substances that our own cells make.

So, how can bacteria in the gut affect the brain? Substances made by bacteria in the gut can get into the blood, just like nutrients in our food travel from the gut into the blood. Also, certain nerves connect the brain and the gut: bacteria in the gut can send signals through those nerves to the brain. Finally, gut bacteria can stimulate immune system cells in the wall of the gut, and the immune cells then can send signals though the nerves to the brain.

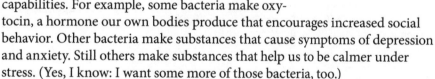

Gut bacteria may influence our emotions, cognition, and more.

Research in the past decade has found that gut bacteria may influence our emotions and cognitive capabilities. For example, some bacteria make oxytocin, a hormone our own bodies produce that encourages increased social behavior. Other bacteria make substances that cause symptoms of depression and anxiety. Still others make substances that help us to be calmer under stress. (Yes, I know: I want some more of those bacteria, too.)

Finally, the gut bacteria also have been shown to influence our vulnerability to certain brain diseases, including Alzheimer's disease, Parkinson's disease, and autism. For example, a substance called synuclein, found in the brains of people with Parkinson's disease, is made by gut bacteria and can travel via nerves from the gut to the brain.

Recognizing the roles that the bacteria (and viruses and other microbes) inside us appear to play in our health, even in our personality, has been one of the most important discoveries of the past 50 years. Yet we are just beginning to understand it, and how to change the microbes within us in ways that will improve our health. It may take another 20 years, but I think we'll figure it out.

Working out your brain

Cardio exercise can build your brain just as it does your muscles.

Cardiovascular exercise, which gets the heart pumping, the muscles moving, and the sweat glands working, is one of the best medicines for overall health. And what's good for the body also benefits the brain. "There is no surefire medical tool that can delay the onset of dementia and other memory problems," says Dr. Julie Brody Magid, Clinical Director of the Memory Disorders Assessment Clinic at Harvard-affiliated McLean Hospital. "Certain drugs may help slow mental decline when symptoms arrive. But cardio exercise has consistently proved to help protect the brain from cognitive decline and perhaps even improve cognitive functioning if issues arise."

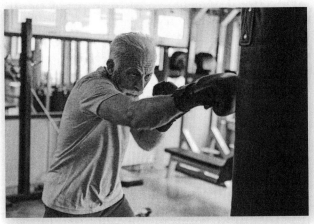

Challenging cardio exercise that includes mental stimulation works out both body and brain.

Popular theories

How does cardio boost your brain? There are many theories. Research has focused on how it can strengthen the heart, promote artery health, improve blood flow to the brain, fight inflammation, and increase key chemicals that encourage new brain cell growth.

For instance, cardio activates a molecule called brain-derived neurotrophic factor (BDNF). BDNF helps repair brain cells and make new brain cells. It's also been associated with a larger hippocampus, the brain region that stores and retrieves memories.

A study published online Aug. 20, 2021, by *Nature Metabolism* found that the hormone irisin, produced by muscles during exercise, protected mice against brain inflammation. The study also suggested that increasing irisin through exercise may help counter the effects of Alzheimer's disease. (While this was only an animal study, the researchers speculated based on previous research that the effect could work with humans.)

Cardio exercise strengthens the heart and improves blood flow throughout the body, including to your brain, specifically its white matter. This helps protect against vascular dementia caused by reduced blood flow to the brain. Better blood flow also can clear toxins from the brain, further protecting against inflammation and promoting neurogenesis—the development of new brain cells.

Type doesn't matter

How much cardio does your brain need? Research continues to explore this question, but it may depend on your fitness level. A 2015 study found that 20 minutes of moderate exercise produced the most significant cognitive boost for nonathletic people. Yet research in the January 2021 *Journal of Sports Science* found that 45 minutes was ideal for

---

Cardio helps even if you have memory issues

It's never too late to adopt brain-protecting exercise, even if you show early signs of memory loss. A study published online March 23, 2021, by the *Journal of Alzheimer's Disease* looked at how cardio exercise affects people with early cognitive decline. Those who followed a yearlong moderate-to-vigorous cardio program scored better on cognitive tests than those who only did a stretching routine. Specifically, they improved their executive function skills, which involve planning and decision making. Most exercisers did brisk walking, but others did swimming, cycling, or ballroom dancing. They followed a 30-minute, three-day-a-week routine for six months and then increased it to five workouts per week.

trained cyclists and triathletes. Until more is known, aim for the recommended federal guidelines of at least 30 minutes of moderate-intensity exercise, five days a week, says Dr. Brody Magid. She suggests that you establish a regimen that is approved by your primary care physician and stick with it.

As for the best type of cardio, again there is no clear winner. However, challenging yourself is vital. "Just like your body acclimates and doesn't get stronger when you do the same workout all the time, your brain also can get too comfortable with routine exercise," says Dr. Brody Magid. She suggests mixing up your cardio workouts with varied intervals and trying new, challenging activities whenever possible. If you

regularly walk, try swimming. If you cycle, try hiking. Also, consider cardio that includes mental stimulation and challenges. "These offer a two-for-one combination of working your thinking skills while you work out your body," says Dr. Brody Magid.

For instance, non-contact boxing forces you to remember various sequences of punches, so you have to concentrate and stay focused. With racquet sports like tennis or pickleball, you to need to react to shots from an opponent and then plan and execute your return. "The bottom line is that when it comes to the brain and exercise, any movement is better than none, and the more you move, the more you boost and protect your brain," says Dr. Brody Magid.

Even light physical activity may help prevent dementia

Small daily activities, such as cleaning the house and running errands, can add up to better brain health.

You don't have to be a marathon runner to help keep your brain healthy. Regular walks through your neighborhood or trips to the grocery store may still reduce your risk of dementia a bit, according to a study published online Dec. 16, 2021, by *JAMA Network Open*.

"We already knew from many studies that moderate- and vigorous-intensity physical activity was associated with a reduced risk for developing dementia," says Dr. Andrew Budson, Chief of Cognitive and Behavioral Neurology at the Harvard-affiliated VA Boston Healthcare System. "What's new in this study is that even light-intensity physical activity was associated with a reduced risk."

About the study

This study was very well designed, says Dr. Budson. Not only was the sample size large—more than 62,000 people—but the researchers used careful criteria to determine whether people truly had dementia, and that they hadn't changed their exercise habits in response to a dementia diagnosis.

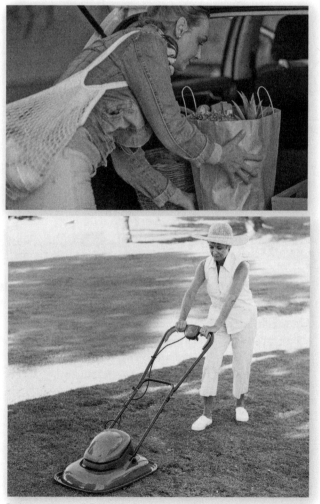

Doing your own light yard work or shopping may help to ward off dementia.

Study participants were age 65 or older and dementia-free at the start of the trial. All had health check-up data in a Korean national insurance database between January 2009 and December 2012. Based on their self-reported activity, researchers divided them into four categories based on how close each person came to meeting the recommended activity range of 150 to 300 minutes per week of moderate-intensity physical activity or 75 to 150 minutes of vigorous-intensity physical activity.

The categories were

- inactive (didn't do any physical activity)
- insufficiently active (did less than the recommended activity range)
- active (met the recommended activity range)
- highly active (exceeded the recommended activity range).

The researchers then followed the participants for about three-and-a-half years. During that time, 3,757 of them were diagnosed with dementia.

Exercise appeared to be linked with individual risk. The more exercise someone got, the less likely that person was to develop dementia. But it wasn't only the active or highly active participants who saw a reduction in dementia risk. Even people in the insufficiently active category still had a lower risk for dementia than the people who were inactive.

Applying the findings

The findings are good news if you feel like you aren't getting as much exercise as you should.

"There are many people who are either unable to or do not wish to perform moderate- or vigorous-intensity physical activity on a regular basis," says Dr. Budson. "This study shows that if these individuals can perform light-intensity physical activity, they can still reduce their risk of dementia. Their risk reduction is not as great as those who exercise more, but it is certainly a risk reduction relative to those who are inactive."

The findings should also motivate you to squeeze more activity into your day whenever you can, he says. "Even small decisions that we make in our daily life can affect our future risk for dementia," says Dr. Budson.

Take a short walk around the block each day, or try to do your own shopping or housework. Also aim to add more steps into your everyday activities. For example, make two trips with the laundry, instead of one. "This study suggests that whether you decide to walk up or down the stairs, versus taking the elevator, makes a difference," he says.

IN THE JOURNALS

Cataract removal tied to lower dementia risk

Struggling with cataracts? Removing those clouded lenses in the eyes might do more than improve your vision. A study published online Dec. 6, 2021, by *JAMA Internal Medicine* found an association between cataract removal and reduced dementia risk.

Researchers followed more than 3,000 dementia-free older adults (who had either cataracts or glaucoma) for about 24 years. During the study period, the risk of developing dementia was 29% lower in people who underwent cataract extraction, compared with people who didn't have their cataracts removed. The risk of dementia didn't change among people who did or did not have glaucoma surgery (which does not restore vision).

The study was observational and didn't prove conclusively that cataract removal protects cognition. However, researchers note that some evidence shows impaired senses (such as poor vision) contribute to social isolation and reduced brain stimulation, which are risk factors for developing dementia. Scientists also speculate that visual impairment may keep people from exercising, and inactivity is another risk factor for dementia.

Turning up the volume on brain health

Hearing loss may be linked to dementia. Here's what you should know about this issue.

Is there a connection between hearing loss and dementia? Researchers have been working intently to answer this question in recent years.

"There are several studies that show an association between hearing loss and cognitive decline," says Dr. Elliott Kozin, assistant professor of otolaryngology–head and neck surgery at Harvard Medical School. But while the two seem to be linked, doctors say it's too early to say whether hearing loss is actually causing cognitive decline.

"As the statistics mantra goes, 'association is not the same as causation,'" says Dr. Kozin, who specializes in the evaluation and treatment of complex ear disorders at Massachusetts Eye and Ear. "There may be additional or multiple unknown risk factors linked to both hearing loss and cognitive decline." One of those factors may be causing both problems.

However, even though a connection hasn't been confirmed, it's important to get tested if you notice signs that your hearing may not be as sensitive as it used to be. There is already ample evidence that hearing difficulties take a toll on your social ties and your quality of life. Simple solutions can help.

Exploring the link

There are some potential reasons why hearing loss and brain changes may be related. First, when you can't hear well, you may not be able to communicate well with others, which may affect your social life. This loss of interaction may reduce your quality of life and affect your cognitive processing, says Dr. Kozin.

"Collectively, these problems are theorized to result in the development of conditions like depression or dementia," he says. It's also possible that hearing loss

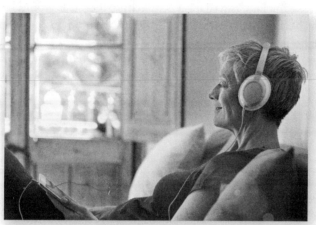

There may be a link between hearing loss and dementia, but researchers need more information to know for sure.

somehow affects the actual structure of the brain, he says. This, in turn, could make the brain more susceptible to the type of damage that is commonly found in people who have Alzheimer's disease.

A modifiable risk factor?

This potential link between hearing loss and changes in the brain has piqued researchers' interest for two reasons.

First, dementia is a growing concern because the U.S. population is aging, and there is a push to identify modifiable risk factors. "The thought is that if we identify factors that lead to a condition, such as dementia, we can act early to prevent it, slow it, and potentially even treat it," says Dr. Kozin. If hearing loss causes changes in the brain, for example, it's possible that fitting someone with a hearing aid might head off cognitive deficits.

"This is an active area of research and is being heavily supported by the National Institutes of Health," says Dr. Kozin. "What is generally needed are high-quality prospective longitudinal studies that compare two groups, those with and without hearing loss, to determine if they develop disorders like dementia. As part of these studies, individuals may be given hearing aids to determine if they mitigate risk of conditions like dementia. These studies are challenging; they require large numbers of patients who are closely followed over a period of time."

Second, if hearing loss is an indicator of dementia, it may help doctors to spot the condition earlier. The hope is that it could one day be used as a way to help diagnose dementia, says Dr. Kozin. It's far too soon to say whether either of these is true, but researchers hope they will someday have an answer.

Understanding hearing loss

In the meantime, Dr. Kozin says people should be alert to hearing deficits. Hearing loss is a common problem among American adults. "An epidemiologic study supported by the National Institutes of Health indicated that 14% of adults experience hearing loss," says Dr. Kozin. While men are twice as likely as women to have difficulty hearing, women are not immune.

The problem becomes more common with age. "Among adults ages 50 to 59 and 60 to 69, one study found that 23% and 39% of adults had hearing loss, respectively," says Dr. Kozin. But it isn't limited to older adults.

"There is no definite age that one may develop hearing loss, as it could be due to many different factors, such as noise exposure and genetics," says Dr. Kozin. Eight percent of adults in their 40s reported hearing problems, according to the same study.

Diagnosing the problem

Many people who have hearing deficits aren't aware of the problem. "Auditory dysfunction results in many different symptoms, such as hearing loss, tinnitus [ringing in the ear], and noise sensitivity. Some individuals may only notice hearing difficulties in noisy environments, such as restaurants," says Dr. Kozin. Other individuals may only be aware due to feedback from friends and family.

While there are no national recommendations that call for hearing screening or testing in adults, get tested if you start experiencing symptoms of hearing loss or if someone points out that you seem to be having difficulty.

"A hearing test is quick and noninvasive. There are many potential treatment options for hearing loss, so testing by a hearing professional may provide actionable next steps," says Dr. Kozin. Addressing the problem is crucial to healthy aging.

"If hearing rehabilitation also addresses cognitive decline, then this would be a 'bonus' benefit; however, the research does not yet support this direct gain, and clinicians should be wary of making these types of claims to patients," says Dr. Kozin.

While the focus of many health initiatives is often

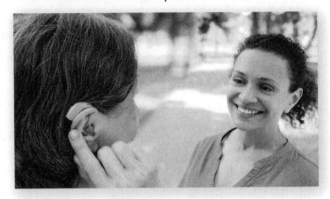

Some simple strategies can help treat hearing loss, so be certain to act quickly if you notice changes.

on things like heart health, maintaining the health of your ears is also important. "We should also be speaking about 'hearing health,' in terms of both hearing loss prevention and treatment. It is well studied that addressing hearing loss will lead to numerous downstream health benefits," says Dr. Kozin. "For this reason, we always recommend hearing protection in noisy environments and some form of hearing rehabilitation strategy if someone has hearing loss."

Are you experiencing hearing loss?

Below are some signs to look for that may signal trouble:
- ▶ an inability to hear in quiet or noisy environments
- ▶ missing words or phrases when people are speaking
- ▶ tinnitus
- ▶ noise sensitivity
- ▶ a sensation of ear fullness
- ▶ needing to turn up the television or music volume.

You may also notice that you feel tired because you need to concentrate intently to follow a conversation.

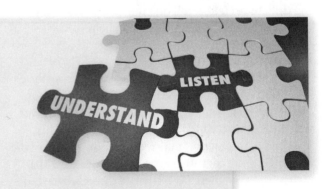

Finding your focus

Trouble concentrating when doing even the simplest tasks? Here are eight tips to keep your attention front and center.

Your brain is a three-pound supercomputer capable of almost unlimited power to learn, remember, and solve problems. Yet, like any other body part, it gradually slows with age. Over time, people may find it harder to perform certain thinking skills, especially the ability to concentrate and focus.

"This can make it challenging to retain essential medical information, manage personal finances, and remember detailed directions," says Joan Gillis, senior clinical team manager of Geriatric Psychiatry Inpatient Services at Harvard-affiliated McLean Hospital. Brains also can get "rusty" as people age, since they are less likely to regularly engage in mentally stimulating activities like working and socializing.

Fortunately, there are ways to keep your attention at full attention. Here are some strategies.

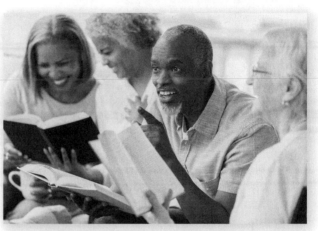

Exercising your brain with mentally engaging activities helps keep your thinking skills sharp.

In the moment

When you feel your attention waning or need to prepare your brain for situations that require a high level of focus, try the following:

Avoid multitasking. "Don't be a mental superhero," says Gillis. "Do one task at a time until it's completed, and then move on to the next one. That way, your mind doesn't have to compete with other stimuli."

Work in blocks of time. Find your ideal time frame for brain work. When you do routine mental activities, like reading a book passage, take note how much time has passed before your attention drifts. "You should be able to find a range where your attention is at its peak," says Gillis. Work within this time segment (set a reminder when time's up), take a break, and then return for another round.

Remove distractions. Turn off your TV and set up website blockers so the Internet won't tempt you. If your smartphone interferes with your ability to stay focused, place it in a drawer, another room, or anywhere that you can't see or hear it while you try to concentrate. You also can adjust your phone's settings to block calls during certain hours. (If you're worried about missing a critical call, you can create a list of contacts who will be allowed to reach you.) If you find that some background noise actually helps with concentration, listen to soothing ambient sounds, like nature settings or white noise.

Take a quick run. A study published online Nov. 22, 2021, by *Scientific Reports* found that just 10 minutes of moderate-intensity running increases blood flow to the prefrontal cortex—the part of the brain responsible for executive function skills, like staying focused on a task until completion. Not a runner? Try a brisk walk—or anything else that gets your body moving and heart pumping.

Build a better brain

These lifestyle habits help maintain a healthy brain and keep thinking skills sharp.

Stay mentally engaged. Like your muscles, your brain needs frequent "exercise" to achieve and maintain peak performance. There are many ways to work out your mind and your thinking skills. For example, do crosswords and jigsaw puzzles, join a book club, take a class, volunteer, or work part-time.

Get enough rest. Aim for seven to nine hours of sleep nightly. Stick to a strict sleep schedule, and get to bed around the same time each night. Speak with your doctor about any medical issues that can cause

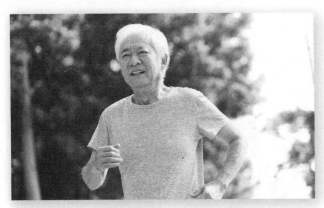

Quick bouts of aerobic exercise increase blood flow to brain regions that help with focus.

sleep problems, such as obstructive sleep apnea, restless legs syndrome, frequent nighttime bathroom trips (often caused by an enlarged prostate), or joint pain.

Check your medication. Many prescription drugs and even some over-the-counter medical products can make you drowsy and less focused. Your pharmacist can review your medications for these side effects; then you can talk with your doctor about switching drugs or lowering doses if needed.

Watch the caffeine. Studies have shown caffeine can temporarily increase attention, but too much can make you jittery and anxious and distract your thinking. The FDA considers 400 milligrams per day—the amount found in about four or five cups of coffee—a safe level for healthy adults, but experiment to find out how much gives you a mental jolt without the jitter.

Be open to mindfulness

Practicing mindfulness is another way to improve focus. One exercise to try is open awareness. The goal is to keep your mind from wandering while doing routine and mundane tasks like eating, showering, cooking a meal, or household cleaning. Here's how to do it:

1. Bring your attention to the sensations in your body, both physical and emotional.

2. Breathe in through your nose, allowing the air to fill your lungs. Let your abdomen expand fully. Then breathe out slowly through your mouth.

3. Carry on with the task at hand, slowly and with deliberation.

4. Engage each of your senses, paying close attention to what you can see, hear, feel, smell, and taste.

5. Try "single-tasking," bringing your attention as fully as possible to what you're doing in a given moment.

6. If your mind wanders away from your current task, gently refocus your attention back on the sensation of the moment.

IN THE JOURNALS

Take short breaks to maximize memory and learning

How do you get to Carnegie Hall? Practice, practice, practice! And a study published June 8, 2021, in *Cell Reports* shows that taking short breaks between practice sessions is also essential to mastering a new skill. In the study, right-handed volunteers agreed to use their left hand to tap out on a keypad a series of six numbers shown to them on a computer screen. Participants tapped the numbers as quickly as they could for 10 seconds, followed by 10-second rest breaks, for a total of 36 training-and-rest periods. Brain waves recorded during the experiments revealed that the brain was rapidly replaying the keypad task dozens of times during breaks. The more the brain did this instant replay—and the faster—the better people performed during practice sessions. Staying mentally engaged helps keep your mind and memory strong. So when taking on new mental challenges—whether you're mastering a physical skill like golf or learning a new language—remember that periods of focused study or practice mixed with rest will boost your proficiency better than marathon sessions.

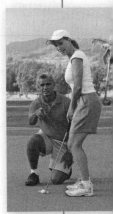

Can brain training smartphone apps and computer games really help you stay sharp?

These programs can be fun, but evidence that they improve or maintain brain health is limited.

"Improve your memory." "Get a personalized brain training plan." "Keep your mind sharp." These are the promises of an ever-growing number of smartphone apps and computer games being sold as a means to help protect and even improve your mind and memory. But is it true? Can electronic products really help your brain health?

"The companies who make these games would like you to think so," says Dr. Andrew Budson, chief of cognitive and behavioral neurology at the VA Boston Healthcare System. And it is theoretically possible that some do—after all, there are hundreds on the market. But the problem is there's not a whole lot of concrete proof that this is the case.

Understanding the research

Research into these apps often hasn't followed best research practices, such as controlling for other factors that may influence the results. And unfortunately, when researchers do use careful research methods, the benefits of using these apps and games often evaporate, says Dr. Budson. That said, there are some studies that have shown positive results, he says.

Researchers from the University of Iowa recently published one such study in *The Journals of Gerontology*. The researchers asked a group of adults to follow a 10-week computerized brain training program and compared them against a control group of people who played traditional computer games.

The researchers found that at the end of the study period, the people in the brain training group were faster at processing information and had better working memory (a measure of how well they could recall information and apply it to tasks), compared with those who played the traditional computer games, says Dr. Budson.

But more commonly, tests of electronic programs seem to fall flat, says Dr. Budson. For example, a recent *International Psychogeriatrics* study of people ages 80 and older, which was structured much like the University of Iowa study, found no improvements in thinking or memory in either the computerized cognitive training group or the control group.

In addition, the Federal Trade Commission has already moved to penalize some app and computer game makers for making claims that it deemed unsubstantiated. In 2016, the regulatory agency fined a number of companies and ordered them to purge their marketing of misleading statements.

In addition to a dearth of research confirming the value of electronic brain-boosting programs, there is some additional evidence linking certain types of screen-based activities to worse brain outcomes. For example, some studies have linked frequent use of social media to a higher risk of memory problems later in life. A 2021 study published in *The Journal of General Psychology* said this may have to do with how scrolling on these sites affects your mood.

"Interestingly, some of the effects of social media seem to be linked to their tendency to increase negative emotions, working against your attempts to maintain a positive outlook," says Dr. Budson.

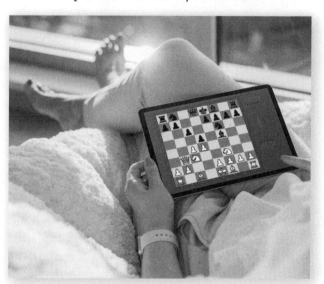

Apps and computer games designed to keep your mind sharp as you age aren't yet backed by strong science.

Strategies to protect the brain

Ultimately, Dr. Budson says that based on the information out there, it appears that while computerized brain training programs may help people get better at specific tasks that they practice using each program, the programs don't seem to help them do better on other, unrelated tasks or improve their cognitive performance overall.

That said, if you're using an app or brain training computer program and you like it, keep doing it, in moderation. Enjoyable activities, says Dr. Budson, can be good for you.

"Consider it a hobby, something you do to have fun, rather than something critically important for your brain," says Dr. Budson.

But don't overlook strategies that have already been shown to help maintain brain health, with physical activity and dedicated time for exercise topping the list. Budson says there are at least six more that should be a priority.

Eat a healthy diet. Adopting a Mediterranean-style diet—heavy on fruits, vegetables, healthy fats, and lean meats, and low in processed and sugary foods—can benefit your brain health.

Ditch bad habits. Illegal drug use, drinking too much alcohol, and not getting enough sleep at night take a toll on cognition.

Take time to socialize. People whose brains age well often have one thing in common: they have strong social ties. A study published in the *Journal of the International Neuropsychological Society* found that among more than 1,000 older adults followed for five years, those who were the most socially active had 70% less cognitive decline compared with their less-social peers. But keep in mind that not all social experiences are beneficial. Negative or stressful relationships have been found to harm cognition.

Turn up the tunes. Listening to music or playing an instrument can benefit your brain, says Dr. Budson. When you listen to music, it engages multiple regions of your brain, activating the parts associated not only with language but also rhythm and memory. In addition, music has mood-altering abilities, which can help get you out of a funk or calm and relax you after a stressful day.

"The AARP surveyed over 3,000 adults ages 18 and older and found that music was associated with self-reported reduced levels of anxiety and depression, very good or excellent brain health, good quality of life, happiness and mental well-being, and the ability to learn new things," says Dr. Budson. Combining music, dancing, and social interactions can bring particularly potent brain benefits, he says.

Be mindful. Taking time out of your day to focus on the present and to reset can bring cognitive

---

IN THE JOURNALS

Waking up one hour earlier than usual may reduce depression risk

The saying goes that early to bed, early to rise makes one healthy, wealthy, and wise. Recent research supports the first part by suggesting people who wake up an hour earlier than usual, without sleeping less, can reduce their risk of major depression. The results were published online May 26, 2021, by *JAMA Psychiatry*. Researchers analyzed data from nearly 840,000 people of European ancestry to look for common variants that influence a person's chronotype, or sleeping time preference. From this, they were able to pinpoint those who were early and later risers. Next, the researchers identified those who had been diagnosed with a major depressive disorder. When they examined all this information, the investigators found that people who were genetically predisposed to getting up one hour earlier in the morning compared with later risers had a 23% lower risk of depression.

These results are consistent with another small study showing improvement in depression scores in people who actually shifted bedtime and wake time to one hour earlier than their usual routine. These researchers acknowledged that a larger clinical trial is needed to determine if this intervention is truly significant.

benefits, primarily because it reduces brain-harming stress. It can also get you into the habit of paying attention to what you're doing—which can help you in numerous ways, among them remembering names, where you parked your car, or where you left your keys. Taking a few minutes each day to do mindfulness training can make a difference. Learn how by signing up for an in-person or online class, or use a smartphone app or computer program.

Look on the bright side. Taking the time to put a more positive spin on your life might help your brain health, says Dr. Budson. A study published in *The Journals of Gerontology* found that positive thinkers appeared to have healthier brains than their pessimistic peers. Data from the Baltimore Longitudinal Study of Aging demonstrated that those who reported positive attitudes about aging had 30% less memory decline than people who held more negative views.

Can medication help us combat Alzheimer's disease?

Scientists are taking aim at plaques, proteins, and inflammation to prevent or slow disease progression.

When the FDA approved the Alzheimer's medication aducanumab (Aduhelm) in June 2021, it set off a firestorm of criticism. Some doctors and their patients celebrated the decision, hailing the arrival of the first Alzheimer's treatment in almost 20 years. The treatment is designed to reduce beta-amyloid in the brain—clumps or plaques of the amyloid-beta protein, a hallmark of Alzheimer's disease.

Other doctors felt the medication was rushed to market without enough evidence that the drug's removal of amyloid plaques reversed cognitive decline. They also expressed concerns about the drug's steep price tag ($56,000 per year), potential side effects of brain swelling and bleeding, and the frequent brain scans required for follow-up. Remarkably, the skeptics included a panel of experts convened to advise the FDA on whether to approve the drug. It is

---

IN THE JOURNALS

Tooth loss associated with cognitive impairment, dementia

Poor oral hygiene is a path to gum disease and tooth loss, and an increasing amount of evidence suggests there may also be a link to cognitive decline. One example, published October 2021 in *JAMDA: The Journal of Post-Acute and Long-Term Care Medicine*, evaluated 14 studies focusing on tooth loss and cognitive impairment among 34,000 older adults. People in the study with more tooth loss had, on average, a 48% greater risk for developing cognitive impairment and a 28% greater risk for dementia, compared with people who had less tooth loss. There was no significant difference in risk for dementia among people who had dentures (possibly because they can chew foods and maintain nutrition, the researchers speculated).

The researchers say mouth bacteria may play a role in brain inflammation, which might promote cognitive problems. The takeaway: Brush your teeth twice a day, floss every day, and see your dentist regularly. It may also protect your brain.

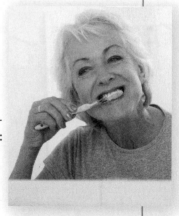

unusual for the FDA to approve a drug against the advice of the experts it has consulted.

Aducanumab is just one drug with the potential to treat Alzheimer's disease. Here are some others, including some being studied at Harvard.

Monoclonal antibodies

Monoclonal antibodies for Alzheimer's (such as aducanumab) are lab-made antibodies designed to stick to amyloid. This signals the immune system to remove the amyloid. There are two types of these drugs. One type targets soluble amyloid-beta (protein fragments that haven't yet formed into plaques).

Clinical trials of one, solanezumab, began in 2014. But by 2016, headlines noted that the drug failed in people with dementia. "We don't think it failed as much as we were too late in the disease process. So we quadrupled the dose and we're trying solanezumab in people ages 65 to 86 with amyloid but no dementia symptoms. We'll get results in 2023," says Dr. Reisa Sperling, lead researcher and director of the

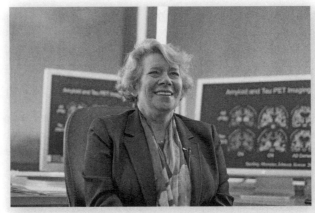

Dr. Reisa Sperling is investigating drugs that aim to remove amyloid from the brain.

Center for Alzheimer Research and Treatment at Harvard-affiliated Brigham and Women's Hospital.

The other type of monoclonal antibody targets insoluble amyloid, which has already formed plaques. (Aducanumab is in this group.) Dr. Sperling is on the team investigating another such drug, lecanemab, in people ages 55 to 80 with either intermediate or high levels of amyloid plaques but no symptoms of Alzheimer's. "We're dosing people on the basis of how much amyloid we see on brain images," Dr. Sperling says, "and the earlier we start, the more chance we may have to prevent the symptoms of Alzheimer's disease." Scientists are still recruiting participants for this trial; if you're interested, visit www.aheadstudy.org.

Other examples of monoclonal antibodies targeting insoluble amyloid-beta include donanemab and

---

A blood test may predict increased risk for Alzheimer's disease

Tests to determine whether people are at risk for developing Alzheimer's disease can be difficult and costly. Some require a spinal tap, and others involve expensive brain imaging studies not done

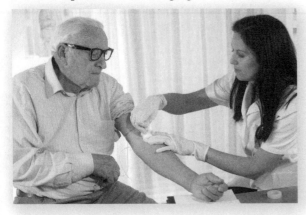

in every hospital. A study published online June 2, 2021, by the journal *Brain* found that a blood test may help to predict an increased risk for Alzheimer's disease. The study followed 159 people who were cognitively normal for two years, and found that higher levels of one blood marker—called P-tau—predicted people who were more likely to develop cognitive decline and brain shrinkage. P-tau is known to be associated with Alzheimer's disease. P-tau levels also were abnormal in 123 people who already had Alzheimer's, but not in people with other kinds of dementia. Measuring P-tau in the blood was as accurate in predicting increased risk as measuring it in the spinal fluid, meaning that a simple blood test could eliminate the need for a spinal tap.

gantenerumab, both of which are now in clinical trials.

Gamma-secretase modulators

The body produces amyloid-beta by cutting it out from larger precursor proteins. "Amyloid precursor proteins are like a long piece of rope; amyloid-beta is a small section in the middle of the rope. You have to cut the long rope twice to get the amyloid-beta section out. The first cut is made by an enzyme called beta-secretase; the second is made by gamma-secretase," explains researcher Rudolph Tanzi, who directs the Genetics and Aging Research Unit and co-directs the Henry and Allison McCance Center for Brain Health at Harvard-affiliated Massachusetts General Hospital (MGH).

Experimental drugs called gamma- and beta-secretase inhibitors interfere with the cutting process and thereby reduce the amount of amyloid-beta produced. Unfortunately, several were found to be unsafe. So

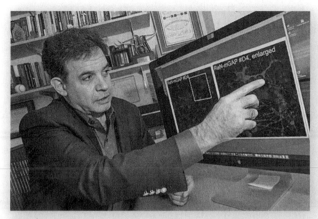

Rudolph Tanzi is studying ways to reduce amyloid production and ward off neuroinflammation.

Tanzi is trying a different approach. "At MGH we are making gamma-secretase modulators that do not inhibit gamma-secretase but instead change where the second cut is made—another way of reducing the amount of amyloid-beta produced. We are aiming at a clinical trial to assess safety over the coming year," Tanzi says.

Additional approaches

Some experimental drugs target other aspects of the Alzheimer's disease process.

Preventing tau tangles. Abnormal tau proteins are another hallmark of Alzheimer's disease. They stick together and turn into fibrous tangles inside brain cells, killing the cells. Many researchers believe amyloid triggers the accumulation of tau. "Once you hit a certain level of amyloid, we think there may be an

---

IN THE JOURNALS

Protein intake associated with less cognitive decline

A Harvard study published in the January 2022 issue of *The American Journal of Clinical Nutrition* suggests that getting enough protein in your diet may be important for protecting your cognition. Researchers evaluated the self-reported dietary habits and health of more than 77,000 men and women who were followed for more than 20 years. Compared with eating carbohydrates, eating protein was associated with lower odds of developing cognitive decline later in life. It didn't take much to make a difference. For example, for every 5% of calories that came from animal protein instead of carbohydrates, there was an 11% lower risk for developing dementia. And for every 5% of calories that came from plant protein instead of carbohydrates, there was a 26% lower

risk for developing dementia. "Beans and legumes had the strongest protective association. Peas and lima beans in particular were associated with a 28% lower risk of cognitive decline for every additional three servings per week," says Dr. Tian-Shin Yeh, the lead author and a postdoctoral research fellow at the Harvard T.H. Chan School of Public Health. The study was observational and doesn't prove that eating more protein will protect your brain. But we already know that proteins are the building blocks of muscles and organs and are essential for tissue and cell repair and the production of important brain chemicals. So be sure to add proteins to your plate at each meal, especially plant-based proteins such as beans, lentils, nuts, and seeds.

explosion of tau tangles, which we call the 'cataustrophe,'" Dr. Sperling says. Experimental medications and vaccines to keep tau from tangling are being studied around the world, though not in large trials.

Stopping inflammation. Tanzi agrees that treatments targeting amyloid and tau may prove valuable if they're started before Alzheimer's symptoms emerge. After symptoms appear, however, he thinks that treatments targeting brain inflammation (neuroinflammation) have the most promise. "Our lab discovered the first Alzheimer's disease neuroinflammation gene in 2008, and there is an ongoing clinical trial to block that gene. Another company has made a drug combination, called AMX035, that also protects neurons against neuroinflammation. It has already proved beneficial in a trial to treat ALS [amyotrophic lateral sclerosis, or Lou Gehrig's disease] run by MGH and is now being considered for approval. It is currently being tested in an Alzheimer's clinical trial at MGH as well." Other scientists are also developing drugs that target inflammation. None is in a large-scale trial yet.

Keys to success

Will any of these experimental medications be the breakthrough treatment we've been waiting for? It's too early to tell. Experts are still debating whether the recently approved drug aducanumab will even be effective.

What's becoming clear to many researchers is that we need to treat brain changes as early as possible in the Alzheimer's disease process, before there's a large buildup of plaques, tangles, and inflammation. "The disease pathology begins silently, a decade or two before symptoms appear, like cholesterol in heart disease. We don't wait for someone to have a heart attack before we treat a high cholesterol level; we lower it earlier in life. That's what we have to do with Alzheimer's," Tanzi says.

And it may take a number of approaches to do the job. "I think anti-amyloid drugs might help somewhat in very mild dementia, but we likely need combination therapy once people have significant symptoms," Dr. Sperling says. "I feel positive we're going in the right direction."

IN THE JOURNALS

Treating insomnia may head off depression

Can treating insomnia prevent depression? A study published online Nov. 24, 2021, by *JAMA Psychiatry* found that it might. The study included 291 people with insomnia. None of the participants (all ages 60 and older) had a history of major depression or any serious health problems at the start of the trial. The participants were divided into two groups. One group received two months of cognitive behavioral therapy for insomnia (CBT-I), an approach that seeks to modify thoughts and habits to improve sleep. The other group spent the same amount of time receiving sleep education therapy (SET), a program that aims to change environmental factors and behaviors that contribute to poor sleep. The researchers then followed both groups for three years to see who went on to develop major depression.

Of the 291 people enrolled in the study, 19 (12.2%) in the CBT-I group and 35 (25.9%) in the SET group were diagnosed with depression. The researchers also found that more people in the CBT-I group than in the SET group saw a lasting improvement in their insomnia. CBT-I participants who saw these sustained sleep improvements were 82.6% less likely to develop depression than the rest of the participants, including all of those in the SET group as well as those in the CBT-I group whose insomnia did not have lasting improvement.

The results support the use of CBT-I to treat insomnia and show a link between the therapy and a lower risk of major depression.

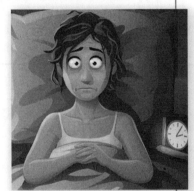

Reducing insomnia using cognitive behavioral therapy might help to reduce the risk of major depression.

Scroll smarter to protect your mental health

While social media networks can build real-world connections, they may have a dark side.

Social media platforms offer a way to connect with others—long-lost friends, busy family members, and neighbors. So, why do you sometimes feel deflated after spending time online?

Social media might not be the problem. The issue might be how you're using it, says Jacqueline Sperling, the co–program director of McLean's Anxiety Mastery Program and an instructor in psychology at Harvard Medical School.

Social media and mood

Research has found associations between social media and negative mental health effects in youth, says Sperling. Although there's less research in adults, some shows similar links, she says.

One November 2021 study, published online by *JAMA Network Open*, found a connection between social media use and depressive symptoms in adults. Researchers looked at Internet survey data collected between May 2020 and May 2021 among more than 5,300 adults (average age about 56). Participants filled out at least two surveys. None of those included in the study reported symptoms of depression in the first survey. But those who used social media were more likely to report an increase in depressive symptoms on subsequent surveys than those who didn't.

"Although the research found associations and not causes, it's possible that some types of social media use are linked with negative effects on one's mood across a wide range of the life span," says Sperling.

A bright side

Although social media may take a toll on your

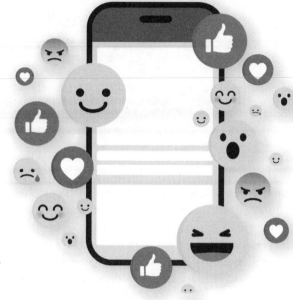

We are all susceptible to a steady onslaught of news, sales pitches, and hacking attempts.

mood, it doesn't always do so, says Sperling. There is evidence that online social interactions even have mood benefits for some users. The question is, why is social media harmful in some instances but not in others?

The difference may relate to whether you engage in active, self-oriented activities or those that are passive and other-oriented, says Sperling.

Activities that are active and self-oriented, such as sending a direct message to a friend or updating a profile picture, are less likely to worsen mood, says Sperling. But the opposite might be true for passive or other-oriented practices, such as looking through social media posts. This type of scrolling creates opportunities for social comparison, she says. Did someone else's photos get more likes? Did their post attract more positive comments? Why do they get to experience exciting travel adventures while you're sitting at home?

If you've noticed that you feel worse after using social media, there are things that you can do to improve your experience without giving it up entirely, says Sperling.

Track your feelings. First, identify how social media use makes you feel, says Sperling. Rate your emotional state on a scale of 0 to 10 before and after using social media. (A 10 signifies the most intense emotion, for example, extremely happy, anxious, or sad.) Also, note whether you engaged in more passive or active use during the session.

If you find that your online time left you feeling more upset, angry, or worried than you were beforehand, it might be time to make some changes, she says. Here are some possibilities:

Frame the experience. People typically don't post the full range of their real-life experiences on social media, says Sperling. People can use filters on photos to make themselves appear more attractive than they are in real life, and they may carefully curate their online image.

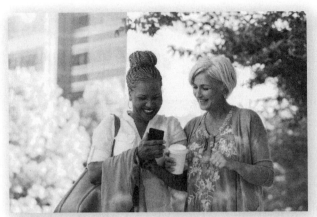

Don't let social media screen time interfere with your real-life, in-person relationships.

When you find yourself feeling jealous, remember that there's likely a lot that you're not seeing. Although someone may post pictures of her recent trip, you won't see the fight she had with her partner at the airport, or the strained relationship she has with the daughter she was visiting. Reminding yourself of this can help limit the urge to compare yourself to others.

Curate your feed. Consider being more selective about what you expose yourself to. For example, do you have a friend whose posts consistently make you feel jealous or angry? Instead of enduring content that bothers you, use the "unfollow" or "mute" option that's available on some social media platforms, such as Facebook, Twitter, and Instagram. This allows you to stay friends, but you don't have to see the person's posts, unless you deliberately view them. Sometimes removing a few problematic people from view makes the experience healthier, says Sperling.

Activate your experience. Instead of passively scrolling, use social media to bolster your real-life relationships. Send direct messages to friends or family members to stay in touch. Also, use social media to identify opportunities to socialize in real life. For example, if you see a post about an upcoming event from a restaurant you follow, invite a friend to attend,

says Sperling.

Choose your battles. Social media sometimes becomes a forum to hash out contentious subjects, and emotions can quickly boil over. Consider having these conversations in person instead of online, says Sperling. Tensions tend to escalate more quickly when people are communicating electronically. People may say things while using a keyboard that they would never say during a face-to-face interaction. If the person you are engaging with isn't a close connection, consider whether it's worth discussing a controversial or emotional subject at all, says Sperling. Sometimes it's better to walk away.

Keep perspective. Be conscious of how much energy you're devoting to social media. Some people spend an excessive amount of time creating the "perfect" post. If this sounds like you, consider setting some limits or modifying your use. For example, if you really like to share photos of restaurant meals that you enjoy, take the picture, says Sperling. But don't post it until you get home. Time spent posting the photo at the restaurant and checking for "likes" takes away from time that is better spent focusing on your dining companion.

Examine your motivations. If your online habits are detracting from your personal relationships, consider the root cause.

"What is it that you're seeking? Are you looking for validation that is missing from somewhere else in your life? Is something missing from your real-life social connections?" asks Sperling. "The answers to these questions may help you take steps to enrich your in-person interactions and rely less on those on social media."

Grieving: A natural process to help heal

The loss of someone can affect your mental and emotional health for months or even years. Here's how to navigate the mourning process.

Grief is an unfortunate reality of life. At some point, almost everyone experiences the passing of a loved one, whether it's a relative, a friend, your spouse, or a beloved pet. The emotional and physical pain that follows can feel debilitating.

"Grieving is a natural process that most people simply have to work through," says Dr. David H. Rosmarin, director of the Spirituality and Mental Health Program at Harvard-affiliated McLean Hospital. "Everyone grieves at their own pace and in their own way, and the process is essential to healing."

Types of grief

Grief can be characterized by feelings of sadness, hopelessness, depression, anger, numbness, and guilt. Prolonged grief also can lead to other problems, like memory issues, pain and fatigue, and obsessive behavior, like becoming overly concerned with mundane matters. There are many categories of grief (some experts place the number as high as 16). But Dr. Rosmarin says most people face one of three types: normal, disenfranchised, or complicated.

The differences between them are sometimes subtle. They often manifest as how people initially react to the loss, the severity of their grief, and its duration. "Each of these three has its own level of difficulty," says Dr. Rosmarin. "Normal is hard, disenfranchised is a bit harder, and complicated is the most difficult."

Here's a look at each one.

Normal. Also known as uncomplicated grief, it's the most common type. Normal grief lasts about six months to two to three years.

Disenfranchised. This kind is not usually acknowledged or socially accepted. It may occur with the loss of a pet, a more distant friend, or even a stranger. "People feel they don't have permission to mourn or that it should be minimized," says Dr. Rosmarin. "Putting this kind of restriction and timetable on grief can make the process last longer and be more severe."

Complicated. In these cases, people have trouble accepting the loss. They shut themselves off from friends and family and experience bouts of depression, loneliness, and paralysis. This makes recovery difficult, and they usually need help from a therapist. Without therapy, complicated grief sometimes lasts several years.

Good mourning

The saying "time heals all wounds" is somewhat true when it comes to grief. For some, it can be a short and relatively painless process. For others, it's a long and agonizing journey. Even when the grieving period has ended, the feelings may reappear during anniversaries, birthdays, or situations that trigger memories of the person.

There's only so much we can do about grief management, says Dr. Rosmarin. "The best way to deal with grief is to look for ways to make the mourning and healing process less challenging." Here are some suggestions.

Accept your grief. Give yourself permission to grieve. "Don't keep it inside and hope it goes away," says Dr. Rosmarin. "Focusing only on external stressors instead of internal feelings, and keeping emotions suppressed, complicates the

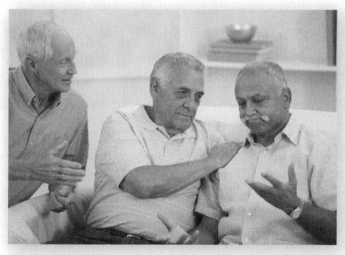

Sharing your feelings with others who have grieved offers needed support and guidance.

grieving process and makes it harder to work through."

Cherish mementos. Keeping tokens of the person is a healthy and normal practice. "It's a way to keep that relationship connection together and his or her memory alive while you grieve," says Dr. Rosmarin.

Embrace the person's community. Reach out to that individual's social circle—family, friends, neighbors, and co-workers—even if you don't know them well. "Learning more about the person from others and sharing stories helps everyone through the process," says Dr. Rosmarin. "Plus, everyone can fill the role of listener, which is so helpful for grieving people."

Talk with others who have grieved. You may know people who have experienced a similar loss. Ask them how they mourned. "Listening to someone else's perspective can offer insight into how to manage your own grief," says Dr. Rosmarin.

Explore spirituality. Spirituality can be a powerful healing tool no matter what form it takes. "Thinking about the natural course of life and death can be quite transformative," says Dr. Rosmarin. "It can even help you better accept the loss by embracing your own mortality."

> ### Different sources that can cause grief
>
> Grief doesn't have to be related to death. It can arise if someone you know suffers a permanent setback, such as from dementia, stroke, or cancer. The ending of a relationship, a move to a new place, or any other kind of personal separation also can cause grief.

Mentally challenging jobs may reduce the risk of dementia

Do you have a mentally stimulating job? It might reduce your risk of dementia later in life, according to an analysis published Aug. 21, 2021, in *The BMJ*. Researchers combined data from multiple studies that examined how work factors related to chronic disease, disability, and death. They found that people with cognitively stimulating jobs had a 23% lower risk of developing dementia compared with those whose jobs were not considered stimulating. Cognitively stimulating jobs were defined as those that allowed people to make decisions independently and required them to perform demanding tasks.

The studies, from the United States and Europe, collected information from people about their jobs. All of the participants were free of dementia at baseline (between 1986 and 2002). Follow-up to identify dementia lasted until 2017. After adjusting for other dementia risk factors, the researchers found that people in the less stimulating jobs were more likely to experience

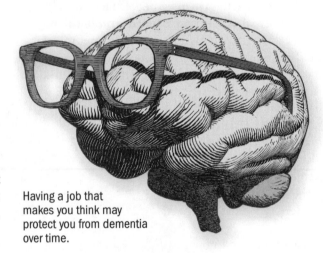

Having a job that makes you think may protect you from dementia over time.

© Jolygon | Getty Images

cognitive decline. However, it's important to note this analysis could not establish whether the job type affected the brain or whether the association reflected other factors. Additional research is needed to shed more light on this issue.

Stuck in a brain fog? Look in your medicine cabinet

Some over-the-counter and prescription drugs can affect memory and cognitive function.

It's an unfortunate reality of aging—those occasional periods of forgetfulness or "brain fog" where you can't think clearly or have trouble multitasking and comprehending information. Older adults may shrug it off as "senior moments," but don't be too quick to blame Father Time for a faulty brain. Your medication may be the real culprit.

"Memory issues can be common side effects for many drugs older adults often take for the first time in their lives," says Dr. Mark Albers, a neurologist with the McCance Center for Brain Health at Harvard-affiliated Massachusetts General

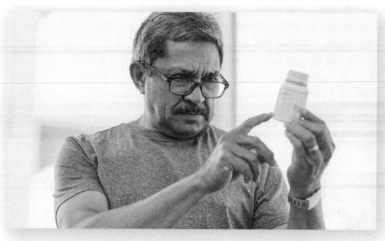

Pain and sleep medications are the drugs most associated with memory problems.

IN THE JOURNALS

Exposure to traffic noise linked to higher dementia risk

Could living by a busy road or near the train tracks put you at higher risk for dementia? A study published Sept. 11, 2021, in *The BMJ* found that people living close to noisy transportation routes for many years appeared to have an elevated risk of dementia, in particular Alzheimer's disease, compared with those who lived in quieter locales.

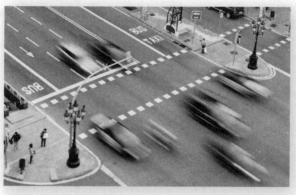

Living near a noisy roadway or train tracks for many years may raise the risk for dementia.

Study authors in Denmark looked at national health registers, which included 105,500 cases of dementia among adults over age 60 from 2004 to 2017. They then looked at estimates of traffic and railway noise from residential neighborhoods throughout the country. After controlling for other factors, such as socioeconomic status, and air pollution they found that people living in areas of high traffic or railroad noise for a decade or longer had a higher risk of dementia in general and a 27% increase in risk for Alzheimer's disease. Roadway noise, but not train noise, was also linked to a higher risk of vascular dementia, a type of dementia caused by reduced blood flow to the brain from plaque buildup in the arteries. Researchers speculated that noise may affect sleep quality or cause an increase in stress that affects brain health. They say the findings show the importance of public programs to lessen noise pollution.

Hospital. "While these drugs don't affect everyone equally, people should examine any new medication or changes in dosage and frequency if they suddenly have problems with memory and thinking."

Multiple factors

There are several reasons medication can affect memory more as you age.

Weak blood-brain barrier. The blood-brain barrier allows blood to carry nutrients and oxygen into the brain while blocking toxins and other harmful substances. This wall weakens with age, and drugs can "leak" into the brain, affecting cognitive functions.

Polypharmacy. Many older adults need multiple medications to treat one or more conditions, a situation known as polypharmacy. It is also common for older people to need to take drugs in higher doses and with greater frequency than younger people.

Sensitivity. Older people tend to metabolize drugs more slowly, making them more sensitive to medications and more vulnerable to side effects.

Drugs of choice

Medications usually affect memory by interfering with how hormones and neurotransmitters transmit signals between brain cells. You often know if a drug causes memory problems soon after taking it, according to Dr. Albers. Some memory issues are temporary or come and go. Others are more frequent and begin to affect quality of life. "It depends on how much you take, how your body metabolizes the drug, and your individual sensitivity," says Dr. Albers. "Problems also could be caused by undesirable drug interactions."

While many medications can cause brain fog and other memory problems, sleep and pain drugs are the most common culprits.

Sleep aids. Over-the-counter sleep aids often contain diphenhydramine, an antihistamine with anticholinergic properties. Anticholinergic drugs are well known to impair cognitive function in older people.

Prescription sleep drugs, such as zolpidem (Ambien), can diminish activity in parts of the brain involved in how events are transferred from short-term to long-term memory, which affects memory recall.

Pain medications. Most of the drugs used to treat chronic pain can cause confusion and memory issues. The list includes opioid analgesics, tricyclic antidepressants such as amitriptyline (Elavil, Endep) and nortriptyline (Aventyl, Pamelor), and gabapentin (Neurontin). The good news is that these problems often go away with modifications. For instance, your doctor might suggest you switch to a different drug, change the dose or frequency, or go off the drug entirely if your health has improved. "Sometimes, just changing when you usually take your medication can make a difference," says Dr. Albers.

If you take multiple medications, the approach may be trial-and-error: your doctor will try modifying one drug at a time, and if your condition doesn't change, will move to the next one and repeat the process.

Track your memory problems

If you suspect a drug is causing memory problems, don't stop taking it on your own. Instead, track your symptoms for one to two weeks and then share the results with your doctor. Make a note of the following:

► when you usually take the drug

► whether you take it with or without food

► what type of memory problems you experience and how long they last

► when the issues usually arise, such as a specific period after taking the drug or when you're trying to complete certain tasks.

Be as detailed as possible. The more information you can provide, the better chance your doctor can identify a pattern to determine if and how a drug may be the problem.

Managing memory slip-ups

Here's how to overcome those annoying everyday lapses.

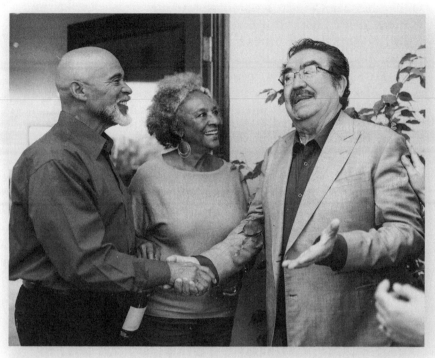

When meeting new people, immediately repeating their name can help you recall it later.

W here did I leave my keys? Did I lock the front door? What is the name of that person I met last night? After a certain age, it seems everyone battles these nagging and sometimes embarrassing memory lapses. "These moments may seem like an unfortunate part of aging, but they can happen to people of all ages," says Lydia Cho, a psychologist and neuropsychologist with Harvard-affiliated McLean Hospital. "But don't let them stress you out or make you question your ability to live an active and engaging life."

While recurring or worsening memory issues always should be checked out (see "When does memory become a problem?" on the next page), everyday lapses can be managed. Here are some tips on how to overcome some common memory situations.

Names

When you meet someone for the first time, make the connection meaningful. "Many times, we forget a name because we didn't notice it being said or don't make an effort to try to remember it," says Cho. Repeat the name back and immediately link it to something that may help trigger recall, such as the person's appearance or job. Or associate the name with someone who has a similar name, like a celebrity, relative, or movie character.

You can also try to connect the name with a rhyming word, a song, or an image. For example, link the name Sandy with the idea of a beach, and imagine Sandy on the beach. Use as much detail as possible—picture her walking along the water's edge or on a beach that's familiar to you.

Finally, write down the name and the person's relation to you (for example, your neighbor's sister) in your smartphone or in a memory notebook specially dedicated to things you want to remember.

Routine tasks

Do you ever question whether you locked a door before bed or turned off the stove after cooking? "We often forget routine behaviors because we are not fully engaged when we do them," says Cho. An excellent way to remind yourself of a completed task is to talk to yourself while doing it. Say it out loud, like "I'm locking the front door," or "I'm putting the clothes in the dryer."

Everyday items

Always put things you regularly use in the same place. For example, set up dedicated areas near the front door, in the living room by your favorite seat, and in the bedroom, and use these spaces for all your vital objects like phone, keys, glasses, and medicine. For objects you don't handle regularly, make a point to focus on the location where you place them and, again, tell yourself out loud what you are doing; for instance, say "I'm placing the scissors in the kitchen drawer below the coffeepot." If you still don't think you'll remember, write down the location, or take a picture with your smartphone.

Online information

Online user names and passwords can easily get forgotten, but it's not safe to write them down where others might find them. Instead, try an online password manager, like LastPass (www.lastpass.com), Dashlane (www.dashlane.com), or 1Password (www.1password.com). You store all your information securely in one place, and it only requires a single password to access from any computer, tablet, or smartphone.

To-do lists

Smartphones also are great for scheduling reminders for tasks and appointments, and their alarms can be set up for one-time or recurring events. You can also email yourself reminders, or leave yourself a note where you are guaranteed to see it, like the refrigerator door, kitchen table, or bathroom mirror.

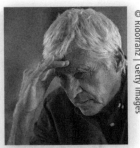

© Ridofranz | Getty Images

When does memory become a problem?

Lifestyle factors like stress, depression, poor sleep, isolation, an unhealthy diet, and lack of exercise can contribute to memory issues. "Examine your situation to determine if any may play a role, and then see if your memory improves when they are addressed," says psychologist Lydia Cho with McLean Hospital. Still, it's best to err on the side of caution and consult your doctor if you or someone else notices memory problems becoming more frequent or severe.

Another approach is to create a visual reminder: put an object associated with the task in a prominent place. For instance, if you need to order concert tickets, leave a picture of the artist near your phone or on your memory table.

The worst habits for your brain

These four areas have the greatest effect on cognitive function.

Many habits contribute to poor brain health, but four areas can have the most influence. They are too much sitting, lack of socializing, inadequate sleep, and chronic stress. "The good news is that they also can be the easiest to change," says Rudolph Tanzi, director of the Genetics and Aging Research Unit and co-director of the McCance Center for Brain Health at Harvard-affiliated Massachusetts General Hospital.

Too much sitting

The average adult sits for six-and-a-half hours per day, and all this chair time does a number on the brain. A study in *PLOS One* found sitting too much is linked to changes in a section of the brain essential to memory. Researchers used MRI scans to look at the medial temporal lobe (MTL), a brain region that makes new memories, in people ages 45 to 75. They then compared the scans with the average number of hours per day the people sat. Those who sat the longest had thinner MTL regions. According to the researchers, MTL thinning can be a precursor to cognitive decline and dementia.

Do this: Tanzi recommends moving after 15 to 30 minutes of sitting. "Set an ongoing timer on your phone as a reminder." Make your movements active. Walk around the house, do push-ups against the kitchen counter, bang out several squats or lunges, or take a quick power walk around the neighborhood.

Lack of socializing

Loneliness is linked to depression and a higher risk for Alzheimer's and can accelerate cognitive decline. A July 2021 study in *The Journals of Gerontology: Series B* found that less socially active people lose more of the brain's gray matter, the outer layer that processes information.

Do this: Sometimes it's a challenge to stay socially engaged, but Tanzi says you don't have to interact with many people to reap benefits. "Find two or three people with whom you basically can share anything," he says. Make this group your social pod. Text or call them regularly or set up a weekly Zoom cocktail hour (alcohol not required). "You want meaningful and mentally stimulating interactions, so choose people you care about and who care about you," says Tanzi.

Inadequate sleep

According to the CDC, one-third of adults don't get enough sleep. Research published in the journal *Sleep* found that cognitive skills—such as memory, reasoning, and problem solving—decline when people sleep

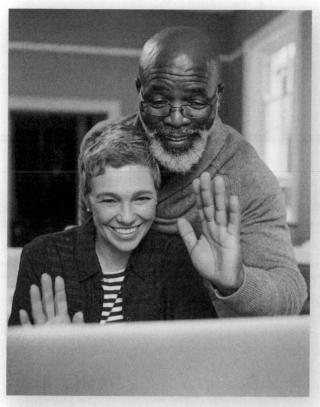

Social engagements like scheduled video chats help to keep the brain engaged.

fewer than seven hours per night.

Do this: Don't focus on getting more sleep. A better approach is to give yourself more time to sleep. "Make yourself go to bed an hour earlier than usual," says Tanzi. "This will help cut down on late nights and give your brain and body extra time to get enough sleep." If you wake up, give your mind time to relax. "Try reading, but avoid watching TV or a laptop, which can be stimulating," says Tanzi. "Even if you are awake for a while, you still have that extra hour to make up for it."

Chronic stress

Chronic stress can kill brain cells and shrink the

Drinking both coffee and tea linked to lower risks for stroke and dementia

Are you a coffee drinker, or are you more of a tea person? Consider being both. A study published Nov. 16, 2021, in *PLOS Medicine* found that having both coffee and tea in the diet was associated with a reduced risk of dementia and stroke. Researchers evaluated the health and self-reported coffee and tea drinking habits of more than 365,000 older adults in the United Kingdom who were followed for 11 years. Compared with people who did not drink any tea or coffee, people who drank two to three cups of coffee as well as two to three cups of tea per day had a 28% lower risk of dementia and a 32% lower risk of stroke during the study period. The combination of both drinks in

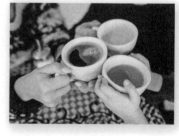

the diet appeared to have a stronger association than just having one or the other. The study is only observational and doesn't prove that drinking coffee and tea prevents stroke or dementia. But we know that the beverages both contain polyphenols—plant chemicals that may help fight chronic inflammation. Chronic inflammation is associated with both dementia and cardiovascular disease.

prefrontal cortex, the area responsible for memory and learning. A major stress trigger for older adults is a "my-way-or-the-highway" approach to everything, says Tanzi. "This high expectation mindset can trigger negative reactions that raise stress levels whenever things don't go your way."

Do this: Be flexible with your reactions. When you sense you are about to get upset, take some deep breaths and remind yourself that you don't always know what is best, and accept that other approaches might be fine. Also, calm yourself by repeating to yourself the mantra, "I'm all right, right now." "Taming your ego can cut off stress before it gets out of control," says Tanzi.

How much sleep keeps cognitive decline at bay?

Getting too much or too little sleep may hurt your brain and lead to memory and thinking impairment, suggests a study published online Aug. 30, 2021, by *JAMA Neurology*. Researchers analyzed the brain images, cognitive test results, and self-reported sleep habits of more than 4,400 older men and women around the world. Sleeping six hours or less per night (short sleep) was associated with impaired cognition, mostly in memory, as well as an increase in amyloid-beta—the protein that can form brain plaque (a hallmark of Alzheimer's disease). Sleeping more than nine hours (long sleep) was also linked to cognitive problems, especially in decision making. And both short and long sleep were associated with higher body mass index (a measurement of body fat), more depressive symptoms, and more napping, compared with people who got seven or eight hours of sleep. The study was observational and can't prove causation, but the findings echo many other studies that suggest too little—and possibly too much—sleep causes cognitive problems.

—

Chapter 3

Blood Pressure and Cholesterol

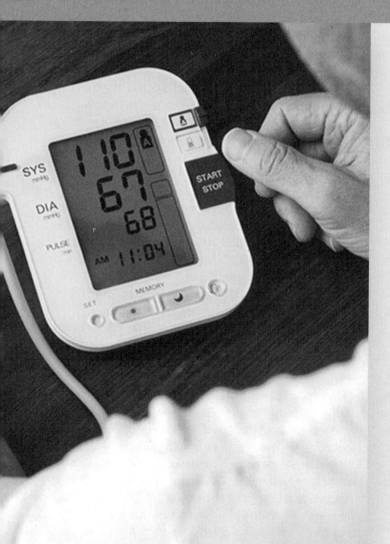

Take Action!
5 Things You Can Do Now

1 **Be cautious when taking pain relievers.** Even acetaminophen may raise blood pressure. (page 54)

2 **Know what to look for in a home blood pressure monitor.** Follow these tips. (page 55)

3 **Measure your diastolic blood pressure.** The number should be low, but not too low. (page 57)

4 **Learn the latest options for lowering LDL.** Two novel drugs may be good choices for some people. (page 59)

5 **Include strength training in your workout.** Like aerobic exercise, muscle-building exercises can help lower blood pressure. (page 61)

Looking past blood pressure numbers

New research suggests an individualized, multifactor approach to treatment may be better.

For many years, numbers have served as the primary indicators for whether you are healthy or at risk of disease.

"Numbers can offer some important information, but decisions about treatment and management shouldn't always revolve around the results of one test or reading," says Dr. Howard LeWine, assistant professor of medicine at Harvard Medical School and chief medical editor for Harvard Health Publishing. This is especially relevant with blood pressure. New research suggests an individualized approach to managing blood pressure that considers other heart health risks, lifestyle habits, and family history may be a better way to ward off heart attacks and strokes.

The cholesterol example

To understand the limits of health numbers—and how individualized treatments can improve outcome—let's take a look at how the approach to cholesterol treatment has evolved.

In 2018, updated guidelines placed the optimal level for "bad" LDL cholesterol at less than 100 milligrams per deciliter (mg/dL). A level of 100 to 129 mg/dL was deemed acceptable, 130 to 159 mg/dL was borderline high, and 160 to 189 mg/dL was high. A reading of 190 mg/dL or higher was deemed very high.

Yet the guidelines also suggested statin therapy should not be prescribed based solely on the cholesterol numbers. Treatment decisions should also consider age, current heart health, a person's 10-year heart attack and stroke risk, and perhaps most important, personal preferences.

For example, a person with an LDL of 140 mg/dL who exercises regularly and has no other risk factors for cardiovascular disease might not need to begin a statin immediately. However, someone with known heart disease or at high risk for it should aim for an LDL of less than 70 mg/dL, which often requires a high-dose statin and sometimes additional cholesterol-lowering therapy.

"The approach now is not just about reducing cholesterol levels to the same fixed numbers for everyone," says Dr. LeWine. "Instead, the goal is to prevent fatty deposits in blood vessels and reduce heart attack and stroke risk with the right cholesterol medications for each individual."

Taking a similar approach

For decades, blood pressure treatment was dictated by a person's numbers, with a blood pressure less than 140/90 millimeters of mercury (mm Hg) considered normal. But mounds of research proved this to be an inadequate goal.

In 2017, the American Heart Association updated its blood pressure guidelines: 130/80 mm Hg to 139/89 mm Hg is now considered Stage 1 hypertension (high blood pressure).

Treatment for Stage 1 is based on your 10-year heart disease and stroke risk. If it's less than 10%, diet and exercise changes could be enough. Anything higher than 10% requires medication and monthly follow-ups.

Blood pressure that reaches 140/90 mm Hg is labeled Stage 2 hypertension, and lifestyle changes and a combination of two drugs from different classes are usually recommended along with monthly checkups. What if your blood pressure is normal (under 120/80 mm Hg) or slightly elevated (120/80 to 129/80 mm Hg)? Here, the guidelines suggest making healthy lifestyle changes as needed and keeping tabs on the numbers every six months to a year.

"While helpful, the guidelines still don't take into account other cardiovascular disease risk factors like family history, diabetes or prediabetes, cholesterol level, smoking, age, and lifestyle," says Dr. LeWine. "Many people may benefit from lowering their blood pressure no matter where it is now."

An analysis in the May 1, 2021, issue of *The Lancet* looked at 48 clinical trials involving almost 345,000 people, average age 65. Researchers found that just a 5 mm Hg reduction in systolic pressure (the top number) resulted in a 13% lower risk of heart failure and stroke no matter a person's prior cardiovascular risk. This was true whether they started with normal, elevated, or high blood pressure. The researchers said this challenges the idea that lowering blood pressure with medication should be guided only by the numbers.

It's all relative

"These findings resonate with me," says Dr. LeWine. But, he adds, "in no way does that mean everyone should try to lower their blood pressure with medication."

Instead, he says that drug treatment decisions should be made based on a person's overall health, potential side effects (such as dizziness while standing), costs, and personal preference, as well as traditional cardiovascular risk factors.

Still, the next time your blood pressure gets checked, it's worthwhile asking your doctor if you should try to lower your number. This may involve just losing a few pounds, eating more plant-based foods, reducing salt intake, or getting more exercise. But it may include adding a low-dose blood pressure pill.

"Exploring these questions and other factors with your doctor can help you both form a strategy that addresses all your concerns," says Dr. LeWine. "Blood pressure numbers are an important piece of information, but they alone should not dictate whether you need treatment or what that should be."

What's the best blood pressure target for older adults?

For people over 60, intensive blood pressure lowering may prevent more heart problems than standard therapy.

Current guidelines from the nation's leading heart organizations say adults should aim for a blood pressure reading under 130/80 millimeters of mercury (mm Hg). However, some doctors believe that target might be too aggressive for older people, who may be more prone to side effects from blood pressure drugs, such as dizziness and falls.

Now, a new study confirms the effectiveness of intensive blood pressure reduction in people over 60. "Not only is a lower target safe, it's also associated with better outcomes in older people," says Dr. Umberto Campia, a cardiologist at Harvard-affiliated Brigham and Women's Hospital.

The study, in the Sept. 30, 2021, issue of *The New England Journal of Medicine*, included more than 8,500 Chinese people ages 60 to 80 with high blood pressure. Half were randomly assigned to a standard treatment group, with a target for systolic blood pressure (the first number in a blood pressure reading) of 130 to 150 mm Hg. For the other half, the intensive

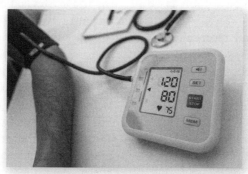

Some physicians say higher blood pressure readings are OK for older people. But lower targets are linked to fewer heart problems.

treatment group, the systolic target was 110 to 130 mm Hg.

Fewer strokes and heart attacks

After a year, the average systolic blood pressure in the standard group was 135 mm Hg, compared with 127 mm Hg in the intensive group. During a median follow-up of just over three years, researchers tracked the participants' rates of serious cardiovascular problems, including stroke, heart attack, heart failure, and atrial fibrillation. The incidence of these problems was 4.6% among those who received standard treatment, compared with 3.5% in those who received intensive treatment. Rates of adverse side effects, including dizziness, fainting, fractures, headaches, and cough, were similar in both groups, although the intensive-treatment group experienced more episodes of abnormally low blood pressure (hypotension).

The findings support those from an earlier trial done in the United States that also documented fewer heart-related problems when doctors aimed for an even lower—120 mm Hg—systolic blood pressure target, Dr. Campia notes. In fact, when researchers analyzed the results only from people ages 75 and older, the heart-related benefits were even more striking. And the rates of side effects were similar to those seen in people with a target of 140 mm Hg.

The historical view

The incidence of high blood pressure clearly rises with age. In fact, the original term to describe high blood pressure seen in aging adults was "essential hypertension," says Dr. Campia. "At the time, the thinking was that high blood pressure was essential to deliver sufficient blood to the brain," he says. With age, blood vessels become stiffer and less flexible. To reach the brain, circulating blood needs an extra "push" in the form of higher blood pressure. That's why some physicians have suggested that for people over 65, systolic blood pressure (the first number in the reading) can be as high as 150 mm Hg.

Increasingly, however, doctors are reconsidering their approach to treating hypertension in older people. "We've learned that high systolic blood pressure in older adults is a major contributor to strokes and heart attacks," says Dr. Campia. The recent findings mean older people should work with their physicians to bring their systolic blood pressure below 130 mm Hg.

Aiming low

People often expect that a single medication will get them to their blood pressure goal, but that's rarely feasible, says Dr. Campia. For example, someone with a systolic blood pressure of 150 mm Hg almost always needs at least two medications. "Even a full dose of a single drug will only lower blood pressure by an average of 5 to 10 points," he says.

Using lower doses of two different blood pressure medications is more effective than maximizing the dose of a single drug. "High blood pressure can result from several different mechanisms, so combining drugs that target different mechanisms typically works better," he adds. The combination approach is also less likely to cause side effects. Moreover, many combinations are available as single pills, which is as easy for patients as taking just one drug.

"We have a broad array of medications to control blood pressure, which means that doctors can usually find the right combination that's safe, effective, and free from side effects," says Dr. Campia.

Your brain on high blood pressure

High blood pressure is not just a heart problem. It also can raise your risk for strokes and cognitive decline.

People think of high blood pressure as a heart problem, as it can raise your risk for a heart attack. But it also can affect your brain health. Blood pressure is the most important factor contributing to brain injury, often in the form of a stroke, according to Dr. Steven Greenberg, a professor of neurology at Harvard Medical School. "Keeping blood pressure low can make brain injury less likely, help conserve brain function, and perhaps slow the natural decline in cognitive function."

Blood pressure and strokes

High blood pressure (hypertension) accelerates the process of atherosclerosis (the buildup of fatty plaque inside artery walls) in both the neck and the brain. The impediment can slow blood flow dramatically, or a blood clot can suddenly form on top of the plaque, cutting off the supply of oxygen and nutrients to part of the brain.

In addition, hypertension increases stroke risk in several ways. It makes you more likely to develop atrial fibrillation, which allows small clots to form in the heart; these can escape and travel to the brain, where they can cause a stroke by blocking blood flow.

These types of strokes tend to affect both medium-sized and large arteries, usually leading to recognizable symptoms, such as sudden weakness on one side of the body or face, difficulty speaking, or inability to walk.

High blood pressure also can damage the smaller arteries in the brain. When blood flow in one of these arteries slows too much or stops altogether, the result can be a small stroke, often referred to as a "silent" stroke because it usually causes no immediate symptoms. Such strokes often occur in multiple parts of the brain.

Cognitive problems commonly develop after a major stroke or repeated small strokes. You might develop problems with learning and retaining new information, short-term memory, and even memory of names, faces, and familiar places.

"This is why prevention is so important," says Dr. Greenberg. "By addressing high blood pressure now, you can hopefully avoid large or small strokes and the memory damage that often comes with them."

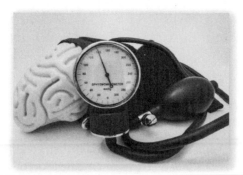
High blood pressure can lead to problems that affect blood flow to the brain.

Conserving brain function

Besides protecting the brain from strokes, lowering high blood pressure can help conserve existing brain function, according to a recent study in the journal *Circulation*.

The study included 199 adults ages 75 and older, with a systolic blood pressure value (the top number. in a reading) of 150 mm Hg or higher, which is defined as Stage 2 hypertension (see "Blood pressure categories").

Their brain scans showed abnormalities in the brain's white matter, which contains nerve fibers that send signals from one part of the brain to another. Such white matter changes, which reflect damaged small blood vessels, have been linked to a propensity for thinking and memory problems.

Half of the participants were given medication to lower their systolic pressure to 145 mm Hg, while the others got drugs to reach a goal of 130 mm Hg or lower. Three years later, brain scans showed

fewer new white matter lesions in people whose systolic pressure was 130 or lower than in those whose target was 145.

Everyone's cognitive skills naturally decline over time. But reducing high blood pressure may slow the process.

A study recently published in *JAMA* looked at 12 studies involving more than 92,000 people with Stage 2 hypertension. All the studies tested participants' cognitive skills, such as concentration, decision making, and learning new information.

At the follow-up (which lasted about four years, on average), the risk of cognitive impairment was about 7% lower among people who took blood pressure drugs compared with those who didn't.

The right number

Current medical guidelines place elevated blood pressure at 120/80 to 129/80 mm Hg and normal as less than 120/80 mm Hg. Which range is best for protecting your brain?

"Because the definitions of normal, elevated, and high blood pressure have gradually dropped over the decades, the recommendation is trending in the direction that the lower the number, the better," says Dr. Greenberg. "Just like with the heart, the best way to protect your brain from high blood pressure is to drive your number down if it's high and keep it as close to a normal level as possible."

Blood pressure categories

BLOOD PRESSURE CATEGORY	SYSTOLIC MM HG (UPPER NUMBER)		DIASTOLIC MM HG (LOWER NUMBER)
Normal	Less than 120	and	Less than 80
Elevated	120 – 129	and	Less than 80
High blood pressure (hypertension) Stage 1	130 – 139	or	80 – 89
High blood pressure (hypertension) Stage 2	140 or higher	or	90 or higher
Hypertensive crisis (consult your doctor immediately)	Higher than 180	and/or	Higher than 120

by **HOWARD LEWINE, M.D.**

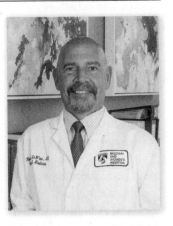

Seasonal changes and blood pressure

Q *My blood pressure stays close to normal except during the winter. Do the seasons affect blood pressure?*

A Yes, seasons can affect blood pressure. Some people with borderline high blood pressure have higher readings during winter. And their pressure can get high enough to need medicine to control it. They might be able to reduce the dosage when spring comes, or stop taking the medication once summer rolls around.

The leading theory about higher blood pressure in colder weather is related to tension in the arteries. When our bodies get cold, blood vessels clamp down to keep in the heat. This raises blood pressure in some people. But other factors might cause your higher winter blood pressure. For example:

Seasonal weight gain. During the winter—especially around the holidays—people often eat more and exercise less, leading to a few extra pounds. Even small gains can cause blood pressure to rise.

Too much salt in your diet. This also raises blood pressure. You're more likely to hang around indoors for longer times come wintertime, which may invite cravings for salty, satisfying foods. Make an effort to stock up on healthier snacks and avoid high-salt processed foods.

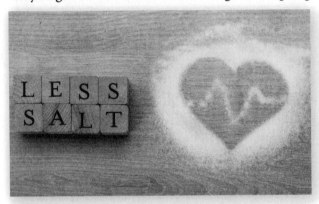

Excess dietary salt can raise your blood pressure.

© AndreyPopov | Getty Images

IN THE JOURNALS

Some blood pressure drugs are linked with better memory

The blood-brain barrier protects the brain from toxic substances. While some medication can penetrate this defensive wall and cause memory problems, certain drugs that treat high blood pressure appear to be associated with better cognitive function. In an analysis published in the August 2021 issue of *Hypertension*, researchers gathered information from 14 observational studies of nearly 12,900 adults ages 50 years and older with high blood pressure. It looked specifically at people who took either ACE inhibitors or angiotensin II receptor blockers (ARBs) to treat their condition. There are many types of drugs within these two classes, some of which can cross the blood-brain barrier.

After three years on their medication, those who took an ACE inhibitor (such as lisinopril) or an ARB (like candesartan) that crosses the blood-brain barrier, scored higher on memory recall tests, when compared with those who took a different drug in the same class that doesn't cross over. High blood pressure is a risk factor for cognitive decline and dementia in older adults, and treatment with lifestyle changes and all types of blood pressure medications can lower the risk. But these findings suggest that certain blood-brain-crossing blood pressure drugs may offer additional brain benefits.

What to do when your blood pressure won't go down

Finding and treating underlying causes and making lifestyle changes will help.

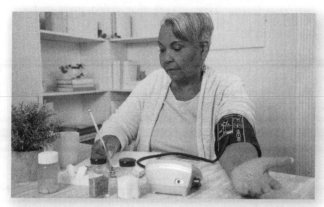

Measure blood pressure at home regularly when you have resistant hypertension.

Many people have high blood pressure in older age, and sometimes it's hard to control. That problem is called resistant hypertension—blood pressure that stays above a set goal despite taking three classes of blood pressure drugs (including a diuretic) at the highest tolerable doses. The condition is a major risk factor for stroke, heart disease, dementia, and more.

What can you do to tame it?

Reassess all medications

Bring your doctor a list of all the medications you are taking, or bring a bag with all the medication bottles. Include over-the-counter drugs, vitamins, and supplements. The list, or bag, of medicines can help your doctor identify drugs or supplements that may be raising your pressure.

For example, taking nonsteroidal anti-inflammatory drugs (NSAIDs) such as ibuprofen (Motrin, Advil) can raise blood pressure. So can decongestants (such as phenylephrine found in many cold medicines), certain antidepressants, and corticosteroids. For example: "Alternative medications or physical therapy to relieve arthritis pain can decrease or eliminate the need for NSAIDs, helping reduce blood pressure in some patients," says Harvard cardiologist Dr. Deepak L. Bhatt, editor in chief of the *Harvard Heart Letter*.

Or the doctor may see that your medicines can be streamlined: fewer pills in total or fewer pills you need to take more than once a day.

Treat underlying causes

Underlying conditions can also keep your blood pressure high (see "What causes resistant hypertension?").

Getting them under control is essential. But figuring out if you have one can take detective work and a thorough physical evaluation.

For example, you may not know that you have a condition that boosts blood pressure, such as sleep apnea—pauses in breathing during sleep. Sleep apnea signs include chronic loud snoring, episodes where you stop breathing briefly (and perhaps gasp for breath), and being very sleepy during the daytime.

A sleep study in a lab or at home (with a portable device) can provide answers.

Make lifestyle changes

You may need to ramp up healthy habits to maximize their effects. Start by eating a plant-based diet that's low in salt; aim for less than 2,300 milligrams (mg) of salt per day. You should also be getting at

What causes resistant hypertension?

Resistant hypertension (high blood pressure that won't go down despite treatment with multiple drugs) has many possible causes. Top reasons include consuming too much salt, which can make blood pressure medications less effective; and missing doses or adjusting them on your own. Other reasons include:

▶ weight gain

▶ sleep apnea

▶ high alcohol consumption

▶ chronic pain

▶ drug interactions and side effects

▶ panic attacks

▶ high levels of the hormone aldosterone (which causes the body to hold on to sodium and water)

▶ kidney problems

▶ eating black licorice (which contains a compound that can increase blood pressure).

least seven hours of sleep per night, limiting alcohol, avoiding smoking, and maintaining a healthy weight.

"Sometimes losing just 5 or 10 pounds can make a meaningful difference in blood pressure for people who are overweight," Dr. Bhatt says.

And if you're not exercising much, it's time to start. Exercise boosts cardiovascular health in many ways. And a small, randomized trial published online Aug. 4, 2021, by *JAMA Cardiology* suggests that aerobic exercise (the kind that gets your heart and lungs pumping) may be another effective treatment for resistant hypertension.

In the study, people who walked, cycled, or both—for 40 minutes, three times per week, for 12 weeks—lowered their blood pressure by seven points in the top (systolic) number of their blood pressure measurement, and five points in the bottom (diastolic) number of the measurement, compared with people who didn't exercise.

What else will help?

If these strategies don't reduce your blood pressure, your doctor may feel it's necessary to prescribe more pills. But don't despair. "No matter what you are taking now, your doctor should be able to make affordable changes in your blood pressure medications to bring down your numbers," Dr. Bhatt says.

The right way to check your blood pressure

Follow these tips to make sure you get an accurate reading—both at home and during health care visits.

Because high blood pressure rarely has any warning signs or symptoms, many people with this stealth condition don't realize they have it. But pressure that measures 130/80 millimeters of mercury (mm Hg) or higher—the official definition of high blood pressure—injures blood vessels, causing them to thicken and stiffen. Left untreated, high blood pressure eventually damages the heart, brain, and kidneys.

That's why every single health care visit should include a blood pressure check. Keep a record of your readings, which can fluctuate due to a range of factors, including exertion or stress. If your readings start trending toward the high range or you've already been diagnosed with high blood pressure, you should get a device for home-based checks (see "Choosing a home blood pressure monitor" on the next page).

"Heart attacks, strokes, and other serious health

IN THE JOURNALS

High-dose acetaminophen may boost blood pressure

Acetaminophen, the popular pain reliever known by the brand name Tylenol, can raise blood pressure when taken regularly, according to a study in the Feb. 7, 2022, issue of *Circulation*.

Earlier research had hinted at this problem, so investigators designed a clinical trial to clarify the risk. They recruited 110 people with high blood pressure and randomly assigned them to take 1,000 milligrams (mg) of acetaminophen or a placebo four times a day for two weeks. (The 4,000-mg daily dose is the generally recommended maximum daily amount for healthy adults.) After a two-week wash-out period, those taking acetaminophen were switched to taking the placebo and vice versa for an additional two weeks. While people were taking acetaminophen, their blood pressure rose by an average of 5 points, the researchers found.

Experts have long known that other common pain relievers—nonsteroidal anti-inflammatory drugs such as ibuprofen (Motrin, Advil) and naproxen (Aleve, Naprosyn)—can also raise blood pressure. The take-home message? If you need a pain reliever, take the lowest possible dose for the shortest possible time.

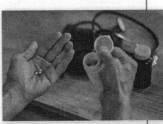

© Dejan Marjanovic | Getty Images

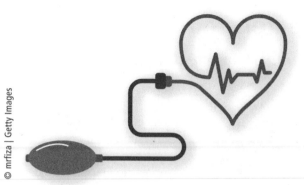

problems correlate far more closely with home blood pressure than with office blood pressure readings," says internist Dr. Katherine Sakmar, assistant professor of medicine at Harvard Medical School. Blood pressure at home better represents what your heart and brain experience most of the time than blood pressure during the 15 to 20 minutes you're in a doctor's office, she explains.

Although automated machines have made checking blood pressure quite simple, it's still important to be aware of factors that can affect the accuracy of the reading, both in health care settings and at home.

At the doctor's office

If you've never had your blood pressure checked in both arms sequentially, ask to have this done at your next health care appointment. If the reading from one arm is higher, that side should be the one upon which to base any treatment and to check in the future, says Dr. Sakmar. (Of note: women who've had a mastectomy should generally have their blood pressure checked in the arm on the side opposite to the breast that was removed.) Bring your home monitor to your next medical appointment to compare its readout with the measurement taken in the doctor's office. If the readings vary by less than 10%, you can consider your home monitor validated, says Dr. Sakmar.

General advice

Many factors (some of which may be connected) can slightly elevate your blood pressure—for example, drinking a lot of coffee, having a full bladder, and crossing your legs. Caffeine is a stimulant that raises the heart rate and also blood pressure. A full bladder and crossed legs can both reduce blood flow returning to your heart; your body's natural response to this is to raise your

blood pressure to make sure your kidneys and brain are getting enough blood, Dr. Sakmar explains.

The following tips can help you get the most accurate blood pressure reading:

- Avoid caffeine, tobacco, and exercise for at least 30 minutes beforehand.
- Empty your bladder.
- Sit with your feet flat on the floor.
- Place the cuff on your bare arm (not over clothing) with the bottom edge about a finger's width above the crook of your elbow.
- Support your forearm by resting it on a table, with your elbow positioned roughly at heart height.
- Sit quietly without talking (or doing anything else such as reading, watching TV, or doing a crossword puzzle) during the measurement.

Current guidelines suggest that people wait one minute, retake the reading, and then average the two numbers. Follow your doctor's advice about when and how often to check your blood pressure at home. To watch a video from the American Heart Association demonstrating the correct technique, go online to https://targetbp.org/tools_downloads/self-measured-blood-pressure-video.

Choosing a home blood pressure monitor

Home blood pressure monitors range in price from about $40 to $100. Look for one that automatically inflates and automatically records the pressure. Many can store readings for a week or two, and pricier ones can wirelessly send the data to an app on your smartphone, making it easier to track your progress over time and share the information with doctors.

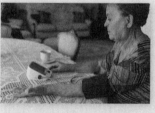

Take care to support your arm when measuring your blood pressure at home.

Skip devices with a wrist cuff or a fingertip sensor, as they're not as reliable as those with an upper arm cuff. Be sure to choose the correct cuff size—the inflatable part should completely cover at least 80% of your bare arm. (A too-small cuff can give a reading that's falsely high.) Ask your physician if you're not sure if you should get a large or extra-large cuff.

Understanding secondary hypertension

Sometimes high blood pressure results from an underlying condition. Should you be checked for these problems?

High blood pressure (hypertension) usually results from a combination of factors, including age, genetics, obesity, a high-salt diet, and lack of exercise. But up to 10% of people with high blood pressure have secondary hypertension, which is a byproduct of another condition or disease.

Most of the time, secondary hypertension is caused by problems with the adrenal glands or the arteries supplying the kidneys. Diagnosing and treating the underlying condition often improves or even resolves a person's elevated blood pressure. But how can you tell if you might have one of these uncommon issues?

"There are four main groups of people in whom you might suspect secondary hypertension as a possibility," says Dr. Randall Zusman, director of the Division of Hypertension at Harvard-affiliated Massachusetts General Hospital. Specifically:

1. People who develop high blood pressure before age 30

2. People who have never had high blood pressure but then develop it "out of the blue," usually after age 70

3. People who experience a sudden rise in blood pressure following many years of stable hypertension that's been well controlled with medication

4. People who have blood pressure above 130/80 mm Hg despite taking four or more medications.

Aldosterone overload

The most common cause of secondary hypertension is hyperaldosteronism, in which one or both adrenal glands make too much aldosterone. This hormone raises blood pressure by telling the kidney to hold

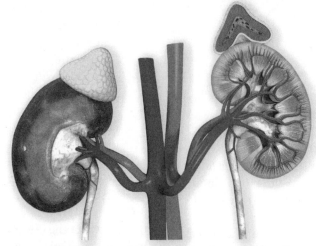

Most cases of secondary hypertension involve problems with the adrenal glands or the renal arteries.

on to sodium and water and sending it back into the bloodstream, boosting blood volume. One common cause is a benign (noncancerous) growth in one adrenal gland. Another is bilateral adrenal hyperplasia, in which both adrenal glands are working overtime, for unknown reasons.

Hyperaldosteronism is uncommon in younger people (group 1) and more likely in those who are middle-aged with poorly controlled blood pressure (group 4). A low potassium level can be a red flag, but most people with hyperaldosteronism have normal potassium levels, says Dr. Zusman.

Narrowed kidney arteries

Renal artery stenosis, a narrowing of the arteries that supply the kidneys with blood, is another common cause of secondary hypertension. This condition typically stems from a buildup of fatty plaque in artery walls, a problem usually seen in older people. But it can also occur in young women with an inherited condition called fibromuscular dysplasia, which is marked by an overgrowth of muscular tissue in artery walls. As a result, doctors are more likely to suspect renal artery stenosis among people in groups 1, 3, and 4.

Less-common causes of secondary hypertension include Cushing's syndrome (which results from overproduction of the stress hormone cortisol by the adrenal glands or from long-term use of steroid drugs) and thyroid disorders (diseases or growths that affect the thyroid gland's production of its hormone). Sleep apnea, a disorder in which you to stop breathing for short periods during sleep, can also trigger rises in hormones that raise blood pressure. (For group 2, any of the problems mentioned so far can lead to secondary hypertension).

Resistant hypertension

Secondary hypertension is common among people with so-called resistant hypertension, which includes people in the fourth group, as well as people who take three different blood pressure drugs at their maximum tolerated doses but still have high blood pressure. Overall, about one in four people with resistant hypertension ends up having an identifiable secondary cause.

However, in many people with stubbornly high blood pressure, the contributing cause isn't a disorder or condition but lifestyle habits, says Dr. Zusman. Often, these people are not taking their medications as prescribed, or they're consuming too much sodium (which counteracts the effects of many blood pressure drugs). Some are taking other medications or dietary supplements that elevate blood pressure.

But when those habits aren't to blame, doctors will look for clues to the other secondary causes, which can be revealed by a physical exam and specialized blood or imaging tests.

Remember: high blood pressure has no symptoms, and secondary causes can strike anyone. So have your blood pressure checked at every health care visit, Dr. Zusman says.

A look at diastolic blood pressure

Aggressively lowering high systolic blood pressure (the top number) can reduce the risk of heart attack and stroke. But how significant is the diastolic (bottom) number?

When it comes to managing blood pressure, doctors tend to focus on lowering the top (systolic) number, and for good reason.

"It's been well established that aggressively treating high systolic pressure can help lower one's risk for a heart attack or stroke," says Dr. Stephen Juraschek, a blood pressure specialist at the Hypertension Center of Harvard-affiliated Beth Israel Deaconess Medical Center.

But what about the bottom (diastolic) number? It also plays an essential role in heart health, although it tends to get overlooked.

Tale of two numbers

The two blood pressure numbers measure the heart at work and rest. Systolic pressure is the pressure in

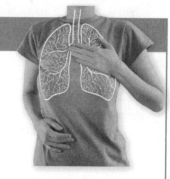

IN THE JOURNALS

Breath training may lower blood pressure

Using a device that strengthens breathing muscles for just five minutes a day may help lower blood pressure, according to a small study. Inspiratory muscle strength training (IMST) uses a small handheld device that provides resistance as you inhale and exhale. It was originally developed for people with serious lung conditions to strengthen their breathing muscles. Researchers tested the device on 36 older adults with elevated blood pressure. Half did high-resistance IMST for five minutes, six days a week, while the others did a low-resistance breathing program for comparison.

After six weeks, systolic blood pressure (the first number in a reading) dropped by an average of nine points among those who did the treatment. This benefit appeared to stem from improvements in blood vessel function and increases in nitric oxide, a molecule that helps widen arteries. According to the authors, IMST may offer benefits similar to exercise but in far less time. Although the training appears to be safe, people should consult a doctor before trying the device. The findings appeared June 29, 2021, in the *Journal of the American Heart Association*.

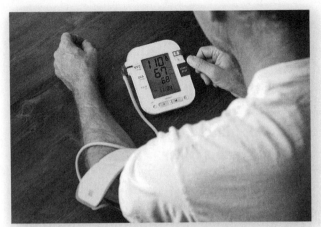

Keeping an eye on both blood pressure numbers can offer the most protection.

the arteries when the heart contracts to pump blood throughout the body. The higher the number, the harder the heart works to pump blood.

Diastolic pressure is the pressure during the resting phase between heartbeats. "This pressure plays a critical role in helping coronary vessels supply oxygen to the heart muscle," says Dr. Juraschek.

According to current guidelines, normal blood pressure is a systolic number less than 120 millimeters of mercury (mm Hg) and a diastolic number less than 80 mm Hg. A systolic number of 120 to 129, with the diastolic measurement less than 80, is deemed "elevated."

When it comes to diagnosing high blood pressure (hypertension), either number can be an indicator if persistently elevated. For instance, you're said to have Stage 1 hypertension if your systolic pressure is 130 to 139 or your diastolic pressure is 80 to 89—or both. Stage 2 hypertension is defined as either (or both) 140 or higher for systolic or 90 or higher for diastolic.

"It's important to keep track of both numbers because in many cases, if the systolic is high, so is the diastolic," says Dr. Juraschek.

Exceptions to the rules

However, there are exceptions. While systolic pressure tends to increase with age as blood vessels weaken and narrow, diastolic pressure declines after age 50.

Why? Arteries become less elastic with age. If they become too stiff, arteries that expand with the systolic push of blood have a harder time springing back between heartbeats, which causes diastolic blood pressure to drop.

Another possible cause of declining diastolic pressure is endothelial dysfunction, a condition where the coronary arteries on the heart's surface constrict instead of opening.

It also is possible to have only a high systolic number, a condition known as isolated systolic hypertension. This is a common type of high blood pressure among older adults. Isolated systolic hypertension happens because less elastic arteries have trouble accommodating surges of blood. Blood flowing at high pressure through these arteries can damage their inner lining, accelerating the buildup of cholesterol-laden plaque. This further stiffens and narrows the arteries, which elevates systolic blood pressure while diastolic pressure remains within a normal range.

Lower but not too low

Is diastolic pressure ever a serious concern? While lower is better for overall blood pressure, you don't want either number to drop too low. A very low systolic blood pressure increases the likelihood for weakness, lightheadedness, and fainting.

Surprisingly, a too-low diastolic number may signal a higher risk of heart issues, according to a study published Feb. 1, 2021, in *JAMA Network Open*. This study included people with high cardiovascular risk who received medication to lower their systolic blood pressure.

The researchers found that among those with systolic blood pressure less than 130, a diastolic blood pressure of less than 60 mm Hg was linked to more heart attacks and strokes. However, those with diastolic values between 70 and 80 mm Hg had the lowest risk of heart disease.

For most older adults, the goal should be to keep the systolic blood pressure close to 120 mm Hg, and perhaps a bit lower, as long as the diastolic pressure stays at 60 mm Hg or higher. Lifestyle changes like reducing dietary sodium, increasing potassium, exercising more, and maintaining a healthy weight are always the cornerstones of treatment, even if you also need medication.

The less common problem is a high diastolic pressure with a normal or slightly elevated top number. The treatment approach here is similar, with lifestyle changes first and blood pressure-lowering drugs when necessary.

The changing landscape of LDL-lowering drugs

For most people, statins are still the best way to lower harmful LDL cholesterol. But two newer drugs may be promising additions or alternatives for those with stubbornly high LDL levels.

There are many reasons why statins rank among the most widely prescribed drugs in the United States. First approved in the late 1980s, statins have a long track record for being effective and safe. These drugs don't just lower LDL cholesterol; they also reduce heart attacks and death from heart disease, the nation's leading killer. Plus, most are available in generic versions and cost only about $11 per year

---

ASK THE DOCTOR

by **HOWARD LEWINE, M.D.**

Do beta blockers interfere with exercise?

Q *I manage my high blood pressure with hydrochlorothiazide (a diuretic) and long-acting metoprolol (a beta blocker). I feel fine, but my heart rate doesn't go up like it used to before I started taking the metoprolol. Does that mean I am not getting as much health benefit whenever I exercise?*

A All beta blockers slow down your heart rate. The slower rate happens at rest and also when you exercise. To get the most from aerobic exercise, you would normally want your heart rate in a moderate-intensity zone for at least 30 minutes most days of the week. Moderate intensity means exercising at a heart rate that is 60% to 75% of your maximum.

An easy formula to find your maximum heart rate is 220 minus your age. So, if you are 60, your maximum heart rate is 160. Therefore, moderate-intensity exercise measured by your pulse is 96 to 120 beats per minute. While this formula usually works well to help gauge aerobic intensity of exercise, it doesn't work for people who take a beta blocker. And unfortunately, there is no simple way to adjust for the slower rate from the drug.

Instead, you can use your breathing to gauge your effort. With moderate-intensity exercise, you should be able to talk, but with pauses to catch your breath.

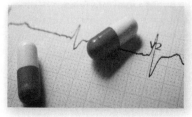

Beta blockers slow heart rates, but they don't interfere with health benefits from exercise.

If you are breathing very hard and unable to speak during exercise, you are at high intensity.

Can beta blockers affect your ability to work out? Studies that have addressed your question have not provided a definitive answer. A competitive athlete's performance likely could be diminished by taking a beta blocker. However, for most of us who exercise to stay healthy, the evidence tilts toward no decrease in benefit, even though you may not hit the standard heart rate goals.

So, your beta blocker won't prevent you from getting the positive effects of exercise. You will still build muscle, keep your bones strong, and lower your cholesterol and blood sugar levels. You'll also improve your heart's efficiency and endurance.

If you recently started the beta blocker, you might feel less energetic and even sluggish during your exercise routine. But over time, you should get back to the same sense of fulfillment from working out. I took a beta blocker when I was diagnosed with hypertension. I didn't like not having my heart rate to guide my workouts. So, I switched to a drug from a different class of medication that doesn't slow heart rate. However, there may be reasons your doctor specifically wants you on a beta blocker. It's a good question to ask at your next doctor visit.

per person, according to a 2021 statement from the American Heart Association.

Yet some people taking the maximum dose of a statin still have higher-than-recommended LDL levels. And a small percentage of people report that they can't tolerate statins. Until recently, the primary alternatives for lowering LDL were ezetimibe (Zetia) and PCSK9 inhibitors, which include alirocumab (Praluent) and evolocumab (Repatha). All three drugs have been shown to also lower heart attack risk. In the past few years, the FDA has approved two new drugs, bempedoic acid (Nexletol) and inclisiran (Leqvio), that further expand the options for lowering LDL.

"But while these two newer drugs may be helpful for some people, we still don't know if they will prevent heart attacks or strokes," says Dr. Jorge Plutzky, director of preventive cardiology at Harvard-affiliated Brigham and Women's Hospital. In most cases,

---

ASK THE DOCTOR

by DEEPAK L. BHATT, M.D., M.P.H.

Yoga and high blood pressure

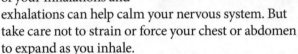

Q *I have coronary artery disease and take medications for high blood pressure. I did yoga when I was younger and would like to resume the practice. Are there any poses I should avoid?*

A Restarting your yoga practice is a terrific idea. Yoga may help lower your blood pressure, especially if you practice often. A recent review and analysis of earlier data published in *Mayo Clinic Proceedings* found that people (most of whom were overweight, middle-aged adults with high blood pressure) who did yoga for an hour about five times a week for 13 weeks had significant reductions in their blood pressure. The improvements were even greater when the yoga practice included breathing techniques and meditation.

While you're doing yoga (as is true for any type of exercise), your blood pressure will naturally rise, especially if you move quickly or hold poses for longer periods of time. Play it safe by restarting with a beginner or gentle yoga class. To minimize possible spikes in blood pressure, move slowly from one pose to the next. If the teacher has you hold a pose longer than 10 seconds, you may want to take a break by moving briefly out of the pose and then back into it. If you feel the need, rest between moves in child's pose (kneeling with your knees apart, belly resting between your thighs, resting your forehead on the ground).

Holding your breath may also elevate blood pressure, so keep breathing—something a good instructor will remind you about periodically during class. Extending the length of your inhalations and exhalations can help calm your nervous system. But take care not to strain or force your chest or abdomen to expand as you inhale.

As for poses to avoid, most people (not just those with heart disease) should be cautious about inversions. These poses, which place the heart higher than the head, require the heart to pump blood against gravity and tend to be more challenging. Some of the more advanced inversions, such as shoulder stand, headstand, and handstand, probably aren't a good idea. However, one common inversion, downward-facing dog (see photo), is generally fine for people with well-controlled high blood pressure, says Dr. Darshan Mehta, assistant professor of medicine at Harvard Medical School and medical editor of the Harvard Special Health Report *Intermediate Yoga*. But it's always best to check with your doctor if you have concerns about specific poses.

Finally, always end your practice with meditation, which is sometimes done while lying on your back, in a pose called savasana. This ritual helps relax your body as your breathing rate and blood pressure gradually drop.

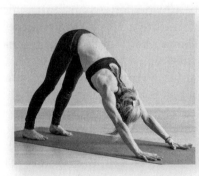

Inversions (such as downward dog) are poses that place the heart higher than the head.

a lower LDL value translates to a lower heart attack risk, but not always, he notes. Results from clinical trials evaluating both drugs are expected within several years.

Who might benefit?

For most people, taking a statin can lower LDL to the recommended target of no more than 100 milligrams per deciliter (mg/dL)—or no more than 70 mg/dL for people with cardiovascular disease or a high risk for it (those who've had a heart attack or have diabetes, for example).

But statins often aren't sufficiently potent for some people, especially those with familial hypercholesterolemia. This inherited condition, which affects about one in 250 people, can lead to LDL levels of 190 mg/dL or

---

ASK THE DOCTOR

by **DEEPAK L. BHATT, M.D., M.P.H.**

Strength training and blood pressure

Q *I take medication for high blood pressure. I've heard that weight lifting can elevate your blood pressure, so should I avoid that type of exercise?*

A If you have well-controlled blood pressure and are otherwise healthy, most types of strength training—which includes weight lifting—are generally considered not only safe but beneficial for your overall health. You should take precautions, however. But let's start with some definitions. Strength training (also called resistance training) refers to any exercise that works your muscles against an opposing force. You can train your muscles using your own body's weight or equipment such as elasticized bands, dumbbells and other free weights, or specialized machines.

These muscle-building exercises may be dynamic or isometric. Dynamic exercises are those in which you move your muscles and joints, such as a biceps curl or a squat. Isometric exercises are performed against an immovable object, such as a wall or the floor, and include things such as planks or wall sits (see photo).

When you perform any type of exercise—whether it's aerobic, strength training, stretching, or even balance exercises—both your blood pressure and heart rate increase to meet the greater demand for oxygen from your muscles. Some research suggests that during exercise, isometric exercise may boost blood pressure more than dynamic exercise, but the evidence isn't conclusive. However,

it's clear that just as with aerobic or endurance exercise (such as walking, jogging, cycling, or swimming), strength training can help lower your blood pressure if you do it consistently.

Most adults should do strength training exercises at least two days a week, according to the federal activity guidelines. Beginners should start with exercise bands or light hand weights. If you're more experienced, weight machines are a good option. Use a weight that's challenging but manageable. The general advice is to start with a single set of eight to 12 repetitions (reps) and then gradually build up to three sets over time. Rest for at least a minute between each set.

However, people who have high blood pressure, especially if it's not optimally controlled, should be cautious about any movements that involve lifting very heavy weights—not just loaded barbells at the gym, but also heavy furniture or boxes of books. That's because the sudden, intense effort can cause your blood pressure to spike—especially if you hold your breath, which people sometimes do in an attempt to increase their effort. During strength training exercises, be sure to exhale as you lift, push, or pull, and inhale as you release. Counting out loud as you lift and release can help you remember to keep breathing.

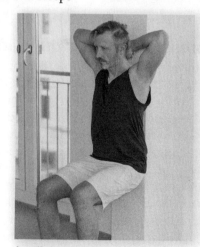
A wall sit strengthens leg muscles by using your own body weight.

© stockfour | Getty Images

higher, Dr. Plutzky says. And some people say they have muscle aches or pain (myalgias) when taking statins. This inability to tolerate statins occurs in about 5% of people in clinical trials but up to 15% of people in the real world, although studies show these symptoms are often not reproducible or actually due to the statin. For people with statin intolerance, doctors may prescribe ezetimibe, which lowers LDL by about 20%.

The newer non-statin drugs have even greater LDL-lowering effects.

Inclisiran. Like the current PCSK9 inhibitors, inclisiran slashes LDL levels by about 50%. Both types of drugs target the protein known as PCSK9, which is made in the liver and regulates LDL. The original PCSK9 inhibitors use antibodies to grab on to and block PCSK9 after it's been made. In contrast, inclisiran interferes with PCSK9's genetic blueprint, preventing the protein from being made in the first place. Another difference: the first two PCSK9 inhibitors must be injected once or twice a month, while inclisiran requires just two injections per year.

Bempedoic acid. Like statins, bempedoic acid comes as a pill and works by interfering in the same cholesterol pathway. But unlike a statin, bempedoic acid changes into its active form only in the liver, raising the prospect of fewer muscle-related side effects, although that remains to be determined, says Dr. Plutzky. Taken alone, bempedoic acid lowers LDL by about 25%. Bempedoic acid is also available in combination with ezetimibe, sold under the trade name Nexlizet. Studies suggest this combination can cut LDL by about 40%.

If your LDL cholesterol is very high, you may need more than one medication to reach a safe LDL level.

Current advice

For people who think they can't tolerate their statin, doctors usually recommend trying a different statin, often at a lower dose. Although PCSK9 inhibitors are a proven alternative, their high cost has limited their widespread use. For those already on ezetimibe, Nexlizet might be a good option because it already includes ezetimibe. It's also more affordable than PCSK9 inhibitors and therefore more likely to be approved by insurers, although findings about the drugs' ability to prevent heart attacks are still pending. While Dr. Plutzky is optimistic about inclisiran, he's looking forward to results from the clinical trials of the drug.

IN THE JOURNALS

Magnesium and blood pressure: What's the evidence?

In January 2022, the FDA announced that companies can make certain health claims regarding the consumption of magnesium and a reduced risk of high blood pressure. However, food companies and dietary supplement makers who want to include such claims on their packaging must add some caveats.

Specifically, the wording has to make it clear that the evidence to support the claim is "inconclusive and not consistent," according to the agency.

If you have high blood pressure, you're better off getting your magnesium from foods that are naturally rich in this important mineral rather than taking pills or eating foods with added magnesium. Good sources of magnesium include unsalted almonds, peanuts, spinach, and black beans. These foods have the added benefit of containing other nutrients (especially fiber) that may lower blood pressure and are also naturally low in sodium. Too much dietary sodium—which can raise blood pressure—has a far greater effect on blood pressure than potentially inadequate levels of magnesium.

Do statins increase the risk of dementia?

The research is mixed, but what's clear is that the benefits of statins typically outweigh the risks in people who need them.

Experts know that statins are good for your heart—they can lower "bad" LDL cholesterol and reduce your chances of having a heart attack or stroke by 25% to 30%. But what effect do statins have on your brain? In 2012, questions surfaced when the FDA issued a warning that statin users had reported short-term cognitive impairment when taking the drugs.

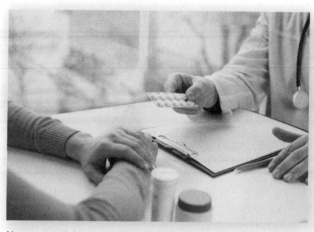

New research has eased concerns regarding dementia risks from statin use.

A study published June 29, 2021, by the *Journal of the American College of Cardiology* (*JACC*) aimed to shed some additional light on this issue. Researchers looked at data on statin use among 18,446 people, ages 65 or older, who had taken part in a large, randomized trial of aspirin. The researchers found that over a follow-up period of almost five years, people who took statins weren't any more likely than non-users to have dementia. The same was true when it came to other changes in cognition, memory, language, executive function, or a measure called psychomotor speed, which measures how quickly someone can process information. They also found no differences between different types of statins.

However, while these findings were good news, they may not be the final word on this issue. Although this particular study found no link between statins and dementia, the research into statins and brain-related effects overall is best described as inconsistent, says Dr. JoAnn Manson, chief of the Division of Preventive Medicine at Harvard-affiliated Brigham and Women's Hospital.

"I think that the relationship between statins and cognitive function remains controversial," says Dr. Manson. "There's still not a clear conclusion whether they help to prevent dementia or Alzheimer's disease, have neutral effects, or increase risk." While the science in this area is a little murky, one thing is clear: "If your health care provider is recommending statins and saying that you are a candidate, the benefits of taking it are very, very likely to outweigh any risks," she says.

Healthy heart, healthy brain?

On the surface, it seems intuitive that statins would reduce the risk of cognitive problems, because many treatments that help your heart can also help your brain, says Dr. Manson. Conversely, high cholesterol levels, high blood pressure, and diabetes are all risk factors for heart disease, as well as for a condition called vascular dementia, in which impaired blood flow to the brain leads to cognitive changes.

"Statins also decrease inflammation, which has been implicated in Alzheimer's disease and some other forms of dementia," says Dr. Manson. Although it seems to make sense that statins would bring brain benefits, the research doesn't always bear that out.

"While you would expect that statin use would reduce the risk of cognitive decline and dementia because statins lower cardiovascular risks and the risk of stroke, it hasn't been clearly shown to be the case," says Dr. Manson. "It's surprising that there's not a clearer reduction seen."

Sorting through the mixed results

Ultimately, when it comes to the research on statins and dementia, there is enough inconsistency in the findings to conclude that statins have minimal if any effect on cognition.

If you take a statin and do experience symptoms,

such as brain fog, confusion, or difficulty concentrating, it might be helpful to talk with your doctor about whether you should lower the dose or switch to a different type of statin, she says.

While the JACC analysis found no cognitive differences between people taking different types of statins, other research has found a higher rate of brain-related side effects related to a category of statins called lipophilic statins, says Dr. Manson. These include

- simvastatin (Zocor)
- fluvastatin (Lescol)
- pitavastatin (Livalo)
- lovastatin (Altoprev)
- and atorvastatin (Lipitor).

Switching to a different type of statin, called a hydrophilic statin—either rosuvastatin (Crestor) or pravastatin (Pravachol)—might be an option to discuss with your doctor, says Dr. Manson. Your doctor might also want to prescribe a non-statin cholesterol medication instead.

It's important to keep in mind that even if you do experience side effects with one type of statin, don't stop taking it without having a conversation with your doctor.

"People shouldn't just stop taking a statin, because high cholesterol is a clear risk factor for heart disease and stroke, in addition to being a risk factor for cognitive decline," says Dr. Manson.

Don't avoid statins if your doctor recommends one

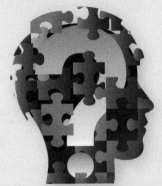

© tonivaver | Getty Images

While the link between statins and dementia risk is inconclusive, Dr. JoAnn Manson, chief of the Division of Preventive Medicine at Harvard-affiliated Brigham and Women's Hospital, says that people shouldn't be afraid to take a statin if their clinician determines that they need one. Some people do hesitate to take statins because they've heard about others who have had symptoms related to statin use, such as brain fog, muscle pain, and liver problems, she says. "But such side effects are rare, and the benefits of statins clearly outweigh the risks in people who are appropriate candidates," she says.

An analysis published July 15, 2021, in *The BMJ* supports that conclusion. Study authors looked at 62 trials that included more than 120,000 participants and an average follow-up of about four years. While the authors found that statin use was associated with a small increase in symptoms such as muscle pain, liver dysfunction, kidney problems, and eye conditions, the significantly lower risk of heart attack, stroke and other vascular conditions outweighed these risks. It's not the first study to examine the risk-to-benefit ratio in people with cardiovascular risk factors.

"Randomized trials have found that side effects are extremely rare, comparing the statin and placebo groups. I think a lot of the concerns about statins are really more about perception than fact," says Dr. Manson. As for the link between statins and dementia, she says there will be much more research on this question in coming years, including randomized trials of statins that look specifically at how they affect the brain.

Tips to help you stay on your cholesterol drug

Low-dose or alternate-day medication schedules and gentle muscle stretches can help.

Statin drugs such as atorvastatin (Lipitor) and rosuvastatin (Crestor) are important medications that reduce high LDL ("bad") cholesterol and significantly lower the risk for heart attack, stroke, or premature death. Despite the drugs' effectiveness,

many people who start a statin discontinue its use.

"It's often cited that 50% of people, a year after starting a statin, are no longer taking it. I find it hard to believe it's that high. But it may be in the range of a quarter to half of people taking statins stop them," says Dr. Christopher Cannon, a cardiologist at Harvard-affiliated Brigham and Women's Hospital.

Statin nonadherence

Statins are often abandoned because of side effects (real or perceived). These can include muscle aches and cramps, an increase in blood sugar, an increased risk for diabetes in people already at high risk for the disease, heartburn, nausea, and in rare cases, liver problems or a potentially life-threatening breakdown in muscle cells that causes kidney damage.

Dr. Cannon says that in blinded studies, about 5%

ASK THE DOCTOR

by HOWARD LEWINE, M.D.

How can I tell if my statin is working?

Q *I recently had a repeat coronary artery calcium scan, and the score was about the same. I take a statin and thought the score would go down. Does this mean the statin isn't working?*

A A coronary artery calcium (CAC) scan measures the amount of calcium in the walls of your heart's arteries. Calcium in the bloodstream makes its way into most of the fatty deposits called plaques that sit in your coronary arteries. So, the amount of calcium in the walls of your heart's arteries reflects how much plaque accumulation you have. While the CAC score provides important information, it doesn't tell the whole story. It can miss the softer uncalcified plaques, which have a more significant influence on heart attack risk.

A CAC scan is quick and easy. You lie on your back with electrodes placed on your chest to record an electrocardiogram (ECG). The CAC scan uses a special CT device that captures many heart images while you hold your breath for 10 to 15 seconds. The images are synchronized with your heartbeat recorded on the ECG. The computer program calculates a coronary artery calcium score. Traditionally, a higher score indicates a greater heart attack risk. But a study published online Aug. 18, 2021, by *JAMA Cardiology* suggests we should rethink how we use and interpret CAC scans.

Researchers enrolled 857 patients with suspected or known coronary artery disease. The patients underwent a baseline CT scan of their coronary arteries, and the test was repeated again two years later.

Of the study participants, two-thirds took a statin, and the rest did not.

The type of CT scan used in this study provides much more detail than a traditional CAC scan. It can show the degree of artery blockages and also the kind of plaque in the arteries. That's important because a soft, fatty plaque with less calcium is more likely to rupture than a hard and heavily calcified one. A ruptured plaque spews out chemicals that trigger blood clot formation on top of the plaques, suddenly blocking blood flow and causing a heart attack.

Over two years, the patients taking statins showed significant transformation of large, soft plaques to smaller plaques with denser calcium deposits. The patients who were not on statin therapy had more of the large, soft—and more dangerous—plaque formations.

Therefore, you should not be discouraged about having the same CAC score as before. You likely have fewer soft plaques now than you would have if you were not taking a statin.

In fact, even if your score had gone up, it would still mean that your statin is both lowering your risk of developing new plaques in your arteries and decreasing your chance of a heart attack.

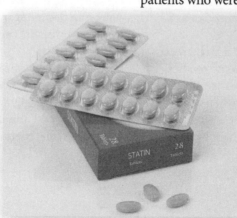

Statin therapy helps to shrink the size of dangerous plaque buildup.

© rogerashford | Getty Images

of statin users experience side effects as a result of an intolerance to the drug, and another 10% experience symptoms that they attribute to the medicine, but which are not actually caused by it. This phenomenon, called the "nocebo" effect, was reflected in a small, randomized trial published Sept. 21, 2021, in the *Journal of the American College of Cardiology*.

Participants followed for one year reported almost as many side effects when they took a placebo (a fake treatment) as when they took a statin.

"People have negative expectations because, unfortunately, there's a lot of false information about statins on the Internet and social media," Dr. Cannon notes.

What you can do

Work with your doctor to see if the following approaches can help you stick with your statin.

Start slowly. Consider a low-dose or an alternate-day-dose strategy to ease into statin use. "This recalibrates expectations and gives people more of an open mind that they can tolerate the statin," Dr. Cannon says.

Try a non-statin cholesterol drug. These drugs don't cause muscle aches the way statins sometimes do. Examples include cholesterol absorption inhibitors such as ezetimibe (Zetia) and bempedoic acid (Nexletol).

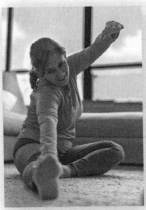

Think about other causes of muscle aches. Is it really the medication causing discomfort, or did you perhaps begin to exercise more when you started the statin, and you have sore muscles as a result?

Consider drug interactions. Some medications can cause adverse reactions when taken with statins, such as certain calcium-channel blockers,

Stretching every day can help you ward off muscle cramps.

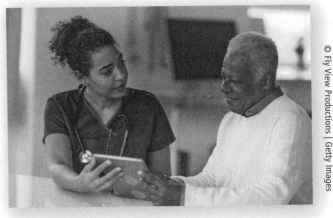

Ask your doctor for tips to help you stay on your cholesterol drug regimen.

including diltiazem (Cardizem), and certain antifungal medications, such as ketoconazole (Nizoral).

Work with your doctor to pinpoint symptom causes. "Sometimes we stop the statin for a month and see if they feel better. Then we start the statin again to see if symptoms come back," Dr. Cannon says.

Take coenzyme Q10. This supplement has mixed results for relieving muscle aches from statins, but Dr. Cannon says it's worth a try. "You can take it and see if it helps. If it doesn't, stop taking it," he suggests.

Check your vitamin D levels. "There's an association between low vitamin D levels and higher muscle aches when you take a statin," Dr. Cannon says. "You'll want to replenish your vitamin D levels if they're low, but no study shows taking vitamin D will relieve aches."

Try gentle stretching. If you're experiencing muscle aches, a program of gentle stretching for all of your muscles (after marching in place or walking for a few minutes) can help. Make it a regular part of your day.

Whatever the cause of the symptoms you may feel when taking statins, work with your doctor to find a solution. "Working together is most important," Dr. Cannon says. "Patients need options, and we need to test things out together."

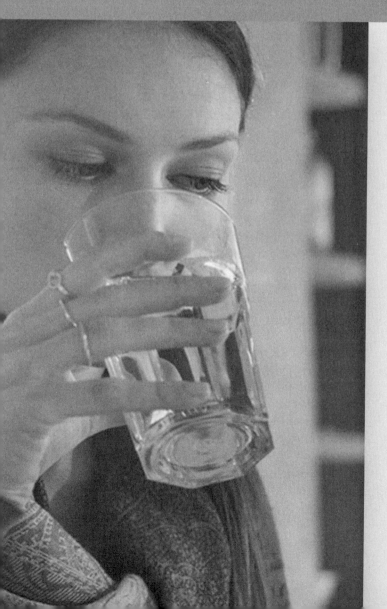

Chapter 4

Cardiovascular Health

Take Action!
5 Things You Can Do Now

1 **Know the warning signs of internal bleeding.** Taking anti-clotting drugs, such as aspirin, increases the risk of bleeding in the digestive tract. (page 68)

2 **Check the details of your family's medical history.** Heart attacks in relatives at an early age boost your risk. (page 69)

3 **Measure your waist circumference.** A large belly raises heart-related risks. (page 75)

4 **Practice stress-busting techniques.** Mental stress can harm the heart. (page 85)

5 **Find out if you qualify for cardiac rehab.** This education and exercise program helps people recover from serious heart conditions. (page 88)

Do you need aspirin therapy?

For most older adults without heart disease the answer is no.

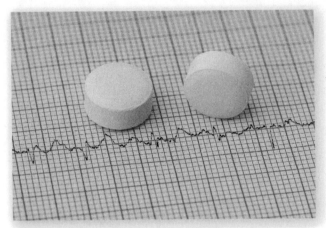

People should weigh the potential risks versus the benefits when considering aspirin therapy.

The medical world agrees that a small daily dose of aspirin can help people with heart disease lower their risk of heart attacks and strokes. But what if you don't have heart disease? Should you take aspirin as preventive medicine? Research suggests perhaps not.

Studies show that for people without heart disease, a higher risk of bleeding may outweigh the benefits of taking aspirin daily. In fact, guidelines from the American College of Cardiology and the American Heart Association recommend against this practice.

"The general recommendation now is that if you have heart disease, then you should probably be on aspirin therapy," says Dr. Christopher Cannon, a senior physician in the cardiovascular division at Harvard-affiliated Brigham and Women's Hospital. "If not, then you need to look at your potential risk for heart disease over the next 10 years and discuss it with your doctor."

Who's taking it?

This advice sounds simple enough. However, many people take aspirin who don't need it, and they often do so without their doctor's knowledge.

A recent survey of 14,000 people ages 40 and older in the *Annals of Internal Medicine* found that about a quarter of those who did not have heart disease took daily aspirin. Of these, about 23% did so without a physician's okay. Even more concerning, nearly half of survey participants ages 70 and older without heart disease took daily aspirin.

"While some people can benefit from aspirin therapy, for others, it may be unwise and potentially dangerous," says Dr. Cannon. "You should never begin taking regular aspirin just because you heard it's good. It always should involve a decision-making process with your doctor."

Your doctor will prescribe aspirin therapy based on your specific needs and your risk for heart attacks, strokes, and bleeding. In general, prescriptions range from a low dose (81 mg) to a full dose (325 mg). Studies have found the benefit is generally similar at both levels. However, the lower amount has been linked with a lower risk of bleeding and therefore is usually the recommended dose.

So, where does aspirin therapy fit into your heart health plan? Here's a breakdown of when you need aspirin therapy, when it may help, and when it's best to avoid it.

Yes, aspirin helps

The people who most benefit from aspirin therapy are those who have been diagnosed with heart disease or who have suffered a heart attack or stroke caused by a blood clot (ischemic stroke). In these people, daily aspirin lowers the odds of a future attack. Aspirin therapy also helps prevent blood clots in the heart arteries for people who have had stent placement or coronary bypass surgery.

Maybe (ask your doctor)

In general, people ages 40 to 70 with diabetes who have a high risk of heart disease should consider aspirin therapy, says Dr. Cannon. High risk means you have at least a 10% chance of having a heart attack or stroke over the next 10 years. (To estimate your 10-year risk, use the calculator created by the American Heart Association and American College of Cardiology, at www.health.harvard.edu/heartrisk.)

People with diabetes and a lower risk for heart disease—less than 10% over 10 years—should discuss their options with their doctor. "Sometimes, the risk of a heart attack and bleeding are about the same, in which case you have to decide with your doctor which risk you want to avoid—a heart attack or bleeding," says Dr. Cannon.

Aspirin therapy may also be appropriate for people deemed to be at high heart risk based on visual evidence of plaque in their arteries. That evidence can come from an imaging test, such as a coronary artery calcium scan, a CT scan, or an ultrasound of the neck arteries. "Here, the benefit of aspirin often outweighs the risk, but whether a person may need aspirin depends on the individual situation," says Dr. Cannon.

There are some gray areas. For instance, some people without heart disease and at low risk for a heart attack or stroke may have already been taking daily aspirin for decades with no bleeding problems. Should they now stop? Others may have a low 10-year risk but slightly high cholesterol or high blood pressure. "In these cases, you need to consult your doctor to discuss individual risks and benefits," says Dr. Cannon.

Best to avoid

In general, people over age 70 without cardiovascular disease should avoid aspirin as a way to prevent a heart attack or stroke. A study published in *The New England Journal of Medicine* highlighted the higher risk of major bleeding when taking daily aspirin without significant health benefit. "Even if you have taken aspirin for a long time as primary prevention of heart disease, you should consider stopping once you reach age 70. But again, check with your doctor," says Dr. Cannon.

The aspirin and clotting connection

Aspirin helps prevent heart attacks and strokes by interfering with how blood clots. When you have a cut that bleeds, cells called platelets gather at the wound site. The platelets help form a plug that seals the opening in the blood vessel, which stops the bleeding. However, there are times when this process causes unwanted clotting. Fatty deposits (plaque) that form in arteries feeding the heart and brain can slow blood flow enough to allow small clots to form. Also, some of these plaques, even smaller ones, can suddenly break open. The broken plaque releases substances that attract blood platelets and can rapidly trigger a clot, block blood flow, and cause a heart attack or stroke. Aspirin makes platelets less sticky, which keeps them from clumping together to form clots. That is the upside. The downside to less clotting is a higher risk of bleeding, especially in the gastrointestinal tract. Another effect of aspirin is that it weakens the stomach's protective lining against stomach acid, making the stomach and intestines more vulnerable to ulcers, which can bleed. Signs of gastrointestinal bleeding include black stools, vomiting with specks that look life coffee grounds, and weakness.

Most people at high risk for bleeding should probably avoid aspirin therapy. That includes those with a history of gastrointestinal bleeding, stomach ulcers, low blood platelets, blood clotting disorders, and people who take nonsteroidal anti-inflammatory drugs for arthritis or other inflammatory conditions.

Does early heart disease run in your family?

Knowing the details can inform your screening and treatment decisions.

Because heart disease is so prevalent, the odds that one or more of your relatives has some type of heart problem are pretty high. But you should pay special attention if someone in your immediate family—a parent or sibling—had a heart attack or related issue at a relatively young age. Known as premature or early coronary artery disease, this condition refers to a heart attack that occurs before age 55 in a man or before age 65 in a woman.

Caused by fatty plaque that narrows arteries feeding the heart, coronary artery disease is responsible for most heart attacks and is by far the most common type of heart disease. But uncommon genetic conditions also can cause the heart to unexpectedly stop beating, known as cardiac arrest in younger people (see "Heart-stopping conditions that strike at an early age" on the next page).

Know your family history

"Understanding the details and circumstances of a close relative's heart condition can make a difference in how you and other family members are evaluated and treated," says Dr. James Januzzi, a cardiologist at Harvard-affiliated Massachusetts General Hospital.

For example, if your brother, sister, or parent had a heart attack during middle age, be extra vigilant about following the American Heart Association's "Life's Essential 8" tips to lower your risk of coronary artery disease (see www.health.harvard.edu/simple7).

Cardiac arrest is more challenging to predict and prevent, but a policy statement recently released by the American Academy of Pediatrics (AAP) may help

---

ASK THE DOCTOR

by DEEPAK L. BHATT, M.D., M.P.H.

Aspirin and bruising

Q *After my recent heart attack, my cardiologist told me to start taking a low-dose daily aspirin. Since then, I've been noticing more bruising on my arms and legs. I'm not bothered by the cosmetic aspect, but I am worried that it means I may be bleeding on the inside.*

A Most bruises happen when a minor blow or injury damages the tiny blood vessels near the skin's surface (capillaries). The trapped blood often appears as a black-and-blue mark that may change colors as it heals. Even slight bumps that you don't even notice can cause bruises.

Aspirin decreases the ability of tiny cell fragments in the blood, called platelets, from clumping together and forming clots. Preventing these clots will help you avoid a repeat heart attack. But it can make you bleed a little more easily, including the below-the-skin bleeding seen in bruises. Small cuts may take a bit longer than usual to stop bleeding. People sometimes also say their gums bleed more easily when they floss or brush their teeth after starting low-dose aspirin. An electric toothbrush can help in that regard.

Likewise, an electric shaver may help you avoid bleeding from razor cuts. Experiencing these types of minor bleeding usually does not mean that more serious internal bleeding is also occurring. But there's always a small risk of internal bleeding when taking aspirin, regardless of

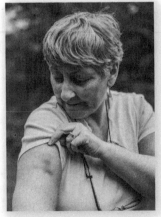

Increased bruising is common after starting low-dose aspirin.

whether or not you notice more bruising.

Aspirin inhibits substances that protect the stomach's delicate lining, which can provoke bleeding in the stomach and intestines. If you notice stomach upset or pain, call your doctor. Taking aspirin with food may help. Older people and others prone to bleeding may want to ask their physician about taking an over-the-counter proton-pump inhibitor such as omeprazole (Prilosec), which can help prevent aspirin-induced stomach bleeding.

More serious bleeding in the gastrointestinal tract can manifest as black, tarry stools. In rare cases, you may vomit dried blood (which resembles coffee grounds) or fresh blood. These situations should be evaluated right away in an emergency room.

The type of bleeding physicians worry about the most is bleeding in the head. Though rare, it poses a high risk of disability and death when it occurs. Some data suggest that controlling high blood pressure might decrease this risk. Follow commonsense approaches to minimize head trauma. Use a seat belt, wear a helmet while biking or skiing, and don't climb up ladders—get a professional to clean your gutters and do other tasks with fall risks.

Always call your doctor's office if you experience bleeding that does not stop. If the bleeding is severe, call 911.

unearth uncommon inherited cases. It calls for screening all children for conditions that can lead to cardiac arrest through questions about fainting, unexplained seizures, chest pain, breathlessness, and whether any family members have a history of heart conditions or have experienced heart-related death before age 50.

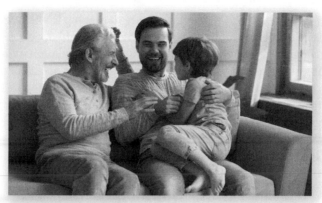

Genes that affect the heart run in families, and lifestyle factors often do as well.

these, such as high cholesterol and high blood pressure, may be linked to genes passed down from their parents. But unhealthy habits—such as smoking and poor eating and exercise habits—also tend to run in families and may contribute to the higher risk.

Most often, inherited risks stem from dozens of mutations in different genes. However, abnormally high LDL cholesterol (190 mg/dL or higher) can arise from a mutation in one of the genes that governs how the body processes cholesterol. This condition, familial

Early heart attacks: Nature and nurture

People who have heart attacks in their 40s and 50s tend to have the same classic risk factors for coronary artery disease as those seen in older people. Some of

Heart-stopping conditions that strike at an early age

Sudden cardiac arrest—when the heart unexpectedly stops beating—can occur in the throes of a heart attack. A blocked artery deprives the heart of oxygen, triggering a potentially fatal heart rhythm. Fortunately, this is the exception rather than the rule: most heart attacks don't cause cardiac arrest.

However, the two conditions are often conflated, says Dr. James Januzzi, professor of medicine at Harvard Medical School. "When someone dies suddenly, the cause is often invoked as a 'heart attack.' But cardiac arrest can occur for a number of reasons," he says. In young people,

possible causes include inherited cardiac abnormalities. One example is congenital long QT syndrome, a rare disorder of the heart's electrical system resulting from mutations in a handful of different genes. A history of unexplained fainting in response to vigorous exercise or sudden loud noises raises suspicion for long QT. Another possibility is hypertrophic cardiomyopathy, which causes a thickening of the heart muscle that sometimes leads to cardiac arrest in young and middle-aged people. Genes that affect the heart run in families and lifestyle factors often do as well.

IN THE JOURNALS

A new way to take aspirin: Liquid-filled capsules

Millions of Americans who take a daily low-dose aspirin to lower their heart attack risk now have a new way to take this popular drug. In March 2021, the FDA approved the first liquid-filled aspirin capsule, Vazalore. The novel formulation is designed to release aspirin in the duodenum, the first part of the intestine. This may help reduce stomach erosions and ulcers that sometimes occur with regular aspirin (also known as plain or immediate-release aspirin). Most of the aspirin sold in the United States is enteric-coated, which is also formulated to protect the stomach. However, the coating reduces aspirin absorption in some people. When compared with regular and enteric-coated aspirin, Vazalore's clot-preventing effects were equal to regular aspirin and faster than enteric-coated formulations. The capsules are available in doses of 81 or 325 milligrams.

hypercholesterolemia, affects about one in 200 people and is one of the leading causes of premature heart disease. It's why the AAP strongly recommends cholesterol testing in children at least once between ages 9 and 11 and again between ages 17 and 21.

Another test cardiologists may recommend for people with a family history of premature coronary artery disease is a measurement of lipoprotein (a), or Lp(a), a substance found in blood that is considered more damaging to the heart than LDL. Because Lp(a) levels are inherited, people with high levels—about 20% of the population—often have a family history of premature heart attack or stroke. Yet many of them have no other traditional risks for heart disease, such as high LDL cholesterol or high blood pressure. New therapies to treat elevated Lp(a) are currently being studied for their potential to reduce heart attacks and strokes, says Dr. Januzzi.

In your eyes: Clues to heart disease risk?

Changes both around and inside your eyes—some visible only with special tests— may be harbingers of heart disease.

Are the eyes a window to the heart as well as the soul? New insights and older observations suggest the answer is yes.

Sudden vision changes such as blurriness, dark areas, or shadows could be a blockage in an eye blood vessel, which can foreshadow a more serious stroke in the brain. And growing evidence hints that subtle, early damage to tiny blood vessels in the eyes may predict cardiovascular disease. Other unusual eye changes also can be clues to possible heart problems, such as small, yellowish bumps around the eyes, or pupils that widen and constrict with the heartbeat (see "A pulsating pupil and a leaky heart valve?" on the next page).

Retina changes reflect heart health

A network of blood vessels, each no wider than a

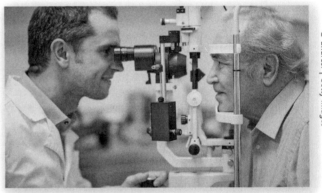

Evidence of cardiovascular disease may be visible during a comprehensive eye examination.

strand of hair, supply blood to the retina, the light-sensitive tissue at the back of the eyeball. "Like arteries

---

IN THE JOURNALS

New treatment for pericarditis approved

Sometimes the lining surrounding the heart (the pericardium) becomes irritated because of an infection, heart surgery, or unknown reasons. This irritation, known as pericarditis, can cause sharp, stabbing pain in the center of the chest. Although it usually disappears within four to six weeks, some people experience repeated attacks. In March 2021, the FDA approved a new drug specifically to treat recurrent pericarditis.

Called rilonacept (Arcalyst), it targets a substance involved in the underlying inflammation that triggers pericarditis. The medication is taken as a self-administered weekly injection. In a clinical trial, the drug helped quell painful symptoms and lowered the risk of future flare-ups. Side effects include redness or swelling at the injection site and respiratory symptoms such as a runny nose and cough.

A pulsating pupil and a leaky heart valve?

When the heart's aortic valve doesn't close tightly (a condition called aortic regurgitation), small amounts of blood leak backward into the heart instead of being pumped into the body. Symptoms typically include fatigue and breathlessness.

In severe cases, another possible sign is a rarely documented eye phenomenon: pupils that dilate and constrict in synchrony with the heartbeat. Called Landolfi's sign, it was first described by Italian physician Michele Landolfi in 1909.

Compared with people who have normal hearts, people with aortic regurgitation have a wide pulse pressure, which means there is an unusually big difference between the two numbers in their blood pressure readings (that is, the systolic and diastolic numbers). The pupil pulsations reflect these large pressure fluctuations.

Illustration by Scott Leighton

throughout the body, these tiny vessels can be damaged by chronic conditions such as diabetes and high blood pressure," says Dr. Nimesh Patel, an ophthalmologist who specializes in retina disorders at Harvard-affiliated Massachusetts Eye and Ear hospital.

Over time, high blood sugar (the hallmark of diabetes) causes the walls of vessels supplying the retina to weaken and leak fluid into the surrounding tissue. This condition, called diabetic retinopathy, can progress, causing further damage that may impair vision. Poorly controlled high blood pressure can cause retinal arteries to narrow or break and bleed into the retina.

While both diabetes and high blood pressure are well-known contributors to heart disease, people may not know they have these conditions if they haven't seen a primary care doctor in years, says Dr. Patel.

"Sometimes, patients come in with vision problems and a retinal photo or exam shows a piece of plaque blocking a retinal artery," he says. Known as a retinal artery occlusion, this condition indicates a greater risk of a stroke in the brain. Blood clots may also form in the veins that carry blood away from the retina. Both conditions—a retinal artery or vein occlusion—are referred to as eye (ocular) strokes.

People who experience eye strokes need further testing, including ultrasounds of the neck to check for a buildup of fatty plaque inside the carotid arteries

and of the heart to check for blood clots.

More subtle changes seen in retina photos may foretell future heart problems. By analyzing the photos with machine learning (combined with health data such as age and blood pressure), several teams of researchers have created algorithms to predict a person's risk of heart attack or stroke. At this point, the models still need to be improved and validated. But advances in both imaging and artificial intelligence mean such tests could be available in the not-too-distant future.

Yellow bumps around the eyes: Xanthelasmas

Some middle-aged and older adults develop soft, yellowish, cholesterol-filled bumps on or around their eyelids, most commonly near the nose (*see illustration*). Called xanthelasmas, these small growths aren't painful and rarely affect vision. But they can be a sign of high levels of cholesterol, triglycerides, or other fats (lipids) in the blood. They're somewhat more prevalent in women than men. People who have them should be sure to get a cholesterol test,

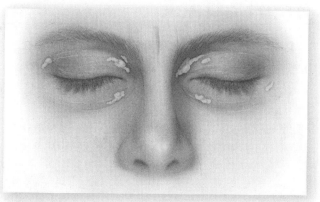

Xanthelasmas, cholesterol-filled plaques, can appear on or around the eyelids.

also known as lipid test or lipid profile.

Xanthelasmas are more common in people with genetic disorders that cause abnormally high cholesterol levels, such as familial hypercholesterolemia, which can cause LDL cholesterol levels of 190 or higher. (A healthier LDL is under 100.)

If your LDL is elevated, regular exercise and a high-fiber, plant-based diet can help lower it. Many people need cholesterol-lowering drugs such as statins, which will sometimes but not always reduce the size of a xanthelasma.

Half of people with xanthelasmas have normal lipid levels, and the growths are simply a cosmetic problem. But people with a family history of early heart disease should make sure their physician knows about this possible sign of heightened cardiovascular risk.

Eye care advice

The American Academy of Ophthalmology recommends:

- People ages 40 to 64 who are otherwise healthy should get a complete eye exam from an ophthalmologist once every two to four years.
- After age 65, you should receive a complete eye exam every one to two years.
- People with type 2 diabetes should get a complete eye exam at the time of diagnosis and then annually after that.

The danger of a "silent" heart attack

Up to half of all heart attacks may go unrecognized—and they are linked to an increased risk of stroke.

Heart attacks don't always cause the dramatic symptoms depicted on TV shows, which

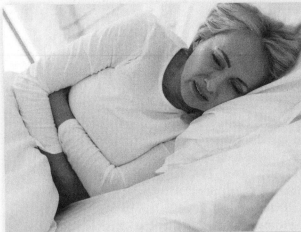

Symptoms such as nausea and fatigue may not be recognized as a potential heart attack.

Is it a heart attack?

The most common sign of a heart attack is discomfort in the center of the chest that spreads through the upper body. But this classic symptom doesn't always occur. Some people experience less typical symptoms, which may be slightly more frequent in women, people with diabetes, and older people.

TYPICAL SYMPTOMS

▸ Pressure or a squeezing sensation in the middle of the chest

▸ Chest pain or discomfort that spreads to the shoulders, neck, and arms

▸ Sweating

LESS TYPICAL SYMPTOMS

▸ Trouble breathing

▸ Weakness

▸ Nausea or vomiting

▸ Dizziness

▸ Back or jaw pain

▸ Unexplained exhaustion

---

often show a middle-aged man clutching his chest in pain. Sometimes, the symptoms are far more subtle, such as unexplained fatigue and weakness, shortness of breath, or nausea (see "Is it a heart attack?").

When that happens, people don't always realize they've experienced a heart attack. But these so-called silent heart attacks may be almost as concerning as heart attacks that are recognized and diagnosed right away. Now, recent research affirms that suspicion (see "Silent heart attacks may signal a higher risk of future stroke" on the next page).

"Doctors have long known that overt heart attacks are linked to a higher risk of stroke. This new study suggests that over the long term, unrecognized heart attacks may pose a similar risk," says cardiologist Dr. Robert Giugliano, professor of medicine at Harvard Medical School.

The heart attack–stroke link

Some of the heightened risk of stroke stems from shared risk factors, including high blood pressure,

Silent heart attacks may signal a higher risk of future stroke

A study published online Aug. 3, 2021, by the journal *Neurology* looked at how heart attacks—including unrecognized "silent" ones—affected a person's risk of stroke. **Who:** 4,224 older adults without a previous heart attack or stroke. All were part of the Cardiovascular Health Study (CHS), which recruited people ages 65 and older from four counties in California, Maryland, North Carolina, and Pennsylvania.

When: Participants were enrolled in the CHS in 1989 and 1990 and followed for a median of nearly nine years.

How: Participants received annual electrocardiograms (ECGs) and twice-yearly phone calls, during which they were asked about any heart-related conditions or hospitalizations.

Key findings: During the follow-up, 10% of the participants had a recognized (overt) heart attack, 9% had a silent heart attack, and 9% had a stroke. After adjusting for blood pressure, diabetes, and other confounding factors, researchers found that silent heart attacks were linked to a higher risk of stroke.

diabetes, and elevated cholesterol levels, all of which leave people more vulnerable to both heart attacks and strokes.

"But sometimes, a heart attack damages muscle in the wall of the heart," says Dr. Giugliano. Damage in the heart's lower chambers (ventricles) prevents the heart from contracting normally, which can lead to formation of a clot that then travels to the brain, causing a stroke.

Diagnosis and treatment

People with diabetes are more likely to have silent heart attacks, perhaps because they're prone to

nerve-related problems that interfere with pain signals. But other people might attribute the discomfort of a heart attack to indigestion, a muscle strain, or an illness such as the flu.

Most unrecognized heart attacks are discovered on an electrocardiogram (ECG), a recording of the heart's electrical activity. Heart muscle damage may create a distinct signature on an ECG. Because this test isn't foolproof, other tests such as a heart ultrasound (echocardiogram) are often needed to confirm the diagnosis.

For people with known heart disease, ECGs are routine. But for everyone else, the recommendations

---

IN THE JOURNALS

A big belly boosts heart risks, even if you're not overweight

Even if your weight is normal, a widening waistline may put you at a higher risk of heart disease, according to a recent scientific statement from the American Heart Association. Fat inside the center of your body (known as abdominal or visceral fat), which encases your organs, is more worrisome than fat found just beneath the skin (known as subcutaneous fat). In addition, fat can also accumulate in the liver, known as nonalcoholic fatty liver disease, which adds to cardiovascular disease risk. According to the statement, published April 22, 2021, in *Circulation*, you should check your waist circumference regularly. To do so, wrap a tape measure just above the upper border of your hipbone. Ideally, your waist size should be less than one-half of your height,

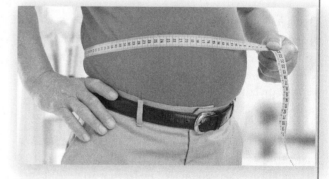

even if your body mass index is in the normal range. (Determine your weight category at www.health.harvard.edu/bmi-calculator.) Regular physical activity and cutting down on simple sugars are the best ways to shed extra belly fat.

for additional testing are still evolving, says Dr. Giugliano. By age 65, you should have at least one ECG; other tests you may need will depend on your cardiovascular risk factors.

Discovering you've had an unrecognized heart attack might feel unsettling, but the information can be useful. Ideally, the knowledge may give you extra incentive to follow a heart-healthy diet and get regular exercise. But medication changes may also be warranted. For example, if your LDL cholesterol is above 70 milligrams per deciliter, you should take cholesterol-lowering drugs (or increase your current dose).

Your physician also may suggest a lower blood pressure goal. If you have diabetes, you may be advised to switch to one of the newer diabetes medications (known as SGLT-2 inhibitors and GLP-1 receptor agonists), some of which also prevent heart attacks and strokes, says Dr. Giugliano.

Look inside your heart

Coronary artery calcium scans can reveal dangerous plaque buildup in your heart's arteries.

The traditional measures to gauge heart disease risk, such as blood pressure, cholesterol, and blood sugar levels, don't always tell the whole story. Sometimes you and your doctor need more information. An increasingly used test to predict your chance of heart attack or stroke is a coronary artery calcium (CAC) scan. It measures the amount of calcified plaque in the heart's arteries, high levels of which suggest higher overall plaque buildup.

"The CAC results can help identify a person's possible risk, even if that person doesn't have obvious risk factors or symptoms," says Dr. Ron Blankstein, associate director of the cardiovascular imaging program at Harvard-affiliated Brigham and Women's Hospital.

Optimal scanning

A CAC scan uses a special CT scanner. You lie on your back with electrodes placed on your chest to also record an electrocardiogram. The scanner takes several pictures of your heart in less than 10 seconds. The scanner emits low-dose radiation similar to that used for a mammogram.

Plaque sometimes calcifies, and the calcium shows up as tiny white specks on the scan. The amount of calcification is scored on a scale from zero to 400 and sometimes higher. In general, the lower the score, the lower the likelihood of a future heart attack or stroke.

"The result can show that plaque buildup is present and offer an estimate of future risk, but does not specifically pinpoint which heart arteries have plaques that are more likely to rupture and cause a heart attack," says Dr. Blankstein.

For example, a score of zero indicates the absence of plaque and a low chance of having a heart attack or stroke over the next 10 years, while a score higher than 400 suggests there is a large amount of plaque and a risk that may be 10 times greater (see "CAC scores").

Your CAC score also can help you and your doctor decide the best course of treatment. "While lifestyle and drug therapies cannot reverse calcified plaques, the CAC score could mean you need additional treatment to stop new plaque formation and keep existing plaques stable to reduce your risk of a heart attack," says Dr. Blankstein.

CAC scores	
SCORE	PRESENCE OF PLAQUE
0	No evidence. Heart attack risk is very low.
1 to 10	A small amount. Heart attack risk is low.
11 to 100	Enough to indicate mild heart disease. Heart attack risk is moderate.
101 to 400	A moderate amount, possibly with some artery blockage. Heart attack risk is moderate to high.
401 and higher	A large amount, with a 90% chance of some artery blockage. Heart attack risk is high.

According to the 2018 American College of Cardiology/American Heart Association cholesterol guidelines, people with a CAC score of 1 to 100, especially those over age 55, should consider statin therapy in addition to lifestyle changes. A moderate or severe amount of plaque—a CAC score higher than 100—suggests the need for even greater efforts to lose weight if needed, eat a plant-based diet, and exercise more. Usually, the high CAC score also means high-dose statin therapy as tolerated, possibly daily low-dose aspirin, and perhaps a lower blood pressure goal, says Dr. Blankstein.

Who should get one?

For people with evident heart disease—like those who've had a heart attack or stent—a CAC scan isn't necessary, since they already need to be on maximal therapy to prevent their disease from progressing.

"A CAC scan is most beneficial for people who have borderline or intermediate risk of atherosclerotic cardiovascular disease [ASCVD] in the next 10 years," says Dr. Blankstein. (You can calculate your estimated 10-year risk of ASCVD using a calculator from the American College of Cardiology, available at www.health.harvard.edu/ascvd.)

People who are unsure of their risk also may benefit from a CAC. For example, this might include someone with good blood pressure and cholesterol levels, but a family history of heart disease (a father, sibling, or uncle who had a heart attack before age 55), or someone with average cholesterol levels and borderline blood pressure who quit smoking five to 10 years ago. Certain conditions also may merit a CAC scan, particularly inflammatory diseases like psoriasis, lupus, or rheumatoid arthritis.

Whether or not you need a follow-up scan depends on your initial score. "If your CAC score is elevated, beginning on the right preventive therapies will be important, and repeat testing is unlikely to be helpful," says Dr. Blankstein. "On the other hand, if your score is zero, it may be reasonable to repeat the test in about four to eight years."

Don't fail your heart health

Here's how to recognize and treat the type of heart failure that's most common in older adults.

Heart failure conjures up the image of your heart suddenly stopping. But it actually means the heart is not pumping as it should. The condition is the leading cause of hospitalization for adults over age 65.

"Heart failure is an abrupt wake-up call for people to address their heart health practices," says Dr. Akshay Suvas Desai, medical director of the Cardiomyopathy and Heart Failure Program at Harvard-affiliated Brigham and Women's Hospital. "Still, heart failure can be prevented in high-risk individuals, and the outlook for those with heart failure continues to improve."

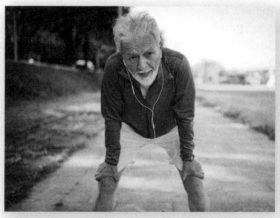

Getting easily winded during normal activity can be a symptom of heart failure.

© MStudioImages | Getty Images

Left-sided issues

Impairments in pumping action can develop in the entire heart or just one side—left or right. Most heart failure is caused by left-sided problems: the left ventricle (the heart's largest chamber) is either too weak or too stiff to pump normally.

To figure out what is happening, doctors usually order an echocardiogram to measure the heart's ejection fraction (EF). EF is a percentage of how much of the blood inside the left ventricle gets pumped out with each contraction.

The left ventricle never pushes out 100% of its

blood when it contracts. A normal heart's EF is 50% to 70%. An EF of 40% to 49% is considered borderline low. Less than 40% is deemed a low or reduced EF. This indicates the left ventricle is too weak to push out enough blood, a problem known as heart failure with reduced ejection fraction (HFrEF).

But when older adults develop heart failure they more often have a normal EF of 50% or greater, called heart failure with preserved ejection fraction (HFpEF). With HFpEF, the left ventricle muscle is too stiff to relax. Ejection fraction is normal, but less blood can enter the chamber in the first place, so less gets pumped out.

What puts you at risk for HFpEF? The usual factors

Different types of tachycardia

Q *What's the difference between supraventricular tachycardia and ventricular tachycardia? How are these problems treated?*

A Tachycardia refers to a rapid heart rate—anything higher than 100 beats per minute (bpm). But supraventricular tachycardia (SVT) tends to be less severe and occurs more often in younger people. Ventricular tachycardia (VT) is more likely in older people with heart disease and can be far more serious. All abnormal heart rhythms are caused by electrical misfires that originate somewhere in the heart. Supra means "above," so in SVT, the errant electrical signals start somewhere above the heart's ventricles (the heart's lower chambers). During a bout of SVT, the heart rate may rise to 250 bpm or higher. But it often returns to a normal rate within a few minutes. If SVT lasts longer, it may cause dizziness or lightheadedness. When that happens, a person can try coughing, gagging, or holding their breath while bearing down as if for a bowel movement, which may help slow down the heart. But if SVT persists, the person may need to go to the emergency room for an injectable medication to slow down the heart.

People with frequent episodes of SVT may take daily medications that slow the heart, such as beta blockers or calcium-channel blockers. Another treatment option is catheter ablation. A doctor guides several catheters through a vein up to the heart, where a pulse of radiofrequency energy destroys the area of tissue responsible for the faulty electrical signals.

In VT, the electrical glitch arises from either the left or right ventricle. If the abnormal rhythm lasts for just a few seconds, it may cause no problems. But with sustained VT (which lasts for more than 30 seconds) blood pressure may drop, triggering dizziness, breathlessness, or fainting. Most of the time, VT is caused by damage from a heart attack, heart failure, valve disease, or inherited heart disorder. VT can also lead to ventricular fibrillation, a life-threatening emergency that can cause the heart to stop (cardiac arrest).

Treatment often requires a jolt of electricity to restore the heart's normal rhythm. This can be done in the hospital with a method called cardioversion, in which medical professionals use a heart monitor and shock the heart using small paddles. Outside medical settings, bystanders can use automated external defibrillators (found in many public places) to treat cardiac arrest. For less extreme cases, other possible treatments include medications or catheter ablation.

People can't always tell the difference between SVT and VT, which is why anyone with an unexplained rapid heartbeat should be evaluated by a doctor.

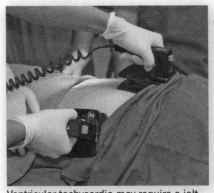

Ventricular tachycardia may require a jolt of electricity to restore the heart's normal rhythm.

Keep a look out for troubling signs

To effectively monitor your heart failure symptoms, you need to know the signs of trouble. Yet, this can be difficult, because symptoms may be mild or come and go. If you have any type of heart failure, weighing yourself at the same time every day is a great way to gauge changes in your condition. Gaining even two to three pounds over 24 hours might be a sign you're retaining fluid and heading in the wrong direction. And don't ignore symptoms like lightheadedness, frequent fatigue, or a new cough. Stay in close contact with your doctor and share any possible signs of symptoms.

are high blood pressure, coronary artery disease, obesity, and diabetes. Less common causes are inherited or acquired heart muscle diseases.

Similar symptoms

Both types of left-sided heart failure have similar symptoms. At first, you might only notice that you're more tired or that you can't walk as fast as you used to. Other symptoms include

- shortness of breath with exertion or when you're lying flat
- swelling in the legs, ankles, or both
- persistent cough
- waking up in the middle of the night short of breath.

"People may dismiss many of these, especially if they don't interfere with daily life, but they need checking out even if the symptoms appear minor or come and go," says Dr. Desai.

Treatment options

Treatment for HFpEF continues to evolve, says Dr. Desai. "We are only now developing specific therapies for the condition. But until more is known, prevention strategies are also the best treatments." This includes addressing weight gain with exercise and diet (especially reducing salt intake), quitting smoking, and curbing alcohol intake.

The mainstays of HFpEF drug treatment are

to reduce fluid in the body with diuretics ("water pills") and to aggressively lower blood pressure with a variety of medications, including ACE inhibitors, angiotensin-receptor blockers, beta blockers, and calcium-channel blockers.

However, Dr. Desai says, new research shows promising results for two additional drug treatments: Angiotensin receptor–neprilysin inhibition therapy uses a medication called Entresto that combines two blood pressure drugs, sacubitril and valsartan.

A study in the Oct. 14, 2021, issue of *The New England Journal of Medicine* found that people with diabetes and HFpEF who took the SGLT2 inhibitor empagliflozin (Jardiance) had lower risks for dying from heart problems or being hospitalized for heart failure. SGLT2 inhibitors are showing promise even for heart failure patients without diabetes.

The FACES of heart failure

To help both patients and doctors quickly spot possible heart failure symptoms, the Heart Failure Society of America came up to a simple acronym: FACES.

Fatigue. A weakened heart can't deliver enough oxygen-rich blood to meet the body's needs, causing a general sense of feeling tired or fatigued.

Activity limitation. Because people with heart failure tire easily, they often struggle to do everyday activities such as preparing a meal or taking a short walk.

Congestion. The heart's poor pumping ability causes blood to back up and fluid to leak into the lungs. The resulting lung congestion can trigger coughing and wheezing.

Edema or ankle swelling. Excess fluid can also collect in the ankles, legs, thighs, and abdomen. All the extra fluid can also cause rapid weight gain.

Shortness of breath. Congestion makes it harder for the lungs to remove carbon dioxide and replenish the blood with fresh oxygen, which makes breathing difficult. Shortness of breath is often worse when people lie down because excess fluid from the lower body moves up toward the lungs.

This unusual syndrome causes your heart to race when you stand up

Postural orthostatic tachycardia syndrome (POTS) involves the nervous system and can cause a constellation of debilitating symptoms.

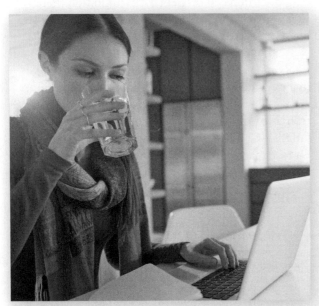
Consuming plenty of water and salt (which helps boost blood volume) is one common treatment for most people with POTS.

When you stand up, gravity pulls blood down into your lower body. Normally, the autonomic nervous system (the body's "autopilot" system) signals the blood vessels in your legs to tighten and your heart to pump a bit faster to send blood back up to your brain.

But sometimes that process goes awry: the blood vessels in the legs don't squeeze enough to ensure sufficient blood flow to the brain, so the heart accelerates even more than usual to compensate. A rapid heart rate—tachycardia—is a key feature of postural orthostatic tachycardia syndrome, or POTS, a mysterious condition that's gained greater recognition in recent years.

Many possible causes

"POTS is not a disease but a syndrome that results from different underlying conditions," says neurologist Dr. Peter Novak, director of the Autonomic Laboratory at Harvard-affiliated Brigham and Women's Hospital. Often, it's difficult to tell what triggers the nervous system dysfunction that underlies POTS.

Researchers suspect that at least half of all cases follow an infection, which then spurs inflammation or an autoimmune response. Common suspects are infectious mononucleosis (mono) and COVID-19, but even a minor sore throat or a gastrointestinal infection could be the culprit.

POTS may result from damage to small nerves that regulate constriction of the blood vessels in the lower body. The syndrome is also associated with high levels of the stress hormone norepinephrine and unusually low blood volume.

Connective tissue disorders such as hypermobile Ehlers-Danlos syndrome are also closely linked to POTS. People with this inherited condition not only have unusually flexible joints, they also have "floppy" blood vessels that make it even harder to pump blood efficiently.

Diagnosing POTS

Most people with POTS don't look sick, and getting diagnosed often proves challenging. POTS affects at least 500,000 people in the United States, most of whom are women of childbearing age. People are considered to have POTS if their heart rate increases by at least 30 beats per minute (bpm) or rises to 120 bpm within 10 minutes of standing up. But POTS can also cause an array of other symptoms, including fatigue, shortness of breath, gastrointestintal upset, headaches, and brain fog, as well as pain in the chest, extremities, or elsewhere in the body. Some of these directly result from decreased blood flow to the brain.

POTS is distinct from a more common condition called orthostatic hypotension, in which blood pressure drops upon standing. In people with POTS, blood pressure may fall after prolonged standing, but in others, blood pressure rises when they stand.

Treating POTS

Treating POTS often involves targeted eating and exercise habits. For most people with POTS, drinking plenty of water (up to 80 ounces daily) and eating lots of salt (3 to 10 grams a day) keeps more water in the bloodstream, enabling more blood delivery to the brain. Certain bottled iced tea brands that are high in sodium are good options, Dr. Novak notes.

A program of graded exercise training can also help. "The best exercises are those that don't require you to be upright, such as using a recumbent bicycle," says Dr. Novak. Swimming is also a great choice because your head stays in the same plane as your body. The intermittent breath-holding during swimming also helps to train your blood vessels to react with more sensitivity, he adds. Doctors may also prescribe a variety of medications that either help improve blood vessel constriction, increase blood volume, or reduce the fast heart rate.

POTS prognosis

About 70% of people with POTS slowly improve over the course of several months, and about half fully recover within one to three years. But the rest have persistent symptoms that linger for a long time, and some get worse. Some even experience levels of impairment similar to people with heart failure. Those who don't respond to lifestyle changes and medication should seek out care from a physician with experience in autonomic disorders.

The 10 rules of a heart-healthy diet

The latest guidelines give you the flexibility to create a healthy diet that fits your lifestyle and needs.

Eating a healthy diet is a cornerstone of treating and preventing heart disease. That's easy to understand, but sometimes hard to implement. There's no one-size-fits-all eating plan that will work for everyone. With that in mind, the American Heart Association updated its dietary guidelines for the first time in 15 years.

Rather than listing dos and don'ts of specific nutrients (such as protein or fat), the new guidelines—published online Nov. 2, 2021, by *Circulation*—focus on healthy eating patterns. As long as you stay within the following rules, you can tailor a heart-healthy diet to your tastes and needs.

Balance your calorie intake with physical activity. Weight gain is a risk factor for cardiovascular disease, and taking in more calories than you burn off leads to weight gain. Talk to a dietitian to find out how many calories you need to eat considering how active you are. It may only require a few tweaks to your diet to have the calories you eat balance the calories you burn during activity. "Maybe you need to reduce fast food and make room for nutritious foods. Or maybe your portions are too large. For instance, your salad might include a cup of beans when a quarter-cup is more appropriate," says Liz Moore, a registered dietitian at Harvard-affiliated Beth Israel Deaconess Medical Center.

Eat a variety of fruits and vegetables. Consuming a rainbow of colorful fruits and vegetables (which are full of nutrients and many types of beneficial plant molecules) is linked to a reduced risk of cardiovascular disease and early death, the guidelines point out. You should get at least five servings per day. Moore says the produce doesn't have to be fresh; it can be frozen or canned. "I prefer frozen, because canned foods have added salt. But you can reduce salt by rinsing canned vegetables."

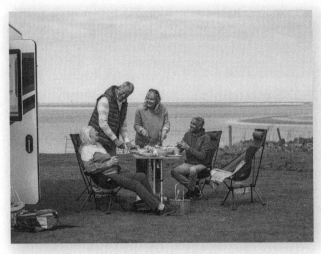

Try to follow the rules of a heart-healthy diet, no matter where you're dining.

Choose whole-grain foods and products. The guidelines stress the importance of eating whole grains (like whole-wheat bread or brown rice) over refined grains (such as white bread or white rice). That's because eating whole grains every day is linked to a reduced risk for cardiovascular disease, heart attack, stroke, and diabetes. "Keep it interesting by trying whole grains that are new to you, such as quinoa, buckwheat, or wild rice. They have B vitamins and protein, and they're not hard to find in most stores," Moore says.

Choose healthy proteins. The guidelines suggest eating mostly plant-based proteins, such as nuts or legumes (beans, lentils), along with two to three servings of fish per week. They're all associated with lower cardiovascular disease risks. And while it's still debated, the recent guidelines recommend replacing full-fat dairy products with low-fat dairy (such as milk or yogurt) for better heart health. If you want meat or poultry, the guidelines urge eating only low-fat cuts and staying away from processed meats of any kind. How much protein do you need? "Don't worry about reaching a number," Moore advises. "Just include protein in every meal, whether it's beans, fish, or low-fat cheese."

Use liquid plant oils instead of tropical oils. The cardiovascular benefits of unsaturated fats from plant oils (like olive, canola, or safflower oil) are especially effective when they replace saturated fats, such as those in red meat and tropical oils (like coconut or palm oil), according to the guidelines. That's not a license to drown foods in plant-based oil; oils are still fats, and fat contains twice as many calories per gram as does protein or carbohydrate. The right amount for you depends on your calorie goals.

Choose minimally processed foods. The guidelines note that eating ultra-processed foods (which are loaded with salt, added sugar, fat, and preservatives) is tied to an increased risk for obesity, diabetes, heart disease, and death from any cause. So as much as you can, avoid processed meats, frozen meals, ready-made baked goods, chips, and other processed foods. Instead, opt for whole foods that haven't been processed and packaged to survive on a shelf for long periods.

Minimize your intake of foods and drinks with added sugars. Consuming sugary foods and drinks has consistently been associated with elevated risks for diabetes, cardiovascular disease, and weight gain, the guidelines report. Scan Nutrition Facts labels for "added sugars" or look for added sugars in the ingredients list (search for names such as glucose, dextrose, sucrose, corn syrup, honey, maple syrup, or concentrated fruit juice). Try to keep them out of your diet as much as possible.

Choose or prepare foods with little or no salt. The guidelines warn that eating too much salt may increase blood pressure, which is a risk factor for heart attack and stroke. Extra-salty foods include restaurant fare and processed foods. But salt hides even in salad dressing and whole-wheat bread. Read food labels carefully to check sodium (salt) levels, and keep your intake below 2,300 milligrams (mg) per day.

Limit alcohol consumption; if you don't drink, don't start. Drinking too much alcohol increases the risk for stroke and dangerous irregular heartbeats, the guidelines warn. Limit yourself to no more than one drink per day if you're a woman and two drinks per day if you're a man.

Use these guidelines wherever you dine. Apply the guidelines to meals you eat in any setting. How does that work if you're at a friend's house or restaurant? "It may be fun, but it's not a free-for-all. You still need to watch your portions," Moore says. "And minimize sauces or ask for them on the side. They're often sources of salt, sugar, and fat. But don't beat yourself up if you break the rules once in a while. Just do a better job at your next meal. Your heart is counting on you."

From the wrist to the heart: A safer route for angioplasty?

In the United States, at least half of all artery-opening procedures in the heart now start at the wrist instead of the top of the leg.

To open a narrowed or blocked artery in the heart, a doctor's first step is to carefully maneuver a slender tube (catheter) through a major blood vessel up to the heart. Traditionally, that vessel has been the femoral artery, the large vessel at the top of the thigh. But increasingly, cardiologists are starting at the radial artery in the wrist instead (*see illustration*).

Called transradial angioplasty, the wrist approach offers several advantages for patients, says Dr. Ajar Kochar, an interventional cardiologist at Harvard-affiliated Brigham and Women's Hospital. "They can sit up right away, which means it's easier to get up, walk around, and eat soon after the procedure," he says. To cover the tiny incision just under the base of the thumb, all they need is a pressure bracelet around the wrist.

In contrast, a puncture site near the groin is associated with more bleeding and may require firm pressure for at least 10 minutes after the procedure, which can be uncomfortable, says Dr. Kochar.

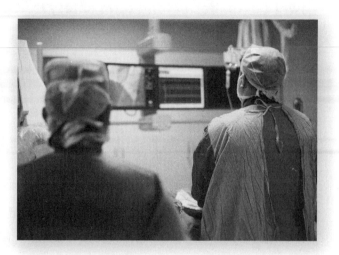

Sometimes, doctors need to place a small stitch or plug to help control the bleeding. Also, you must lie flat on your back for hours afterward, which can be difficult if you have hip or back pain, lung disease, or heart failure, he adds.

Bleeding problems

The bleeding isn't just a nuisance. It can be a serious problem, especially for people at high risk for complications. That includes older, frail people (especially women) and those who take anti-clotting drugs for other heart conditions, such as atrial fibrillation. Sometimes, damage to the femoral artery causes blood to seep into the area behind the pelvis and abdomen, which—in rare cases—can be fatal. That risk, while uncommon, is significantly reduced with the radial approach, says Dr. Kochar. Most bleeding that occurs near the wrist is easy to see and control.

Size and access issues

The femoral approach does have advantages: It's a larger artery, which makes catheter maneuvering a little easier. Also, the vessel provides a direct route to the heart. But in people who are very overweight, the femoral artery may be hard to reach under layers of fat. And bulges of cholesterol-laden plaque inside this artery and the aorta can create roadblocks for angioplasty tools.

The radial artery sits close to the skin, so it's easy to reach, even in people who are overweight. Also, arm arteries are far less likely than leg arteries to develop fatty deposits. While these smaller arteries

During angioplasty, starting at an artery in the wrist instead of the leg is often safer and less costly.

Illustration by Scott Leighton

© U.Ozel.Images | Getty Images

are more prone to spasm, or clamp down, during the procedure, a mix of medications that help relax arteries can minimize this problem, says Dr. Kochar. In addition, the ulnar artery, which runs along the top of the arm, provides a backup blood supply to the hand, if needed.

Lower costs, better long-term safety?

Studies comparing the two different approaches clearly show lower rates of bleeding and related complications with transradial angioplasty. Those benefits also translate to lower costs because people can leave the hospital sooner. That might be because bad bleeding can prolong the length of the hospital stay and lead to additional complications, such as with kidney function.

Past and present trends

Pioneered in the Netherlands in the early 1990s, transradial angioplasty has long been the preferred approach in many European countries and Japan. In the United States, the switch to the radial technique has been slightly slower. However, over the past decade, the use of radial artery heart procedures has grown rapidly. "In 2015, only about 15% of angioplasties were done through the wrist, but that figure is now around 50% to 60%," Dr. Kochar says.

About two-thirds of angioplasties are done on an urgent basis to treat a heart attack, so people usually don't have a say in the matter. But if your physician recommends the procedure, ask if a transradial approach is appropriate. Because everyone's situation is unique, follow his or her advice regarding the best option for you.

Drug therapy needs time to treat heart-related chest pain

Chest pain brought on by exertion (angina) affects about one-quarter of people with stable coronary artery disease. Now researchers have found that many of these individuals can eliminate their symptoms by following conservative drug therapy and do not need a stent or bypass surgery. The findings were published online July 15, 2021, by *Circulation*. The researchers looked at more than 32,000 people, average age 64, with stable coronary artery disease, defined as people who had a heart attack at least three months ago or who have other evidence of significant plaque blockage. Approximately 22% had chest pains or other symptoms caused by coronary artery blockage, like shortness of breath or sudden weakness with exertion. They took at least one anti-anginal drug, such as a beta blocker or a calcium-channel blocker, and usually a statin and aspirin.

After a year, about 40% of this group saw their chest pain symptoms disappear with just medication. The percentage continued to climb annually for five years. A vast majority (85%) never needed a stent or bypass surgery. Another bright spot: those whose symptoms were resolved within

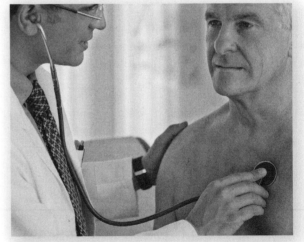

Medication can ease chest pain from coronary artery disease.

a year did not have a higher risk of heart attack or heart-related death than those with stable coronary artery disease who never had chest pains. While this was only an observational study, the findings suggest that doctors and patients give drug therapy adequate time to be effective rather than immediately opt for a stent or bypass.

Under pressure: How stress may affect your heart

In some people with heart disease, mental stress can curtail blood flow to the heart, boosting the risk of a heart attack.

If you're suddenly thrust into a stressful, anxiety-provoking situation, your heart may speed up and your blood pressure may rise. But if you have heart disease, emotional stress may also hinder blood flow to parts of your heart. This phenomenon, called mental stress ischemia, may more than double the risk of a heart attack, according to a new study (see "Mental stress and the heart: A closer look").

The study—the largest and most diverse of its kind to date—helps illuminate the connection between stress and heart disease, which was first described over a century ago. "The findings clearly show that mental stress ischemia is an important

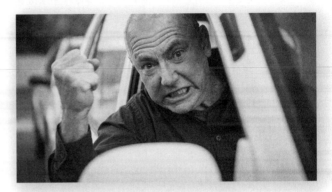

Mental stress may affect the heart's smallest blood vessels, called the microvasculature.

health problem," says Dr. Ahmed Tawakol, director of nuclear cardiology and co-director of the cardiovascular imaging research center at Harvard-affiliated Massachusetts General Hospital.

The fact that this study includes a sizable number of women is important, he adds. Mental stress ischemia appears to be caused in part by changes in the wall and inner lining of the heart's smallest blood vessels. Known as microvascular disease, this problem tends to be more prevalent in women than in men. (However, narrowing of the large arteries of the heart is a more common cause of chest pain in both women and men.)

Understanding microvascular disease

Picture the blood supply to the heart as a tree, where the large blood vessels on the heart's surface are the tree trunk and major branches, Dr. Tawakol says. As they dive into the heart, the large vessels branch into smaller and smaller arteries. The heart's tiniest vessels (microvasculature) are like the tree's twigs or even the veins on a leaf, with

Mental stress and the heart: A closer look

Emotional or mental stress triggers physical changes throughout the body, and the heart is no exception. About one in six people with heart disease experiences decreased blood flow to the heart (ischemia) at times of mental stress. But does mental stress ischemia raise the risk of heart attacks and related problems? A study published Nov. 9, 2021, in *JAMA* explored this question.

Who: 918 people with heart disease with an average age of 60. About one-third were women and 40% were Black.

How: All participants underwent two separate tests to see how stress—physical and mental—affected blood flow to the heart. For most, the physical test was a conventional exercise stress test done on a treadmill; about 30% instead received a medication to stress the heart. For the mental stress test, participants were given a topic and had two minutes to prepare a three-minute speech to deliver to an audience of at least four people.

What: About one-third of the participants had ischemia on the exercise stress test, while 16% experienced ischemia during mental stress. Ten percent had ischemia during both tests.

When: Over the following five to six years, researchers tracked participants' rates of heart attacks, heart failure hospitalizations, and death from cardiovascular disease.

Key findings: Compared with people with no ischemia, those with mental stress ischemia were twice as likely to have a heart attack or heart failure during the follow-up period. Those with both physical and mental stress ischemia had four times the risk. The risk increased only slightly among people with just physical ischemia.

the leaves representing areas of heart muscle. "If you look up into a tree and see disease in one of the large limbs, the leaves at the end of that branch will be affected," explains Dr. Tawakol. "But you might also see disease in the vessels of a leaf—and that leaf will still be affected, even if the large, supporting branch looks okay."

In some people with heart disease, both the larger and smaller arteries are diseased or dysfunctional. They might experience chest pain during exercise as well as during mental stress. Earlier studies have shown that people with both microvascular disease and narrowing of the coronary arteries face the highest risk of future heart problems, says Dr. Tawakol. In this study as well, those with the highest risk were the people who had both mental stress ischemia as well as exercise-induced ischemia.

Unanswered questions

While this study sheds light on how mental stress affects the heart, many questions remain. For example, would it be helpful to screen people for mental stress ischemia? Advanced heart imaging tests are now making it easier to detect subtle changes in blood flow throughout the heart and can detect microvascular disease as well as narrowing of the large coronary arteries. Such tools could potentially further our understanding, Dr. Tawakol says. But a more important question is whether people can do anything to blunt the negative effects of mental stress on their hearts.

To find out, he and colleagues are conducting a study in which volunteers (with and without heart disease) will follow an eight-week Stress Management and Resilience Training (SMART) program. Developed at the Benson-Henry Institute for Mind Body Medicine at Massachusetts General Hospital, the program teaches people self-care practices to better manage stress. A central focus involves learning to evoke the relaxation response—a simple, mind-calming practice that counteracts the body's response to stress.

Participants will undergo specialized brain and heart imaging tests before and after the training. "We suspect the training will tilt the balance to cause less sympathetic nervous system activity—the fight-or-flight response—in response to stressful events," says Dr. Tawakol. That, in turn, may reduce inflammation and other harmful effects of stress on all parts of the cardiovascular system, all the way down to the tiniest vessels.

Results from the study aren't expected for at least several years. But other than a small time investment, there are no downsides to practicing stress-busting techniques on your own. The Harvard Special Health Report *Stress Management* (https://www.health.harvard.edu/sc) provides details and advice.

Staving off heart problems in your 80s and beyond

Prevention and treatment strategies are similar to those for younger people, with a few added nuances and advice.

Older Americans are the fastest-growing segment of the population in this country—including the "oldest old," or people ages 85 and older. With advancing age comes an increased likelihood of health problems, including those affecting the heart. But does preventing and treating heart disease in octogenarians differ from what's recommended for younger people?

For the most part, the advice is very similar, says Dr. Patrick O'Gara, a cardiologist at Harvard-affiliated Brigham and Women's Hospital. "There's a clear benefit to treating high blood pressure, elevated LDL cholesterol, and diabetes in people in their 80s and older to lower their risk of heart problems," he says.

As with younger people, medications are often required to meet recommended blood pressure and other targets. But lifestyle habits that lower heart-related risks should still be the central focus.

Stay active

Sticking to a program of regular physical exercise is probably the most important of those habits because it improves a range of risk factors, says Dr. O'Gara. Physical activity can improve your mood and the quality and duration of your sleep, which benefits heart health.

Walking or other activity that raises your heart rate helps to keep blood pressure in check. Exercises that strengthen your core (such as wall push-ups) can improve your balance and prevent falls. Among people 65 and older with coronary artery disease, the incidence of falls is 34%, compared with 12% in older adults without heart problems, according to one study.

Like falls, frailty—a syndrome marked by weakness, fatigue, and wasting—becomes more common with age.

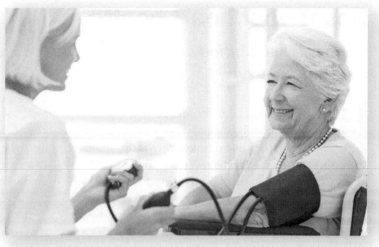

Keeping tabs on your blood pressure can be even more important for people in their 80s or older.

Medication adjustments

Another issue common in older adults is polypharmacy, defined as taking five or more medications. Around age 70, it's a good idea to review all your medications with your physician to see if any adjustments are warranted, says Dr. O'Gara. For example, many otherwise healthy people started taking a daily low-dose aspirin in middle age to ward off a heart attack. But once you reach age 70, the risk of bleeding may outweigh any protection against heart attack or stroke if no evidence of atherosclerosis exists. Bleeding can range from minor (such as bleeding gums or increased bruising) to more serious complications, including bleeding in the stomach, small intestine, and in rare cases, the brain.

Bleeding risk is also a concern for people taking anti-clotting medications, which are prescribed to treat atrial fibrillation, a heart rhythm disorder that raises the odds of stroke. Once you reach your 80s, it might make sense to lower the dose of your anti-clotting drugs to minimize bleeding risk. Weight loss and worsening kidney function, which sometimes occurs with age, affect the dosing of some of these medications.

Although a blood pressure reading of 120/80 or lower is now considered normal, that target might be too aggressive for some people, especially those in their 80s and older. "The older you are, the less forgiving your body becomes. That can leave you more susceptible to side effects such as dizziness or lightheadedness from blood pressure drugs," says Dr.

O'Gara. If that starts happening to you, work with your doctor to dial back your dosage.

Intervention timing

Another consideration for octogenarians involves when to undergo an invasive heart-related procedure, such as aortic valve replacement. In the past, the general practice was to wait until a person's symptoms became so debilitating that quality of life suffered. But sometimes, waiting too long meant the person became so old and frail that valve replacement surgery was too risky. Now, a less invasive alternative—transcatheter aortic valve replacement, or TAVR—has become more widely available, which has expanded eligibility for older people. But there's also a growing trend to do TAVR sooner rather than later, at what Dr. O'Gara calls "the golden moment." That's the age at which a person will likely recover easily from the procedure and still have a good decade ahead.

Longevity advice

Dr. O'Gara has a few patients who are over 100, although one recently passed away at the age of 108. Aside from good medical care, is there anything special about these centenarians that contributes to their longevity? "They exercise, do volunteer work, and have access to other types of social activities and interactions that give them a sense of purpose and belonging in their community," says Dr. O'Gara.

Reset your heart health

Cardiac rehabilitation and cardiovascular wellness programs offer a second chance.

Heart disease can take decades to develop, with years of poor lifestyle habits contributing to the problem. By the time damage shows up, it may seem like there's no way to reverse it. But a number of programs—typically offered in group sessions, in an outpatient hospital or community setting—can help you change unhealthy habits, reduce heart attack risk, and boost your longevity. Here's a look at some of the available programs.

Cardiac rehabilitation

Cardiac rehabilitation ("rehab") is a medically supervised three-month program for people who've had a heart attack, heart bypass surgery, a heart or a heart and lung transplant, stenting to open arteries, or valve surgery, as well as those with chronic chest pain (angina) or certain kinds of heart failure.

A team of doctors and other experts assess participants' health needs and develop individualized treatment programs that focus on exercise, a heart-healthy diet, weight control, stress reduction, sleep, and medication adherence. Groups meet for education and training several times per week, for three months. "We give you the tools to make lasting change. For instance, we work with you to overcome barriers, such as how to cope with arthritis that's keeping you from exercising," explains Dr. Romit Bhattacharya, a preventive cardiologist at Harvard-affiliated Massachusetts General Hospital (MGH).

Experts also guide participants' progress and monitor their exercise sessions. "You have an exercise physiologist there with you, so you learn what it feels like when you're safely pushing the limits and when you should pull back. That helps address the fear element about whether you're overdoing it," Dr. Bhattacharya says.

It adds up to proven benefits. Evidence suggests that people who attend cardiac rehab reduce their risk of heart attack by 31%, and that people who complete all 36 sessions (typically in three months) reduce their risk of death by 47% compared with those who only complete one session. Cardiac rehab also improves overall physical function and reduces chest pain.

Cardiovascular wellness programs

Cardiovascular wellness programs are for people who don't qualify for cardiac rehab but want to improve their heart and blood vessel health. They're offered at hospitals, academic centers, private doctor practices, fitness centers, and even community centers.

Programs vary greatly in their approaches, expertise, topics, and length. Some are similar to cardiac rehab, with a team of health professionals who provide months of health monitoring and training. An example of that is MGH's Cardiac Lifestyle Program. It's for people who have an abnormal heart rhythm, certain kinds of heart failure, obesity, diabetes, or at least one heart disease risk factor (such as elevated weight, blood sugar, cholesterol, or blood pressure).

Other programs are open to anyone and have just one or two experts who focus on a few areas of health. These programs may last for a couple of weeks or even just one session.

Who pays for these programs?

Costs vary by program and provider. For people with qualifying conditions, insurance (including Medicare) covers the costs of cardiac rehab and a similarly classified program called the Ornish Reversal Program, offered at certified hospitals and clinics across the country. Depending on the provider, the Ornish program is also open to anyone who wants to

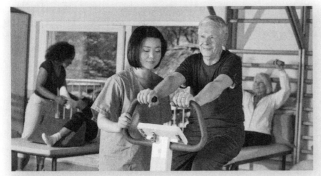

Experts supervise a heart-healthy exercise program in cardiac rehabilitation.

improve cardiovascular health and is willing to pay for it out of pocket (for about $7,000 to $10,000).

Other programs, such as MGH's Cardiac Lifestyle Program, are partially covered by insurance. And some others are free or have a minimal charge. Make sure the program is clear with you about what services it offers, how much it costs, how many experts are involved, and how often and where your group will meet.

Program barriers

Despite the benefits of these programs, many people don't use them. "By some estimates, only 10% to 34% of people who qualify participate in cardiac rehab," Dr. Bhattacharya says. "It's often because of the diagnosis. For instance, only 10% of patients with heart failure are referred to the program, and less than 3% attend. Prevention is something that doesn't get as much of a spotlight as it should."

Other barriers to these programs include transportation issues, fear of being too unfit to take part, and unconscious bias in referrals. "Women and minorities, and people with limited English language skills, are less likely to be referred or participate," Dr. Bhattacharya says. He stresses that we need to change this thinking. "These programs are not yet 'democratized' and made available to as many people as they should," Dr. Bhattacharya notes. "But it could be that everyone would benefit from a group-based program to live the healthiest life they can."

Abdominal aneurysms: Uncommon but potentially dangerous

Learn when and why you should be checked for an abdominal aortic aneurysm.

An aneurysm—an abnormal bulge or balloon-like pouch in an artery—can form in different places in the body and the brain. But most arise in the body's largest artery, the aorta, as it passes through the center of the body (*see illustration*). These abdominal aortic aneurysms (AAAs) occur in up to 7% of people ages 50 and older, most commonly in older male smokers.

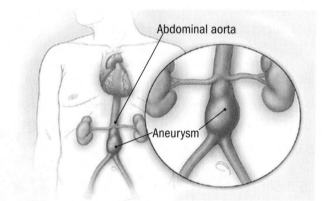

Abdominal aneurysms usually form near the center of the body, below the kidneys.

Labels on illustration: Abdominal aorta; Aneurysm

Most of the time, these bulges stay small, grow slowly, and pose little risk. But a small number expand quickly and may rupture with little warning. The resulting massive bleeding inside the abdomen is usually fatal. "Unfortunately, abdominal aneurysms don't cause any symptoms until they're about to rupture or are rupturing," says Dr. Marc Schermerhorn, chief of vascular surgery at Harvard-affiliated Beth Israel Deaconess Medical Center.

Located deep inside the body just on top of the spine, this section of the aorta is about 2 centimeters (cm) wide. During routine physical exams, primary care providers usually can't feel small aneurysms in the abdominal aorta, and even a large aneurysm is easy to miss, says Dr. Schermerhorn. That's why people at greatest risk for an AAA should be screened with a one-time abdominal ultrasound—a simple, painless test that takes about 30 minutes.

Who should be screened?

The screening test for an AAA is fully covered by Medicare Part B for
- anyone with a family history of AAA
- men between ages 65 to 75 who have smoked at least 100 cigarettes at any point during their lives.

Illustration by Scott Leighton

However, few people seem to be taking advantage of this free screening. If you qualify and your physician hasn't recommended the test, ask him or her to order the screening, says Dr. Schermerhorn.

Why aneurysms form

Cigarette smoking is a potent risk factor for many diseases, and AAAs are no exception. Even men who smoked only casually for a brief time when they were younger face a heightened risk, says Dr. Schermerhorn. "The effect triggered by smoking can happen during your 20s but not show up until years later," he says.

The more you smoked, the higher your risk. Quitting after you're diagnosed definitely helps, since people who continue to smoke tend to fare much worse than those who stop, he adds. High blood pressure can also increase the odds that an aneurysm will grow and rupture.

Monitoring AAAs

If your screening test detects a small aneurysm (a diameter of less than about 4 cm), it should be rechecked every two years. If the aneurysm expands to 4 cm, annual checks are recommended, and every six months if it grows larger than 4.5 cm. Dr. Schermerhorn urges his patients not to worry too much about small aneurysms.

"We want people to be just concerned enough to show up for their next surveillance test," he says. Most never reach a size that would require an intervention, but surveillance can detect the rare cases that warrant treatment.

The risk of a rupture rises as an aneurysm grows larger. If that happens, it usually causes a sudden, sharp pain in the back, or sometimes in the front of the belly. Occasionally, the pain radiates to one side (usually the left) or toward the groin. Many people with AAAs also have chronic low back pain, but the pain associated with a rupture feels new and different, says Dr. Schermerhorn.

Treating an AAA

If an AAA grows large enough, the risk of a rupture outweighs the risk of repairing it. For men, that's about 5.5 cm; for women, about 5 cm. However, the person's overall surgical risk and how quickly the aneurysm has grown are also important considerations. A CT scan of the abdomen provides a more detailed look of the aneurysm, which helps surgeons determine the best treatment option. Some AAAs are repaired with open surgery, but most are done with a minimally invasive technique: the physician threads a catheter through a vessel in the upper leg up to the aorta and places a fabric-coated metal cage to reinforce the bulging portion.

ASK THE DOCTORS

by **HOPE RICCIOTTI, M.D., AND TONI GOLEN, M.D.**

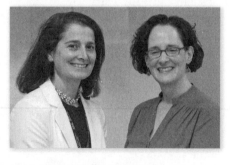

Is there such a thing as a silent stroke?

Q *I've heard of silent heart attacks, but is it also possible to have a stroke and not know it?*

A Yes, it's possible. In fact, a statement issued by the American Stroke Association and American Heart Association estimated that as many as a quarter of octogenarians may have experienced one or more strokes without symptoms. These events are often detected only when a person undergoes brain imaging for another reason. How is this possible? A silent stroke is most often caused by reduced blood flow in one of the smaller arteries that feed the brain. It can occur without noticeable symptoms if it affects a part of the brain that doesn't control major movements or vital functions.

This means it won't produce traditional stroke symptoms such as weakness in your arm or leg or garbled speech. A silent stroke may also produce symptoms you mistakenly attribute to something else, such as garden-variety clumsiness or random memory lapses. Similar to reducing the chance of a major stroke, addressing cardiovascular risk factors, such as high cholesterol and high blood pressure, also lowers the risk of having silent strokes.

Stroke prevention in atrial fibrillation: Beyond anti-clotting drugs

Procedures that block or remove the source of dangerous blood clots in the heart may be an option for growing numbers of people.

More than five million Americans have atrial fibrillation, a heart rhythm disorder commonly known as afib. During a bout of afib, the heart's upper chambers (atria) suddenly start to quiver ineffectually. When that happens, blood tends to pool—and possibly form clots—in a small pouch that protrudes from the top of the left atrium. This ear-shaped sac is called the left atrial appendage (LAA).

About 90% of blood clots in the heart form in the LAA. These clots can escape the heart and travel to the brain, blocking blood flow and causing an ischemic stroke. Most people with afib take anti-clotting medications that help prevent these strokes. However, some people develop serious bleeding problems while taking those medications. Also known as

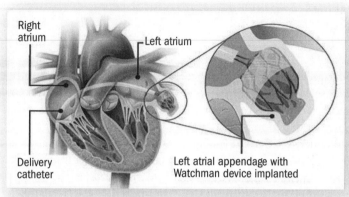

A Watchman device blocks the opening to the left atrial appendage, which helps prevent strokes caused by atrial fibrillation.

Labels: Right atrium; Left atrium; Delivery catheter; Left atrial appendage with Watchman device implanted

blood thinners, these drugs are especially risky for older people who are vulnerable to head injuries from falls, increasing the risk of bleeding in and around the brain.

"Both of these groups of people are possible candidates for procedures that close off the left atrial appendage," says Dr. Thomas Tadros, a cardiologist at Harvard-affiliated Brigham and Women's Hospital. Anyone with afib who's had a stroke despite being on an anti-clotting drug might also benefit, he adds. The usual procedure involves delivering a device that blocks the opening of the LAA.

A device that traps clots

One device, the Watchman, was approved by the FDA in 2015. As with many heart devices, it's

---

IN THE JOURNALS

Anger or emotional upset may trigger stroke

One in 11 stroke survivors felt angry or upset in the hour before their stroke symptoms began, according to a large international study published Dec. 1, 2021, in the *European Heart Journal*. The study included 13,462 people from 32 countries who'd had a stroke. During their first three days in the hospital, they filled out extensive questionnaires about their medical history and what they'd been doing and feeling before their stroke. According to the study authors, anger or emotional upset was linked to an approximately 30% higher risk of having a stroke within one hour of experiencing those emotions. Another potential stroke trigger revealed by the study was heavy physical exertion, although the evidence was less convincing. The findings lend further support to the link between mental stress and cardiovascular health.

deployed through a catheter that a cardiologist snakes through a leg vein up to the heart. The tiny, basket-like device is then placed over the opening of the LAA (see illustration on the previous page).

"People need to keep taking anti-clotting drugs for about six weeks until a layer of cells grows over the device. But after that, they can stop those drugs," says Dr. Tadros. Early studies showed the Watchman prevented strokes in people with afib about as well as warfarin (Coumadin). At the time, warfarin was still widely used to prevent clotting but has now been largely replaced by newer drugs known as DOACs (see "Anti-clotting drugs").

More recent trials compared DOACs to the closure devices, including the Watchman and a similar device called the Amulet, which was FDA-approved in August 2021. The rates of strokes, bleeding, and cardiovascular death were similar regardless of approach. Larger studies are currently under way.

Other research using data from Medicare suggests that for patients, the Watchman is less expensive than the average cost of anti-clotting medications and the drugs' bleeding-related complications within five years. Newer iterations of the device are more flexible and come in a wider range of sizes, making them easier to position, says Dr. Tadros.

People who get an LAA closure device usually receive general anesthesia and stay overnight in the

Anti-clotting drugs

Some people with afib take warfarin (Coumadin) to prevent blood clots, but most take one of these direct oral anticoagulants, known as DOACs:

▶ apixaban (Eliquis)

▶ dabigatran (Pradaxa)

▶ edoxaban (Savaysa)

▶ rivaroxaban (Xarelto).

hospital. But they rarely need any pain medications and can return to doing most regular activities right away, with the exception of running or doing heavy lifting in the first few weeks, Dr. Tadros says.

Surgical options

Some people with afib need open heart surgery to address another problem, such as narrowed coronary arteries or a failing heart valve. For them, removing or closing the LAA during the surgery can reduce their risk of a stroke by about 30%, according to a large international study published in *The New England Journal of Medicine*. However, people in the study were supposed to continue taking anti-clotting medications after surgery; the stroke-prevention benefit is intended to add to the protective effect of the drugs, not to replace it.

The take-home message

About one in seven strokes are caused by afib, and these strokes tend to be more severe than strokes with other underlying causes. People with afib who are doing well on warfarin or a DOAC should feel confident that these drugs—when taken consistently—cut their stroke risk by about two-thirds. But those who've already had a stroke while on anticoagulants, have bleeding problems, or are prone to falls may want to discuss LAA closure options with their cardiologist.

Hospitalization after a ministroke? Not necessarily

For preventing a future stroke, special clinics that test for the underlying causes of stroke seem to be just as effective.

A temporary disruption in blood flow to part of your brain, often called a ministroke, can alter how you move, speak, or see. Also known as a transient ischemic attack, or TIA, this unsettling event may last just a few minutes or many hours (see "Spot a stroke" on the next page). Once the symptoms

subside, you may feel perfectly normal and be tempted to forget it ever happened.

But nearly one in six people who experience a TIA has a full-blown stroke within the next three months—sometimes with devastating effects. Anti-clotting medications are usually started right

SPOT A STROKE

LEARN THE WARNING SIGNS AND ACT FAST

B E F A S T

© elenabs | Getty Images

 Loss of balance, headache, dizziness

 Eyes: Blurred vision

 One side of the face is drooping

 Arm or leg weakness

 Speech difficulty

 Time to call for ambulance immediately

away in people with a suspected TIA or stroke, but they should also undergo testing as soon as possible to uncover the underlying cause.

While there's no consensus on how and where such testing should occur, TIA patients have traditionally received it during a brief hospital stay after being seen in the emergency department. But new research suggests that people who are evaluated at specialized outpatient clinics fare just as well as those who are hospitalized (see "Follow-up care after a ministroke").

"It's encouraging to know that we're on the right track in developing these TIA clinics," says Dr. Christopher Anderson, chief of the Division of Stroke and Cerebrovascular Diseases at Harvard-affiliated Brigham and Women's Hospital. "If you arrive in the emergency room at midnight and receive a TIA diagnosis and a reassuring preliminary workup, doctors at facilities with access to a TIA clinic can schedule all the necessary follow-up tests to be done within the next three days," he explains. Stroke risk is highest within the first week after a TIA.

At the TIA clinic

The specific tests people receive depend on their medical history.

Follow-up care after a ministroke

Does it matter where you receive your follow-up evaluation after a transient ischemic attack (TIA, or ministroke)? To find out, researchers pooled findings from 71 studies published between 1981 and 2018 involving more than 226,000 people with TIAs.

They determined that the risk of a subsequent stroke—a serious concern after a TIA—was not higher among people evaluated in special TIA outpatient clinics compared with people evaluated in a hospital. Not surprisingly, people treated in emergency departments who received no further follow-up had a higher risk of a future stroke. The findings were published Jan. 5, 2022, in *JAMA Network Open*.

Factors that boost stroke risk after a TIA

Doctors use the ABCD2 score to assess a person's risk of having a stroke after a TIA. People with a higher point total—usually 4 and above—may need to be hospitalized after a TIA.

RISK FACTOR	POINTS
A=Age. Age 60 or older	1
B=Blood pressure. Systolic blood pressure above 140 or diastolic pressure over 90	1
C=Clinical features	
Trouble with speech but no weakness	1
Weakness on one side of the body	2
D1=Duration	
Symptoms lasting 10 to 59 minutes	1
Symptoms lasting 60 minutes or more	2
D2=Diabetes	1
TOTAL	

But they usually include a heart ultrasound (echocardiogram) to check for blood clots or heart abnormalities, cardiac monitoring to check for atrial fibrillation (a rapid, irregular heart rhythm that raises stroke risk), and imaging tests of arteries in the brain and neck. The results guide targeted stroke-prevention treatments, which can reduce the risk of a future stroke by as much as 80%.

"Initially, doctors were worried they might be missing problems that could occur soon after a TIA that would be picked up more effectively in a hospital," says Dr. Anderson. But it's now clear that many people are fine to go home after the emergency visit and receive these tests promptly in an outpatient setting. TIA clinics are more convenient and less costly for patients, and hospitals can keep their beds available for people who are more seriously ill, he explains. However, people with health problems that put them at high risk for a stroke are still admitted to the hospital after a TIA, he adds. To help predict this risk, doctors use the ABCD2 score, among other criteria (see "Factors that boost stroke risk after a TIA").

At present, many community hospitals don't yet have access to TIA clinics, so they end up admitting TIA patients to the hospital to make sure speedy workups don't fall through the cracks. But increasingly, these smaller hospitals are partnering with larger academic centers with TIA clinics, which should expand access to more people in the future, says Dr. Anderson.

Chapter 5

Smart Eating

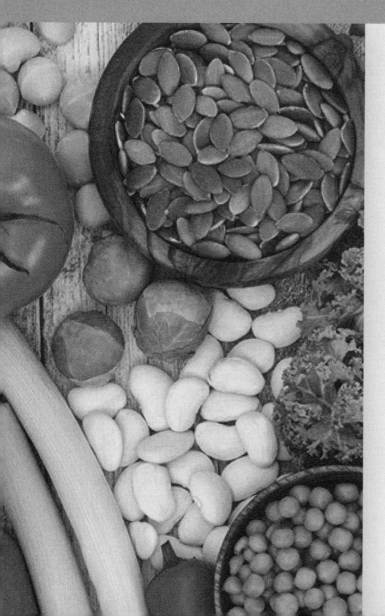

Take Action!
5 Things You Can Do Now

1 **Stock your pantry and fridge.** Always keep these healthy, inexpensive staples on hand. (page 97)

2 **Choose frozen vegetabes wisely.** Avoid those with calorie-rich creams and dressings. (page 99)

3 **Eat more low-glycemic foods.** These slower-digesting carbs help manage appetite. (page 102)

4 **Put whole grains in your soup.** Brown rice or quinoa can add to the nutrients in your bowl. (page 103)

5 **Have a healthy morning meal.** Try nut butter on whole-grain toast. (page 117)

Why is eating healthy so hard?

Everyone knows they should eat healthier. So why do they have a difficult time doing it?

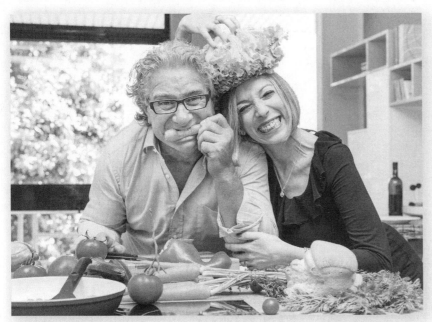

Maintaining an adventurous spirit about food can make healthy eating fun and exciting.

The average person could probably recite the recipe for healthy eating: more fruits and vegetables, less red meat and processed foods. It sounds simple enough. Yet Americans still struggle to follow a healthy diet. Heart disease remains the leading cause of death, and obesity rates have grown from 30.5% in 2000 to 42.4% in 2018.

Adopting a healthy diet can help combat both of these, but only an estimated 22% of Americans follow the American Heart Association's dietary recommendations. So, if we know how to eat healthy, why doesn't everyone do it? Part of the problem lies in people's misguided assumptions. Many still view healthy eating as being too restrictive—low fat, low calorie, low sugar.

Then there are the perceptions that healthy foods are expensive and recipes complex. "The overall message is that healthy eating takes too much work and that healthy food is not tasty," says Teresa Fung, an adjunct professor of nutrition at Harvard's T.H. Chan School of Public Health.

Making the changes

How can you overcome these misconceptions about healthy eating? First, review your usual dietary habits. For a week, write down what you eat for every meal and snack, including the amount and the timing. "An honest evaluation can give you a clear idea of where you need to improve," says Fung. Next, adopt some small changes that can help fill in the gaps and expand your current good eating habits. Here are some suggestions.

Don't be too ambitious. You don't have to make multiple significant dietary changes at the same time to reap health benefits. "Change one thing in your diet for three to four weeks," says Fung. "Once it becomes a staple of your diet, move on to another area and repeat the process." For instance, if you drink soda three or four times per week, cut it back to twice a week, and drink a mixture of seltzer water and juice the other days. Eventually, drink soda once a week, and then try for none.

Adopt a vegetarian day. Once a week, go vegetarian for the entire day and eat nothing but fruits, vegetables, and whole grains (with perhaps a touch of low-fat dairy or eggs), and no processed foods. "This can help you recognize the types and amounts of foods you need to eat without the overwhelming pressure to do it all the time," says Fung. You may discover that vegetarian options are more appetizing than you expected. As you get more comfortable, increase it to twice a week, or even more often.

Expand good habits. For instance, if you eat a daily serving of whole grains, add another one to an everyday meal by substituting it for something less healthy. This helps choosing healthy foods feel more automatic and less like a chore.

Cook something new. If dealing with recipes, ingredients, and cooking feels intimidating, focus on creating just one new meal per week, which can help make preparing meals less daunting. "There are many easy, healthy recipes on the Internet," says Fung. "Find something that uses ingredients you like that requires only a few steps or minimal cooking skills."

Enlist your friends and family. Everyone has a favorite dish, so ask around for suggestions. "This can help with the boredom of eating the same types of foods," says Fung.

Try new foods. During your next grocery store trip, buy something you rarely, if ever, eat. When at a restaurant, order a dish made with a new-to-you food. Also try more global cuisines like Greek and Indian. "The more you experiment, the more you can expand your palate and give yourself opportunities to eat healthier foods," says Fung.

And don't forget to always approach healthy eating with an adventurous spirit. "Healthy eating is not a one-day thing," says Fung. "Make it an exciting part of your life, where you are open to trying new foods, ingredients, and dishes, all of which can make healthy eating fun."

Smarter food shopping

How to get the most out of your food budget while investing the most in your health.

Good nutrition doesn't have to be expensive. In fact, it's just the opposite. Some of the healthiest foods at grocery stores also are some of the least costly. "You don't have to spend a lot of money to supply your refrigerator and pantry with the healthiest foods for regular meals, so you will rely less on takeout and unhealthy snacks," says Elisabeth Moore, a registered dietitian with Harvard-affiliated Beth Israel Deaconess Medical Center. "If healthy food is more available and ready to eat, you will eat more of it."

Thoughts about food

Healthy shopping comes down to following some basic strategies. Here are Moore's tips for choosing the best foods at the lowest prices.

Make a plan. Write down what you need, from the basics to ingredients for specific meals. Place sticky notes on your fridge and write down items you need throughout the week so you don't have to come up with a complete list all at once. Another option: take photos of the inside of your fridge and pantry with your phone to use as a visual reference when you're at the grocery store.

Shop on the same day each week. A simple routine eliminates the need for extra trips to the store, which may tempt you to buy food that's not on your list. "If life gets in the way and you need to change this up, still make sure you stick with a list and a plan," says Moore.

Work around the perimeter. This is where you'll often find the healthiest, least processed options, like fresh produce, dairy, and frozen foods. However, it

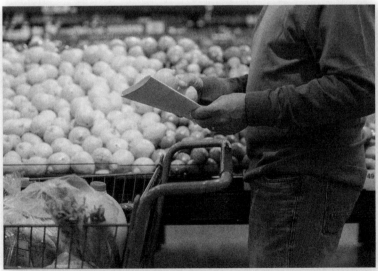

Bringing a detailed list to the store helps you avoid costly impulse purchases.

depends on the store's setup. "For the inner aisles, stick with those stocked with canned vegetables and whole grains," she says.

Become a comparison shopper. Whether you're most concerned about sodium, fiber, sugar, or calories, reading and comparing nutrition labels can help you make better decisions. "If you're trying to manage your weight, pay particular attention to calories and the serving size listed," says Moore.

Buy in bulk. Shelf-stable items like grains, rice, nuts, and dried beans are cheaper in bulk or large containers. For instance, a pound of rice may cost $1.60, but a 5-pound bag might cost $4, which breaks down to 80 cents per pound.

Buy generic or store-brands. These are cheaper in part because less money is spent on advertising and creating attractive packaging for them.

Don't throw away money

Another way people waste money is by not properly caring for fresh fruits and vegetables. "So often we leave them in the refrigerator, forgotten, and then they get tossed into the trash—along with the money you spent," says Moore. Here is how to keep these foods around longer.

Know your fruits. Some fruits continue to ripen with time (called climacteric) while others do not ripen after harvesting (called non-climacteric).

Climacteric fruits include apples, apricots, avocados, bananas, cantaloupe, mangoes, nectarines, peaches, pears, plums, and tomatoes. "Store these on your counter at room temperature until they reach the desired ripeness, or refrigerate them if not used right away," says Moore.

Non-climacteric fruits include bell peppers, berries, cherries, citrus (oranges, lemons, limes, grapefruit), cucumber, eggplant, grapes, and watermelon. "You can refrigerate them immediately to keep them fresh," says Moore.

Prep your veggies. Prepare vegetables as soon as you purchase them. Wash, chop, and dry them. Then store them in labeled containers in clear view. Immediately stuffing them into the produce bins of your refrigerator increases their risk of being forgotten.

Consider frozen over fresh. For regular staples, opt for frozen versions, which are on par nutrition-wise with their fresh counterparts, says Moore. "However, avoid brands with added sauces, creams, or flavorings." Much frozen produce is good for months up to a year. Label each package with the date it was stored.

In terms of organic produce, Moore says it's a personal preference. "Nutrition experts will give you different answers on the potential health benefits of organic foods," she says. "If they are not affordable, it's always better to eat non-organic varieties than none at all."

by HOPE RICCIOTTI, M.D., AND TONI GOLEN, M.D.

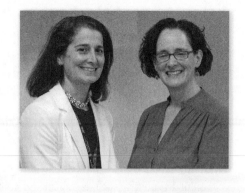

I recently became vegan. Should I be concerned about iron-deficiency anemia?

Q *I've decided to stop eating animal products. I've had anemia in the past. How can I ensure that I'm getting enough iron in my diet?*

A Your body needs adequate iron to produce healthy red blood cells, which transport oxygen throughout your body. When iron levels drop too low and red blood cell production is low, it leads to anemia, which triggers symptoms such as fatigue, dizziness, pale skin, low body temperature, and headaches, among others.

Not only is meat high in iron, but it contains a type that's easy for your body to absorb, making it an important dietary source for many people. If you are eliminating meat from your diet, it is a good idea to be vigilant to ensure that you are getting enough of this important nutrient from other sources. Your body doesn't absorb iron from plant-based sources as readily as it does from meat, so you may need to incorporate more iron-rich foods into your daily diet. Some sources to consider are beans, such as lentils; dark leafy vegetables, including spinach; iron-fortified breads and cereals; and tofu. If you are concerned about your intake, speak with your doctor. She or he can let you know if you are getting enough and may recommend a supplement if you're not. Keep in mind that it is possible to get too much iron, so finding the right balance is important.

Food shortcuts for busy nights

With a little searching, you can find foods that are both easy to prepare and nutritious.

Short on time? Tired of cooking? Looking for a way out of making dinner tonight? At the end of a long day, it may be tempting to order takeout. But it's far less expensive and healthier to eat at home.

To make the job easier, try out some quick-prep, fast-cooking options from your local super-market, says Kathy McManus, director of the Department of Nutrition at

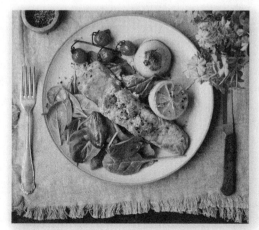

A piece of fish grills up quickly for a busy weeknight meal.

Harvard-affiliated Brigham and Women's Hospital. The trick is to know where to look and what to look for. Below are some ideas to get you started.

Try precooked protein. When it comes to a stress-free dinner, your first thought may be to grab a rotisserie chicken off the shelf and head home, ready to slice and eat. But those grocery store favorites are often loaded with excess salt and saturated fat, says McManus. A better option is to check the refrigerator or freezer section for pre-cooked

How to spot the best quick options in the supermarket

Shopping for foods that are convenient and also nutritious requires some label reading, says Kathy McManus, director of the Department of Nutrition at Brigham and Women's Hospital. Always check for the following:

Excess sodium. You don't want foods with a lot of added sodium. Look for entree items that have less than 400 milligrams per serving.

Sugar. Added sugar can be hiding in places that you wouldn't expect it, such as sauces. Be certain to look at the label and steer clear of overly sweet options.

Other unhealthy additions. Frozen vegetables, fish, and chicken are great, but skip those that are topped with sauces or dressings that jack up the calories, sodium, and saturated fat. Look for unseasoned foods, such as plain shrimp or chicken, and then add your own spices for flavor.

TIP: Don't have time to make salsa? Many grocery stores have fresh options that are lower in sodium than most jarred varieties.

Tips for fast cooking

Laid-back cooking is easier if you plan ahead and have the right tools. Here are some strategies for whipping up an easy dinner.

Invest in appliances. Indoor countertop grills, slow cookers, and pressure cookers can speed cooking or eliminate some of the work involved. A piece of fish or chicken cooks on the grill in a matter of minutes, says Kathy McManus, a nutritionist at Brigham and Women's Hospital. Or toss some ingredients into the slow cooker in the morning, and it will make dinner for you by the evening. "I like to use carrots, broccoli, onions, cauliflower, and chunks of sweet potato along with ground turkey or chicken to make a simple stew," says McManus.

Work ahead. Making a big batch of soup or chili on the weekend can give you something to heat up and eat all week. To save time, buy pre-chopped vegetables. Also mix up your favorite dressings or homemade sauces in batches so they are ready to go on busy nights.

Pressure cookers are designed to reduce cooking time, which can help you make a nutritious meal quickly.

Augment prepared meals. If you can find a prepackaged meal in the freezer section that is low in sodium and saturated fat, you can use it as a base for an easy dinner when you are in a pinch. Very often these meals skimp on vegetables. Add your own to improve the nutritional value, says McManus.

chicken breasts or chicken pieces. (See "How to spot the best quick options in the supermarket.") They're quick to heat and perfect tossed into a salad (pick up a bagged salad mix to make it faster), folded into fajitas, or simply served alongside a side dish.

Go fish. The seafood section is another place to stop for fuss-free dinner options. Buy a bag of frozen shrimp and toss a handful into a pan with some veggies and a few spices, and you've got a meal in minutes, says McManus. Frozen or fresh fish fillets are another fast-cooking option. Just season the fish with your favorite spices.

Consider vegetarian alternatives. Instead of a fast-food burger, try a meatless patty from your freezer case. They only take a few minutes to grill up on a busy night. Putting your burger on a bun? Find one that's 100% whole wheat. Or put your patty on a whole-wheat pita or on a couple of slices of whole-grain bread. Another great option is vegetarian "chicken" strips, says McManus. They're quick and can be paired with a salad or some veggies for an uncomplicated meal.

Crack open a can. While nutrition experts generally advise you to avoid shopping in the center of the store, where the processed foods live, there are some healthy options in the canned food aisle. Canned tuna or salmon is a nutritious addition to a hearty dinner salad. And low-sodium canned beans can be spooned into soup, a salad, or your favorite taco recipe. Taco salads are also easy to make at home. Add black beans, some low-fat Monterey Jack cheese, and chopped tomatoes to a package of mixed salad greens, says McManus. Top it with some seasoning, salsa,

© robynmac | Getty Images

and plain Greek yogurt (a great substitute for sour cream).

Grab some grains. Round out your meals with prepackaged pouches or frozen bags of plain, precooked grains, such as brown rice. Simply heat and use them to accompany your favorite stir-fry, or add them to your plate as a side dish. Also consider a whole-wheat or bean-based pasta as another undemanding dinner option, says McManus. For a healthy pasta sauce, cook up some chopped vegetables in a pan with some olive oil and add a can of low-sodium diced tomatoes.

Here are some other nutritious options that McManus suggests:

Make your own pizza. Grab a premade, whole-wheat pizza crust and top it with fresh tomato sauce or fresh tomatoes, low-fat shredded cheese, and your favorite veggies.

Have breakfast for dinner. A vegetable omelet is a nutritious dinner. Simply cook some spinach, chopped onions, and red bell peppers (or any of your favorite veggies) in a pan with eggs. Serve with fresh salsa on top.

Dig up a potato. Check your produce aisle for a fresh sweet potato you can cook in the microwave. Add some broccoli or other vegetables to fill out your plate.

Instead of chopping your own vegetables, look for frozen options, which include everything from broccoli or peas to stir-fry mixes. "I like frozen, shelled edamame," says McManus. Or try precut vegetables from the produce aisle. Prepackaged coleslaw is an easy side dish, but add the mayonnaise at home so you can control the amount, says McManus.

Stir-fry supper

A stir-fry is a great way to get a healthy dose of vegetables. If you add a little lean protein, a flavorful sauce, and serve your stir-fry over steamed brown rice, you've got a well-balanced meal. It's also quick to make if you use precooked brown rice. Experiment with different ingredient combinations to find your favorite.

Broccoli, red bell peppers, and onions are popular vegetable choices, but you might also try snow peas, bok choy, cabbage, or mushrooms. For protein, diced chicken breast or shrimp are good options, or go vegan and use tofu instead. Some research suggests that eating soy-based foods such as tofu may lower heart disease risk. To enhance the flavor and texture of the mild, white curd,

sprinkle cubes of tofu with low-sodium tamari (a Japanese form of soy sauce) and toss with a little cornstarch before frying.

When stir-frying, it's best to use oils that can withstand high heat, such as peanut or avocado oil. But other vegetable oils, such as canola or sunflower, work as well. To add extra flavor, top your stir-fry with chopped, toasted unsalted peanuts or sesame seeds.

If you need inspiration or advice about the cooking technique, you can find hundreds of stir-fry recipes online. Here's one that features tofu from the Nutrition Source, courtesy of the Harvard T.H. Chan School of Public Health (www.health.harvard.edu/gb).

What are postbiotics?

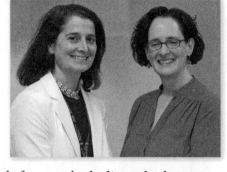

Q *I know about prebiotics and probiotics, but I recently heard the term postbiotics. Can you explain what they are?*

A As you may already know, probiotics are living microorganisms found in certain foods, such as yogurt, sauerkraut, and some cheeses, which are crucial to good digestion. When you eat these foods, it helps your digestive tract and overall wellness by promoting a healthy balance of beneficial bacteria and other microorganisms in your gut microbiome, a collection of 100 trillion tiny critters living in your intestines.

Prebiotics act as food for the probiotics. Foods with healthy amounts of fiber, such as beans, whole grains, and certain vegetables, break down in your body to create substances that help probiotics to grow and thrive within your gut.

So, what are postbiotics? This term refers to the waste left behind after your body digests both prebiotics and probiotics. Healthy postbiotics include nutrients such as vitamins B and K, amino acids, and substances called antimicrobial peptides that help to slow down the growth of harmful bacteria. Other postbiotic substances called short-chain fatty acids help healthy bacteria flourish.

You can increase the amount of useful postbiotics in your system by increasing your intake of fermented foods, such as kefir, tempeh, and kimchi. Focusing on getting enough of the foods that promote a mix of healthy gut bacteria may help improve your overall health.

IN THE JOURNALS

High-glycemic diets could lead to big health problems

A diet consisting primarily of foods high on the glycemic index (GI) can increase your risk of cardiovascular disease and death, suggests a study that looked at the eating habits of almost 138,000 people around the world. The GI is a scale that ranks the amount of carbohydrates in food from zero to 100. The higher the number, the faster the carbohydrates are digested. Eating high-GI foods can cause blood sugar levels to rapidly rise—triggering the pancreas to release more insulin—and then quickly fall. This can promote cravings and overeating. Repeating this cycle frequently may lead to weight gain and insulin resistance, factors associated with type 2 diabetes and higher cardiovascular risk.

Researchers collected data on which foods the people in the study ate, how much, and how often. They organized the mentioned foods into seven categories and gave each category a GI score. At a follow-up nine years later, the investigators found that people who ate high-GI diets had suffered more heart attacks, strokes, and death than those who ate lower-GI diets. This was true regardless of whether people had cardiovascular disease at the start of the study. The results were published online April 8, 2021, by *The New England Journal of Medicine*. Healthier, low-GI foods have a score of 55 or lower; medium-GI foods are 56 to 69; and high-GI foods are 70 to 100. You can find the GI score of many common foods at www.health.harvard.edu/glycemic.

Soup up your meals

A veggie-rich, broth-based soup can warm you up and help you get more nutrients into your day.

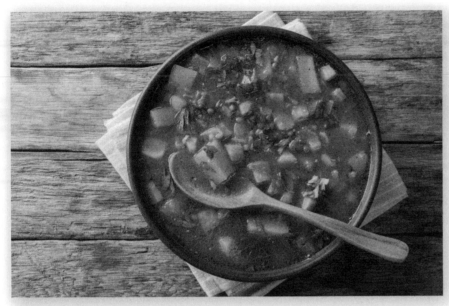

Soup can be a great way to get some added nutrition into your diet. Just add veggies, whole grains, protein, and low-sodium broth.

There's no food more comforting on a chilly winter day than a steaming bowl of soup. With the right ingredients, it can also be an easy way to boost your intake of vegetables and important nutrients. "Soup is a fabulous way to add nutrition," says Debbie Krivitsky, director of nutrition at Harvard-affiliated Massachusetts General Hospital Cardiovascular Center.

Many soups are low in calories—after all, they consist largely of water—but even so, they are often very filling. A study published by the *European Journal of Clinical Nutrition* found that people who ate a smooth soup actually felt full for longer than people who ate a solid meal. This may be because soup is high in volume, which made their stomachs physically fuller. Soup also seemed to affect blood glucose levels differently than the solid meal, which may have increased satiety.

The recipe for a nutritious soup

It's easy to build a highly nutritious soup by focusing on four main components, says Krivitsky.

1. Choose the right base. Use broth, not cream, as the foundation of your soup. "Look for a low-sodium chicken broth with between 140 and 200 milligrams of sodium per serving," says Krivitsky.

2. Go green (and red and yellow). A nutrient-rich soup contains lots of vegetables. "It's an opportunity to eat the rainbow. Vary the colors of your vegetables to add nutrition to your dish," says Krivitsky. Add whatever type you like, whether it's leeks, carrots, or celery.

3. Build it up. After vegetables, add your protein of choice, such as beans or chicken. A quick option is precooked chicken that you can just cut up and toss into the pot.

4. Make it whole. Slipping in whole grains can

Top off your soup

Take your soup to the next level by adding some homemade croutons. Here's how to make them:

- ▶ Cut a whole-wheat baguette into one-inch cubes and spread the cubes on a cookie sheet.

- ▶ Spritz the cubes with olive oil.

- ▶ Sprinkle them with garlic.

- ▶ Put the cookie sheet in the oven at 350° until the croutons are golden brown.

Or make grilled cheese croutons by putting cheese (try a light or reduced-fat cheddar) between two slices of whole-grain bread and grilling it in a pan. Once it's toasty and brown, cut it into cubes and use it to top tomato soup.

Mix-and-match soup

Below is an easy soup recipe that you can customize to fit your preferences and nutritional goals. "These vegetable soups are great because they're so versatile," says Debbie Krivitsky, director of nutrition at Massachusetts General Hospital Cardiovascular Center. To change it up, simply swap in different vegetables—such as zucchini, turnips, broccoli, or bell peppers—for the carrots or green beans. Instead of potatoes, try a whole-grain pasta, barley, quinoa, or brown or wild rice. And if you want to add some protein to the meal, simply toss in some tofu or beans.

Ingredients:
1 tablespoon olive oil
3 medium leeks, sliced
1 clove garlic, minced

pinch of salt
2 medium carrots, chopped
2 cups cut (¾-inch) green beans
2 potatoes, cubed
8 ounces low-sodium vegetable broth
4 cups chopped tomatoes, with their juice
1 cup corn

Heat the olive oil in a stock pot. Toss in the leeks, garlic, and salt and sauté over medium-high heat for five to six minutes. Add the carrots, green beans, and potatoes. Cook for an additional four to five minutes, stirring frequently. Add the low-sodium vegetable broth and bring to a simmer. Stir in the tomatoes and corn. Cook for an additional five minutes. Adjust the seasoning as desired.

round out the nutritional value of your meal. Grains, such as whole barley, farro, and brown rice, can add texture. They are also a good source of nutrients and prebiotics, which are foods that help to promote a healthy balance of beneficial bacteria and other microorganisms in your gut.

Pair your soup with a sandwich or a salad for a simple dinner.

Craving a creamy soup?

Creamy soups can be a nutritious option if you make a few adjustments.

Use

▶ fat-free milk instead of cream

▶ olive oil instead of butter

▶ low-sodium chicken or vegetable stock instead of a higher-sodium variety.

How many fruits and vegetables do we really need?

Here are the numbers to hit and some ways to sneak more fruits and vegetables into your diet.

We often talk about how diets rich in fruits and vegetables are good for your health. But how much do you need to average per day to reap real rewards? An analysis from Harvard indicates that a total of five servings per day of fruits and vegetables offers the strongest health benefits.

About the study

The research, published online March 1, 2021, by

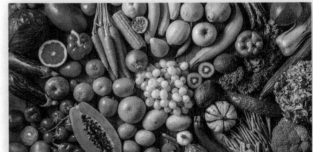

© MEDITERRANEAN | Getty Images

You need to eat two fruit and three vegetable servings every day to maximize health benefits.

the journal *Circulation*, pooled self-reported health and diet information from dozens of studies from around the world, which included about two million people who were followed up to 30 years.

Compared with people who said they ate just two servings of fruits or vegetables each day, people who ate five servings per day had

- a 13% lower risk of death from any cause
- a 12% lower risk of death from heart disease or stroke
- a 10% lower risk of death from cancer
- a 35% lower risk of death from respiratory disease, such as chronic obstructive pulmonary disease.

"Fruits and vegetables are major sources of several

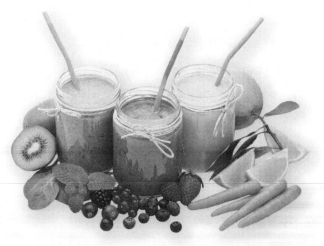

Leafy greens, berries, carrots, and citrus may have the most health benefits (and they're great in smoothies).

ASK THE DOCTOR

by **HOWARD LEWINE, M.D.**

Is extra-virgin olive oil extra healthy?

Q *I know olive oil is part of a heart-healthy diet, but is extra-virgin olive oil healthier than regular olive oil?*

A Many studies continue to confirm the health benefits of the Mediterranean diet, which cuts the risk of heart disease and stroke. The diet's nutritional benefits probably come from various sources, but the generous use of olive oil appears to be a key contributor.

Regardless of the type, olive oil is high in mono-unsaturated fatty acids, containing about 75% by volume. When substituted for saturated fat, mono-unsaturated fats help lower your "bad" LDL cholesterol. The health benefits of olive oil have been attributed to its antioxidant and anti-inflammatory properties. In fact, observational studies have shown a link between lower risks of cardiovascular disease, some cancers, and even dementia in people who consume higher amounts of olive oil than those who use little or none.

Still, extra-virgin olive oil does offer something extra that

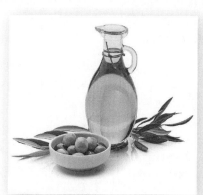

All kinds of olive oil offer similar health benefits.

regular olive oil does not. Extra-virgin olive oil is pressed mechanically from ripe olives and processed without high heat or chemical solvents. This protects chemicals in the oil called phenols. In contrast, regular, highly processed olive oils lose these chemicals.

Small laboratory-based experiments suggest that higher concentrations of phenols may provide extra antioxidant effects. Even so, there are no definitive studies that show extra-virgin olive oil has a greater ability than refined oil to prevent heart problems, cancer, or other diseases.

Keep in mind that olive oil is not the sole healthy ingredient in a Mediterranean diet. Think of it as just one aspect of the Mediterranean style of eating, which includes plenty of fruits, vegetables, and nuts; whole grains; and limited amounts of red meat.

Fruit and vegetable servings

FRUIT (AND SERVING SIZE)

- Apple (1 fruit)
- Apricots (1 fresh, ½ cup canned, or 5 dried)
- Avocado (½ fruit or ½ cup)
- Banana (1 fruit)
- Blueberries (½ cup fresh, frozen, or canned)
- Cantaloupe (¼ melon)
- Grapefruit (½ fruit)
- Grapes (½ cup)
- Orange (1)
- Peaches or plums (1 fresh or ½ cup canned)
- Pear (1 fruit)
- Prunes or dried plums (6 prunes or ¼ cup)
- Raisins (1 ounce)
- Strawberries (½ cup fresh, frozen, or canned)

nutrients that are strongly linked to good health, particularly the health of the heart and blood vessels: potassium, magnesium, fiber, and polyphenols [antioxidant plant compounds]," explains Dr. Daniel Wang, lead author on the study and a member of the Faculty of Medicine at Harvard Medical School and Brigham and Women's Hospital.

Your daily goals

The most effective combination of fruits and vegetables among study participants was two servings of fruits plus three servings of vegetables per day, for a total of five servings daily.

The biggest health benefits came from eating leafy green vegetables (kale, spinach) and fruits and vegetables rich in vitamin C and beta carotene (citrus, berries, carrots). "These are primary sources of antioxidants that may play a role in preventing cancer," Dr. Wang says.

Interestingly, eating more than five servings of fruits or vegetables per day didn't seem to provide additional benefit in lowering the risk of death. Neither did eating starchy vegetables like peas, corn, or potatoes, or drinking fruit juices.

Also, understand that we're talking about how much you eat on average. If during any particular day you have no fruit and vegetables, that's fine: you won't keel over. You can add a little more than usual on other days to raise your average for the week. And you don't need to make major changes to your typical meals: just minor changes. For example, breakfast could be a bowl of cereal with some blueberries, or perhaps eggs and sautéed tomatoes, onions, and spinach.

VEGETABLE (AND SERVING SIZE)

- Broccoli (½ cup)
- Brussels sprouts (½ cup)
- Cabbage (½ cup)
- Carrot juice (2–3 ounces)
- Carrots (½ cup cooked, ½ raw carrot, or 2–4 sticks)
- Cauliflower (½ cup)
- Celery (2–3 sticks)
- Corn (1 ear or ½ cup frozen or canned)
- Eggplant (½ cup)
- Kale, mustard greens, or chard (½ cup)
- Lettuce (1 cup iceberg, leaf, romaine)
- Mixed or stir-fry vegetables (½ cup)
- Onion (1 slice)
- Peppers (3 slices green, yellow, or red)
- Salsa, picante or taco sauce (¼ cup)
- Spinach (½ cup cooked or 1 cup raw)
- Squash, dark orange (winter) (½ cup)
- Summer squash or zucchini (½ cup)
- String beans (½ cup)
- Tomato or V-8 juice (small glass)
- Tomatoes (2 slices)
- Tomato sauce (½ cup)
- Vegetable soup (1 cup)
- Yams or sweet potatoes (½ cup)

Lunch could be a salad with your favorite fruits and vegetables (perhaps kale and spinach salad with grapefruit chunks, red peppers, carrots, and pine nuts), a cup of yogurt with strawberries, or a smoothie with kale and mango.

At dinner, include a side salad or a large side of vegetables such as steamed broccoli or yellow squash and zucchini. If you haven't had a chance to eat enough vegetables throughout the day, make your main meal a large salad with lots of colorful vegetables and some chunks of protein, such as grilled chicken or fish.

For dessert: fresh or frozen fruit is a delicious and healthful treat, especially with a dab of frozen yogurt.

Squeezing in five servings per day

If five servings per day is the goal, how much, exactly, is a serving? We spell that out for a wide variety of fruits and vegetables (see "Fruit and vegetable servings" on the previous page). This can guide you in planning meals that include your favorites. Aim for a wide variety of fruits and vegetables to get the best mix of vitamins, minerals, and other beneficial nutrients in your personalized five-a-day plan.

Stone fruits

Peaches, nectarines, apricots, peaches, plums, and cherries are all considered stone fruits because they all contain large, hard seeds or pits. They're all decent sources of fiber, vitamins A and C, and potassium. While they're all delicious eaten out of hand, you might also want to try them in recipes like these:

Peach salsa: Dice two ripe but still slightly firm peaches and two medium tomatoes. Mix with a little minced red onion, jalapeño pepper, cilantro, garlic, and lime juice to taste. Serve with grilled fish or chicken, or on tacos and other Mexican food.

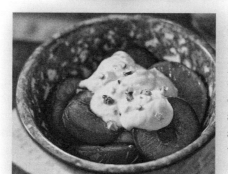

Grilled nectarines: Cut nectarines in half and remove the pits. Brush both sides with a neutral oil (such as canola) and sprinkle with a little brown sugar. Grill until lightly browned, turning once or twice, for 3 to 5 minutes. Enjoy as a side dish or dessert, or in a salad with arugula, toasted pine nuts, and crumbled feta cheese.

Roasted plums: Place halved, pitted plums on a baking sheet and toss with a little canola oil. If desired, drizzle with a little honey and a sprinkle of cinnamon. Roast at 375° F for about 30 minutes, or until soft.

Serve topped with Greek yogurt.

Are these "healthier" choices really better for you?

Our food expert breaks down which better-for-you options are truly superior and which ones you should avoid.

If you've spent any amount of time at the supermarket lately, you've seen a host of products promoted as healthier alternatives to some more traditional favorites. These products often substitute plants or poultry for red meat, or fruit for sugar. But are they really better for you?

It can be difficult to tell, so we asked Kathy McManus, director of the Department of Nutrition at Harvard-affiliated Brigham and Women's Hospital, to give us her thoughts on which swaps to go for and which ones to avoid.

Pork sausage vs. chicken sausage

Is chicken sausage better? Yes. "I would definitely give the edge to the chicken sausage," says McManus. It's significantly lower in saturated fat. It's also 50% lower in sodium and is lower in calories—yet it has the same amount of protein.

McManus added that she also looks at whether products are consistent across a category, or if there is a lot of variation between brands. The chicken sausage consistently performed better in most cases, she says. In addition, some brands of chicken sausage, unlike the pork products, were also free of artificial flavors and nitrates and nitrites (preservatives that have been linked to a higher risk of cancer).

However, while chicken sausage might be a better type of sausage, it's still sausage, says McManus. "We're still concerned about eating too many processed meats." And sausage, even the chicken variety, is definitely a processed meat.

A better option: Reduce your intake of sausage or eliminate it entirely. "My recommendation is to cut down on these products in general," says McManus.

Veggie chips/sticks vs. potato chips

Are veggie chips better? No. It sounds too good to be true: bags of crispy chips that are really vegetables in disguise. Some brands are made from sliced-up sweet potatoes, yucca, and parsnips. But the truth is, aside from a few brands containing a little more potassium, veggie chips are pretty much a

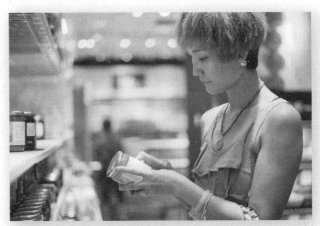

Take time to read nutrition labels to determine if "healthy" products are truly better options.

nutritional equivalent to their fried potato cousins. "There's just not a tremendous amount of difference here," says McManus. "An ounce of potato chips has 150 calories. While they're not particularly high in saturated fat, they do have a moderate amount of sodium."

Some brands of veggie chips might have slightly fewer calories and less saturated fat than traditional potato chips, but not by enough to make a substantial difference. "You're not getting a huge bang for your buck," she says. "Ultimately there's no real advantage to eating veggie chips. Don't fool yourself that veggie sticks or veggie chips are healthier."

A better option: If you're looking for a snack, reach for real vegetables to dip in hummus or yogurt dip. Or slice up an apple and eat it with a tablespoon of peanut butter. These snacks can also weigh in around 150 calories, but they have a far better nutrition profile and a lot more fiber.

Sugar vs. monk fruit sweetener

Is monk fruit sweetener better? Yes.

Monk fruit (sometimes referred to as Buddha fruit) originated in Southeast Asia. "It's been around forever, but the FDA didn't approve its use as a sweetener until 2010," says McManus. The sweetener is made by removing the seeds and skin of the monk fruit and crushing it into juice, which is dried and powdered.

Monk fruit powder is incredibly sweet—100 to 250 times sweeter than sugar—so you only need small amounts of it. This means you can sweeten your food with amounts that are extremely low in calories or calorie-free, says McManus. This gives it the edge over sugar, which has 45 calories per tablespoon.

Monk fruit sweetener consists mainly of a type of sugar known as fructose, but it also contains glucose. Table sugar, or sucrose, is about half fructose and half glucose.

The FDA has approved monk fruit sweetener as generally safe, but if you do choose to use it, know that there are no studies that have looked at long-term effects of using this sweetener over time. "If you want to use a small amount it's probably okay. But we haven't studied it for very long," says McManus.

Ultimately, everyone should make it a goal to reduce the amount of sugar and sweeteners in their diet. Using sweeteners of any kind may stimulate cravings for more sweetness, she says.

A better option: Try to get sweetness from whole foods, such as berries and melons.

Soda vs. seltzer

Is seltzer better? Yes.

There's little question that sugary soda is a dietary disaster. The average 12-ounce bottle contains as much as 12 teaspoons of sugar, so with zero sugar, seltzer is the clear winner in this category. Unlike a can of soda, which adds on average 150 calories to your daily diet, most brands of seltzer don't have any calories and are also free of artificial sweeteners and sodium. (Be sure to read the label to make sure that this is the case.)

"The best thing people can do is to get away from drinking soda," she says. In this case, it's definitely better to make the switch.

A better option: When in doubt, always reach for water, which is always the best choice.

Cauliflower pizza crust vs. regular wheat crust

Is cauliflower crust better? Not unless you need a gluten-free option.

"There is some difference between cauliflower crust and a traditional wheat pizza crust," says McManus. Most cauliflower crusts contain cauliflower, eggs, cheese, and a few spices. Some contain brown rice flour, cornstarch, and tapioca. Many are gluten-free. The calorie counts vary but are close to traditional wheat pizza crust, at about 170 calories per portion. Both cauliflower and traditional crust have about a gram of fiber, but a premade wheat crust at the grocery store can be little higher in sodium, says McManus. Although they are nutritionally similar, if you need a gluten-free option, the cauliflower crust is a better choice.

A better option: The best thing you can do if you are having pizza is to try to make your own crust,

---

Is it healthy? 7 things to look for on a nutrition label

Serving size. When comparing products, be certain that you are comparing apples to apples, and not a 4-ounce serving of one product to an 8-ounce serving of another.

Calories. How many calories does one product have compared with another?

Saturated fat. Always check to see how much saturated fat is in each product and select the one with the lesser amount. Don't just look at total fat, because there are a number of healthy fats, such as those found in olive oil, fresh avocado, or peanut butter. For this reason, it's not helpful to focus on the total amount of fat.

Sodium. Most people should eat less than 2,300 milligrams of sodium each day. Comparing the amount of sodium in different products can help you keep your daily number down.

Fiber. Pay attention to fiber, and in this case, the more the better. Products like breads, crackers, and cereals that are higher in fiber are typically going to be better for you.

Sugar. Look at the labels to check for added sugar. Zero added sugar is best, but the lower, the better.

The ingredients list. Fewer ingredients are preferable. In general, something that doesn't have a ton of ingredients is going to be less processed and contain less extra stuff that you really don't need.

Nutrition Facts

Serving Size 2/3 cup (51g)
Servings Per Container About 9

Amount Per Serving	Cereal	Cereal with 1/2 cup Skim Milk
Calories	240	280
Calories from Fat	70	70

	% Daily Value**	
Total Fat 8g*	12%	12%
Saturated Fat 2.5g	13%	13%
Trans Fat 0g		
Cholesterol 0mg	0%	0%
Sodium 50mg	2%	5%
Total Carbohydrate 37g	12%	14%
Dietary Fiber 3g	12%	12%
Sugars 13g		
Protein 4g	8%	16%
Vitamin A	0%	4%
Vitamin C	0%	0%
Calcium	2%	15%
Iron	6%	6%

using whole-wheat flour. "If 100% whole wheat doesn't taste as good to you, even a 50/50 blend of whole-wheat and white flour is a good option," says McManus. But keep in mind that most often the problem with pizza is what you put on it.

Try to avoid high-fat cheeses, pepperoni, and sausage. "My suggestion is to use a simple tomato sauce with canned tomato and fresh basil and garlic. Alternatively, you can top your pizza with some tomato slices. Finish it off with part-skim mozzarella cheese and your favorite veggies," she says.

Pork bacon vs. turkey bacon

Is turkey bacon better? Maybe.

The reason for the uncertain verdict on turkey versus pork bacon is the large disparities between individual products. "I did find a fair amount of variation between the different types of bacon that are available," explains McManus. One more expensive brand of turkey bacon had 1.5 grams of saturated fat and 190 milligrams (mg) of sodium—far less than an inexpensive brand, which had 5 grams of saturated fat and 500 mg of sodium. In addition, some brands of turkey bacon contained problematic ingredients such as nitrates and nitrites, while others did not.

"Don't just pick up a product and assume that all things are equal," she says. In some instances, pork bacon may be lower in saturated fat and sodium than a particular brand of turkey bacon.

A better option: Don't eat bacon at all. "Turkey or pork, bacon is still a processed meat," says McManus. Processed meats have been linked to a higher risk of cardiovascular disease and cancer. "If you have to have bacon, save it for a special occasion, but don't put it on the weekly menu," she says.

Plant-based meat alternatives: How do they stack up?

Meatless burgers may be better for your heart than regular hamburgers, especially if you pair them with sides and drinks that are healthier than typical fast-food fare.

The original veggie burgers, made from a mix of grains, beans, nuts, and vegetables, date back to the 1970s, when vegetarian diets were still on the fringe. Today, popular fast-food outlets sell meatless burgers that mimic real beef much more closely than those early versions. And plant-based diets (which aren't necessarily vegetarian but lean that way) are now practically mainstream. The ample evidence linking red meat to a higher risk of heart disease and cancer has encouraged many people to steer away from meat and other animal-based foods. However, two of the newer meatless burgers, the Impossible Burger and the Beyond

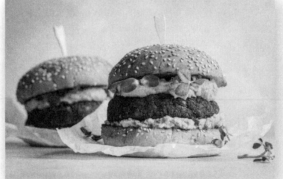

© vaaseenaa | Getty Images

Burger, are heavily processed and contain about the same amount of saturated fat as traditional burgers, along with more sodium (see "Burger battles: A nutrient comparison" on the next page). So are they actually better for you than beef?

A better burger?

So far, the evidence is limited. But according to one small study, substituting plant-based meat alternatives for the real thing appears to improve some heart-related risk factors, says Dr. Frank Hu, professor of nutrition at the Harvard T.H. Chan School of Public Health. "Blood levels of TMAO, an emerging risk factor for

Burger battles: A nutrient comparison

Here's how the newer, meatless burgers stack up nutritionally against beef burgers and other veggie burgers. Beyond Burgers contain protein from peas, mung beans, and brown rice, while Impossible Burgers feature protein from soy and potatoes.

ONE BURGER	CALORIES	TOTAL FAT (GRAMS)	SATURATED FAT (GRAMS)	CHOLESTEROL (MILLIGRAMS)	SODIUM (MILLIGRAMS)	CARBOHYDRATE (GRAMS)	FIBER (GRAMS)	PROTEIN (GRAMS)
Impossible Burger (4 ounces)	240	14	8	0	370	9	3	19
Beyond Burger (4 ounces)	230	14	5	0	390	7	2	20
85% lean ground beef (4 ounces)	240	17	6	80	0	0	0	21
Amy's All-American Veggie Burger (2.5 ounces)	130	4	0	0	430	13	4	11
Boca Burger (2.5 ounces)	110	4.5	1	5	460	7	5	13

cardiovascular disease, were lower when people in the study switched from red meat to a plant-based meat alternative," he says.

Trimethylamine N-oxide, or TMAO, is produced when your body digests red meat. Elevated blood levels appear to boost inflammation, blood clotting, and heart attack risk, says Dr. Hu. The study, recently published in *The American Journal of Clinical Nutrition*, included 36 people who were assigned to eat at least two daily servings of either meat or a plant-based alternative for eight weeks. Then they switched to the opposite diet for another eight weeks. After finishing the meat substitute phase, participants had lower LDL cholesterol values in addition to lower TMAO. They were also a couple of pounds lighter on average than after the real meat phase.

Still, we need longer, larger studies of plant-based meat alternatives to better understand how they may affect people's health, Dr. Hu says. With any highly processed food (especially those that contain many different ingredients), it's hard to tease out which factors might be beneficial or detrimental. Also, it's important to focus more on the overall dietary pattern rather than on a single food in a person's diet.

A healthier homemade version

"The problem with burgers is that people tend to eat them in a fast-food setting, so the burger—even if it's made from plants—is served on a refined-grain bun and often eaten with French fries and a sugary soda," says Dr. Hu. If you're trying to cut back on red meat but yearn for a tasty burger, buy a package of one of the new plant-based meat options (which are widely available in supermarkets) to make at home, he suggests. Serve with your favorite fixings on a whole-grain bun, paired with homemade sweet potato oven fries and a flavored sparkling water. You can also use these meat alternatives in other recipes that call for ground beef, such as spaghetti sauce, chili, or casseroles.

There's good evidence supporting the cardiovascular benefits of a plant-based diet that features lots of unprocessed foods (such as beans, grains, and nuts) as well as minimally processed foods (such as tofu, whole-grain bread, and peanut butter). For now, it's not clear that processed, plant-based meat alternatives are just as heart-friendly. But if you eat them instead of regular meat, that's probably a positive choice.

What's your daily budget for saturated fat?

Find out if you're eating too much of this artery-clogging fat—and how to replace it with more heart-healthy choices.

Guess which has more saturated fat—a serving of meat lasagna or a jumbo blueberry muffin? You might assume it's the lasagna, because two key ingredients, meat and cheese, are common sources of saturated fat. In fact, both the lasagna and the muffin contain about 6 grams of saturated fat—about one-third of the recommended daily amount for most people.

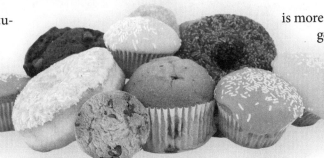

Baked goods may contain high amounts of saturated fat, which can raise LDL cholesterol.

"Muffins, cookies, pie, and other treats you pick up in the bakery section of most major stores often contain butter, lard, vegetable shortening, or tropical oils such as palm or palm kernel oil, which are high in saturated fat," says registered dietitian Kathy McManus, director of the Department of Nutrition at Harvard-affiliated Brigham and Women's Hospital. And while most packaged products feature ingredient lists and a Nutrition Facts panel, that information isn't always easy to find for bakery items.

Why limit saturated fat?

What's more, a lot of people are still a bit confused by the Nutrition Facts panel, she adds. They don't realize that it's important to check the amount of saturated fat (not just the total fat) in the foods you eat.

To be clear: There's no need to avoid saturated fat completely. But eating too much can raise the amount of harmful LDL cholesterol in your blood. That, in turn, promotes the buildup of fatty plaque inside arteries—the process that underlies most heart disease.

How much is too much? The Dietary Guidelines for Americans recommend limiting calories from saturated fat to less than 10% of the total calories you consume each day. The American Heart Association is more conservative, suggesting a limit of 5% to 6%. But McManus and many other nutrition experts recommend 7%. That limit is based on the typical amount of saturated fat in a Mediterranean-style diet, which is known for its heart-protecting qualities, she says.

Stick to a budget

To get an idea of your own target, see "Saturated fat: Know your limit." Then check out "Saturated fat in selected foods" on the next page to see how much common foods contain. Many simple swaps can trim your saturated fat intake, such as choosing skinless

Saturated fat: Know your limit

For heart health, experts recommend that you limit the amount of saturated fat you eat to 7% of your total daily calories. Here's how to calculate it:

1. Use the USDA's www.myplate.gov/myplate-plan to calculate your daily calories (click on Get the Widget, then click Start under the Get Your MyPlate Plan).
2. Multiply that number by 0.07 to find 7%.
3. Divide that number by 9 (the number of calories in one gram of fat) to get grams of saturated fat.

The average recommended calorie intake for women is 2,000 per day, which comes out to about 16 grams of saturated fat. For men, the respective values are 2,500 and about 19.

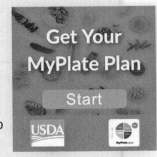

Get Your MyPlate Plan

Start

USDA

Image: USDA.GOV
© Wavebreakmedia Ltd | Getty Images

chicken breasts and low or nonfat versions of cheese and yogurt. If you don't eat meat, maybe go ahead and have some whole-milk yogurt. Just try to stick within your daily budget for saturated fat, McManus says. You can look up the saturated fat content of foods with free apps such as Lose It! or MyFitness-Pal (which you can access on a computer if you don't have a smartphone). Or you can check CalorieKing (www.calorieking.com), which includes popular brands from stores and fast-food restaurants.

Healthier replacements

"But the most important point about saturated fat is how you replace the calories you lose by cutting it from your diet," says McManus. Research clearly shows that the healthiest option is to replace saturated fat with unsaturated fat, which includes both monounsaturated and polyunsaturated fat. Most liquid oils made from vegetables, nuts, and seeds (olive, corn, peanut, walnut, safflower, soybean, and canola, for example) are good choices. So are avocados, nuts, and nut butters. Try a few of her suggestions to add healthy unsaturated fats to your diet:

- Top toasted whole-grain bread with mashed avocado or nut butter (made with peanut, almond, or a more exotic nut, such as cashew or hazelnut).
- Stir-fry a colorful mix of your favorite vegetables in peanut, olive, or canola oil (try a mix of broccoli, green beans, and red and yellow peppers).
- Roast root vegetables (such as sweet potatoes, beets, and parsnips) that have been coated with olive oil.
- Toss your salads with a homemade vinaigrette dressing, prepared with either a neutral-flavored oil (such as grapeseed) or a toasted nut oil, such as walnut or pistachio.

Saturated fat in selected foods	
FOOD	GRAMS OF SATURATED FAT
Cheddar cheese, 1.5 ounces	8.2
Jumbo blueberry muffin, 5.8 ounces	6
Yogurt, Greek, plain, full fat, ¾ cup	5
Ground beef, 85% lean, 3 ounces, broiled	5
Mozzarella cheese, part-skim, 1.5 ounces	4.8
Fast-food hamburger, single patty with condiments	4.8
Cheese pizza, 1 slice	4.7
Vanilla ice cream, ½ cup	4.5
Bacon, 1 ounce, cooked (3 slices)	4
Pork sausage, 1-ounce patty, cooked	2.4
Half-and-half, 2 tablespoons	2.1
Chicken breast with skin, 3 ounces, roasted	1.8
Egg, 1 large	1.6
Eye of round steak, 3 ounces, grilled	1.5
Chicken breast without skin, 3 ounces	0.8
Yogurt, Greek, plain, nonfat, ¾ cup	0
Nondairy creamer, 2 tablespoons	0

Sources: USDA FoodCentral, CalorieKing

by ANTHONY L. KOMAROFF, M.D.

Does a low-salt diet really improve your health?

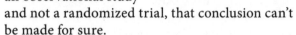

Q *My doctor has been on my case to cut down the salt in my diet. But I like salt, and I hear that not all medical studies show that a low-salt diet really improves your health. Can you unconfuse me?*

A You're right—the value of a low-salt diet for the average person has been controversial. Many studies have shown that a low-salt diet improves cardiovascular health. However, the studies have had limitations: some involved relatively few people, and some measured how much salt people say they eat but not how much salt they actually eat. A study from Harvard published online Nov. 13, 2021, by *The New England Journal of Medicine* overcame both of these problems. The study involved nearly 11,000 people who were followed carefully for almost nine years.

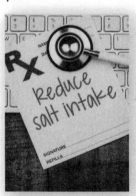

Doctors recommend using a salt substitute.

Researchers measured the amounts of two types of salt the people actually ate: common table salt (sodium chloride) and another mineral often used as a salt substitute (potassium chloride). People who consumed the most sodium chloride had a 60% higher risk of a major cardiovascular event (a heart attack, a stroke, cardiac stent placement, or bypass surgery) compared with those who consumed the least.

In contrast, people who consumed the most potassium chloride had a 31% lower risk of a major cardiovascular event compared with the people who consumed the least. In short, this study seems to say that it would be healthy to substitute potassium chloride for common table salt. However, because this is an observational study and not a randomized trial, that conclusion can't be made for sure.

Fortunately, a randomized trial published online by the same journal Aug. 21, 2021, came to a clear conclusion. Nearly 21,000 people in China were randomly assigned, over the next five years, to use a salt substitute that mixed potassium chloride and sodium chloride, or to use regular table salt (all sodium chloride).

The study participants all were ages 60 or older, had experienced a stroke in the past, and had high blood pressure (hypertension). In the group that used the salt substitute, the risks of another stroke, a major cardiovascular event, and death were 12% to 14% lower, compared with the group that used regular table salt. We can't know if the same would have been true in younger people, people who are not Chinese, or people who had no history of a stroke or other cardiovascular disease.

Controversial medical issues are rarely completely settled by new studies, because all studies have limitations. Nevertheless, I regard these two studies as providing strong evidence that a diet with a high content of sodium chloride should be avoided, and that we should probably be using salt substitutes containing potassium chloride more often. I will be. One caveat: People with kidney disease and those taking heart or blood pressure medications should check with their doctor before making the switch.

© CatLane | Getty Images

Spice up your cooking to cut down on salt

Herbs, spices, and other flavor-boosting techniques can help you eat less sodium, a proven strategy to lower blood pressure.

High blood pressure—one of the key drivers of heart disease—improves when people eat less sodium, a main component of salt (see "How salt affects your blood pressure" on the next page).

One simple way to skimp on salt is to enhance your food with other flavors, including spices, herbs, aromatic roots (such as onions, garlic, and ginger), citrus, and vinegars. Two additional tips to optimize flavor: choose the freshest possible foods, and use appropriate cooking techniques, says Dr. Rani Polak, founding director of the Culinary Healthcare Education Fundamentals (CHEF) Coaching program at the Institute of Lifestyle Medicine at Harvard-affiliated Spaulding Rehabilitation Hospital. "If you can combine these techniques together, your food will taste so amazing, you won't want to add extra salt," he says.

Herbs and spices

In addition to distinct flavors, fresh herbs can provide fragrance and color. Delicate herbs such as basil, cilantro, mint, oregano, parsley, and dill can enliven a variety of dishes. Add one or a combination of several favorites to a simple vinaigrette that you can toss with grains, vegetables, or legumes (beans and peas) or drizzle over grilled fish or chicken. Hardier herbs such as rosemary, sage, and thyme pair well with roasted root vegetables such as potatoes, carrots, and beets. For soups and stews, dried herbs work well.

Spices may offer more than a flavor boost, as these pungent plants contain compounds with antioxidant and antiplatelet properties that may benefit cardiovascular health. Studies have found that people who like spicy foods tend to eat less salt and have lower blood pressure. One possible explanation: capsaicin (the chemical responsible for the spicy-hot flavor in

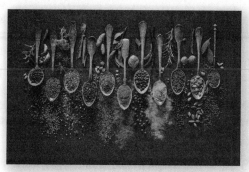

Many international cuisines feature flavorful blends of different herbs and spices, such as garam masala and za'atar.

chili peppers) may alter how the brain processes salty flavors, leading to lower salt intake.

But if you're not a fan of the mouth-tingling heat of chilis, there's a world of other spices to enjoy. Indian cuisine is famous for garam masala, a blend of spices that often contains coriander, cumin, cinnamon, cardamom, cloves, and fennel.

Za'atar is a Middle Eastern spice mix featuring dry hyssop (an herb similar to mint) combined with cumin, coriander, sesame seeds, and sumac, a red, tangy spice with a slightly sour flavor.

Chinese five-spice blend is a mix of star anise, fennel, Sichuan pepper, cinnamon, and cloves. However, you may want to try single spices in different dishes to better appreciate the unique characteristics of each one, says Dr. Polak, who is a trained chef. His current favorite: crushed coriander seeds, which he recently added to a simple salad of finely grated beets with a dressing of olive oil and fresh lemon juice.

Aromatic roots

Regular white or yellow onions are a staple ingredient for many cooks, but don't overlook leeks,

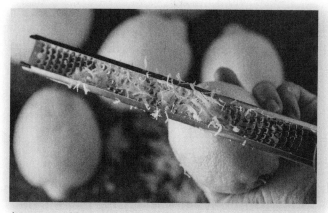

Lemon zest (the outer peel) and juice can add extra flavor to foods.

shallots, or scallions, which have slightly different flavor profiles. Fresh, raw garlic can be quite pungent, but cooking sliced or minced garlic will mellow its flavor. Roasting whole garlic bulbs softens both the texture and taste, creating a paste you can spread on crackers or breads or add to savory dishes. Freshly grated ginger root imparts a warm, spicy flavor to recipes and is popular in many Asian cuisines.

Citrus fruits and flavored vinegars

Both the juice and the zest (peel) of lemon, limes, and oranges can give foods a fresh, sharp taste. Lemons and other sour substances are literally mouthwatering—they increase saliva production, which helps you to better perceive flavors in foods. Using lemon juice and zest can replace up to 75% of the sodium in different recipes for vegetables, fish, and meats without sacrificing flavor, according to one small study.

Chefs often recommend squeezing a lemon wedge on all manner of foods just before serving. For a different sour twist, experiment with different types of vinegars. In addition to red wine, cider, and balsamic vinegars, try rice wine vinegar, sherry vinegar, or a vinegar infused with fruits (such as raspberries or strawberries) or herbs (such as tarragon or basil). Use them in salad dressings or stir into soups or stews near the end of cooking.

How salt affects your blood pressure

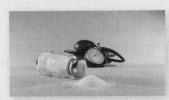

The less salt you eat, the lower your blood pressure, according to a study that pooled findings from dozens of clinical trials published since the early 1970s. The trials lasted between four weeks and three years and included more than 10,000 people in total. Their sodium intakes (manipulated by diet changes, supplements, or both) ranged from 0.4 grams to 7.6 grams per day. (On average, Americans consume more than 3.4 grams of sodium daily.) The studies also measured 24-hour urinary sodium levels to confirm how much the participants were consuming. Every 1-gram drop in daily sodium excretion was linked to a 2.4-point drop in systolic blood pressure (the first number in a reading) and a 1-point drop in diastolic blood pressure (the second number), the researchers found. The study appeared in the April 20, 2021, issue of *Circulation*.

IN THE JOURNALS

Keep heart disease at bay with a salad a day?

Eating just one cup of leafy green vegetables a day may lower your heart disease risk, suggests a study published online April 21, 2021, by the *European Journal of Epidemiology*. The study included more than 53,000 people who took part in the Danish Diet, Cancer, and Health study over a 23-year period. When the study began, their average age was 56, and none had heart disease. Researchers found that people who ate the most nitrate-rich vegetables (especially leafy greens such as spinach and lettuce) had a 12% to 26% lower risk of cardiovascular disease over the course of the study. One cup of greens per day appeared to be the optimum amount, as people who ate higher amounts didn't further lower their risk. The heart benefit may stem partly from the slightly lowered blood pressure observed in those participants.

During digestion, nitrate found in foods is converted into nitric oxide, a compound that relaxes and widens blood vessels. While these observational findings can't prove that leafy greens lower heart disease risk, they jibe with findings from similar studies.

Shopping and cooking tips

Late summer is an ideal time to find locally grown produce at farmers' markets. "Carrots that came out of the ground just a few days ago taste so much better than baby carrots that have been sitting in a plastic bag for months," says Dr. Polak. Fresh, perfectly ripened vegetables and fruits are often delicious raw or prepared very simply, so you can really appreciate their flavors, he adds. For sturdier vegetables such as squash, sweet potatoes, broccoli, and cauliflower, cooking techniques such as sautéing or roasting in a little bit of olive oil helps to caramelize the natural sugars, creating more flavor.

Build a better breakfast

Go beyond toast and coffee and include more heart-healthy nutrients in your morning meal.

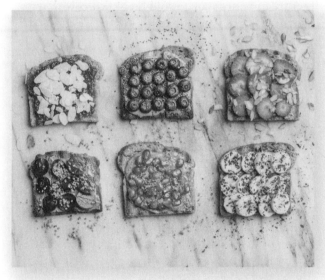

Nut butters and fruits are nutritious, filling, and tasty additions to whole-grain toast.

Many studies have linked eating breakfast to better health, including a lower risk of heart disease. But does breakfast itself deserve the credit—or do habitual breakfast eaters have other healthy habits that explain the association?

It's hard to say for sure. But nutrition experts agree that having breakfast is a good opportunity to eat some of the nutrient-rich foods you need for keeping your heart in good shape. "The message is similar for everyone: Eat more whole grains instead of refined carbs, and choose healthy protein sources with more unsaturated fat and less saturated fat," says Linda Antinoro, a dietitian at Harvard-affiliated Brigham and Women's Hospital.

Toast toppers

If toast is your thing, make sure you're using

IN THE JOURNALS

Adults who skip morning meal likely to miss out on nutrients

Your mother probably said breakfast is the day's most important meal, and a recent study suggests why she might have been right. Researchers examined the nutritional data and eating habits of more than 30,000 adults. Those who regularly skip breakfast miss getting vital nutrients, such as calcium, vitamin C, and fiber found in typical breakfast foods like fortified cereal, fruit, and milk. They also are less likely to get the recommended daily amounts of folate, iron, and vitamins A, B_1, B_2, B_3, and D. The study found that breakfast skippers had an overall lower-quality diet compared with those who always eat breakfast. They also were more likely to snack during the day and consume higher amounts of added sugars, carbohydrates, and total fat. The results were published online April 30, 2021, by *Proceedings of the Nutrition Society*.

Healthy egg muffin cups

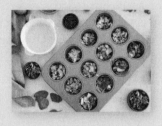

Preheat oven to 350° F. Spray a 12-cup muffin tin with nonstick cooking spray. Whisk together 10 eggs with a few pinches of salt. (Optional additions include ground black pepper, onion powder, and paprika.) Chop up your favorite vegetables, such as broccoli, tomatoes, and onions (about 1 cup in total). Grate ½ to 1 cup of hard cheese, such as cheddar or Parmesan. Divide the vegetables, cheese, and eggs evenly into the 12 muffin cups. Bake 20 to 25 minutes or until set. Store in the refrigerator for four days or in the freezer for up to one month.

whole-grain bread. Even if the label says multigrain or 12-grain, it's not necessarily whole grain. Look for the term "100% whole grain" or "100% whole wheat." To stave off midmorning hunger pangs, add some protein. Try nut butter (peanut or almond are popular choices) or part-skim ricotta cheese. Slice a banana, apple, or pear on top, or have a piece of fruit on the side.

The ever-popular avocado toast is another healthy choice, since the pale green flesh of this fruit is packed with healthy fats and fiber. "But a whole avocado may have close to 400 calories, so just use a half," advises Liz Moore, a dietitian at Harvard-affiliated Beth Israel Deaconess Medical Center. To boost flavor, she suggests adding a squeeze of lemon juice and a sprinkling of black pepper, garlic powder, and sunflower seeds.

Cereal selections

Oatmeal is a great choice because this whole-grain cereal helps lower LDL (bad) cholesterol. Skip the individual instant oatmeal packets, which are often

loaded with sugar. Just mix ⅓ cup of regular rolled oats with ⅔ cup of low-fat milk and heat in the microwave for two minutes. Another option is overnight oats: combine the oats and milk in a jar, shake, and leave in the refrigerator overnight; you can warm it up (or not) in the morning.

You can dress up oatmeal in a variety of ways by adding nuts, seeds, fresh or dried fruit, and cinnamon. Try different combinations, such as walnuts, flaxseeds, and blueberries, or pistachios, chia seeds, and chopped dried apricots.

Many popular ready-to-eat cereals, including granola, are high in sugar, so they're not ideal options, says Moore. "But if you miss the taste and texture of your favorite cold breakfast cereal, try adding a few tablespoons on top of your oatmeal," she suggests.

Eggs with the right extras

Decades ago, eggs were assumed to increase heart disease risk because of their high cholesterol content. But we now know that for most people, dietary cholesterol doesn't affect blood cholesterol nearly as much as the total mix of fat in the diet does. The ideal mix includes mostly polyunsaturated and monounsaturated fat, with limited amounts of saturated fat. The modest amount of fat found in eggs is mostly unsaturated. In addition, two large observational studies found that in healthy people, eating up to one egg a day might not be associated with a higher risk of heart disease.

Part of the problem with eggs can be the company they often keep. "People tend to eat eggs with bacon or sausage plus white toast with butter," says Antinoro. Those side dishes are the least healthy parts of that meal, she notes.

Instead, both she and Moore recommend pairing eggs with vegetables. An easy way to do this is to make egg muffins, which you can freeze and quickly reheat in the microwave (see recipe).

Smart snack strategies

Paying closer attention to your snacking habits can help you control your weight and blood sugar—two key factors for a healthy heart.

If you're trying to improve your diet, between-meal snacks can either help or hinder your efforts. Several simple strategies can keep you on track, whether you're trying to manage diabetes, ward off heart disease, or lose weight. Perhaps the most important tip is to upgrade the quality of your snack choices. "Many people favor starchy snacks, such as chips and bread," says Marc O'Meara, a dietitian at Harvard-affiliated Brigham and Women's Hospital. Many of the veggie chips people believe are healthy are just potato chips with vegetable powder added for flavor and color, he notes.

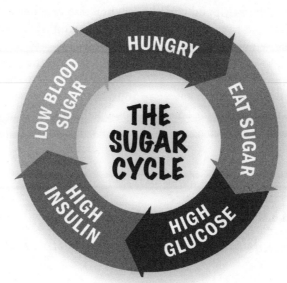

Consuming sugary foods and drinks triggers the sugar cycle.

Better balance

You're better off choosing more nutritious carbohydrate-based foods, such as fruit or whole-grain crackers, and to balance them with a little bit of protein or healthy fat. Doing so will release the carbohydrate into your bloodstream slowly over a longer time. That gives your body more time to burn the calories, and you're also more likely to feel full and satisfied until your next meal.

When you eat low-quality carbs like candy or potato chips, you're often hungry again within an hour (see "The sugar cycle"). You then end up eating even more calories, which are then stored as fat, foiling your attempts to lose weight and control your blood sugar, O'Meara explains. Snacks can help you get the recommended five servings of fruits and vegetables daily, a goal most Americans don't meet. But instead of having a whole apple or banana, have just half, and pair it with a small handful of nuts, such as unsalted almonds or peanuts (for other ideas,

see "Healthy snack suggestions"). If you need a portable snack, all-natural bars made with dried fruit, nuts, and dark chocolate can be a good option. Look for brands made with whole foods, not highly processed products.

Hunger—or habit?

By curbing hunger between meals, snacks may help prevent overeating during meals. When people get too hungry before dinner, they're often tempted to get quick but high-calorie take-out meals instead of spending

Healthy snack suggestions

Choose whole, minimally processed foods that contain healthy sources of fats, carbs, and protein. For example:

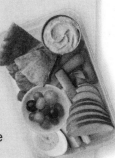

- ▶ ½ cup plain, low-fat Greek yogurt topped with fresh or frozen berries

- ▶ ¼ cup of trail mix made with nuts or seeds, dried fruit, and dark chocolate

- ▶ ¼ cup hummus with 1 cup fresh vegetables, such as baby carrots, broccoli florets, and cherry tomatoes

- ▶ Peanut, almond, or sunflower butter on sliced apple, pear, banana, or whole-grain crackers

- ▶ Low-fat cheese cubes (about the size of three or four dice in total) with an apple or a small bunch of grapes

- ▶ ½ cup shelled edamame (fresh green soybeans, sold shelled or in pods, usually in the freezer section).

the time to cook a healthy, homemade meal, says O'Meara. But sometimes, people snack out of habit rather than hunger, he says. For instance, maybe you treat yourself to a cookie every day at 3 p.m. But there are probably days you aren't actually hungry, because you had a filling lunch or skipped your workout. "Before you grab a snack, ask yourself, 'am I really hungry, or am I just following a routine?'" says O'Meara.

Many people snack after dinner. But if you eat a well-balanced dinner around 6 or 7 p.m., it takes about four hours for your body to digest that food. That means you shouldn't be hungry again before you go to bed at 10 or 11 p.m.

Mindless snacking while watching television is very common, so try to watch less. Enjoy your favorite show, but once it's over, stop. Don't stay on the couch or your favorite chair—move to another part of your house that's far away from the kitchen. Do another activity, such as reading or a hobby, during which you won't be tempted to nosh, O'Meara says.

Another trick he recommends that you can use any time of the day is to sip a hot beverage instead of having a snack. "A mug of herbal tea or decaf coffee fills you up and blunts your appetite," says O'Meara. This practice may even encourage weight loss, according to some research.

A healthier butter for your heart?

Products with plant stanols are an alternative to butter, but the health claims might not stand up.

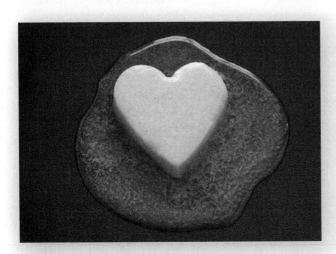

Plant stanols may not make a better butter.

Nutrition experts often advise limiting your daily intake of butter, which is high in saturated fat, in order to keep your arteries clear. Are butter substitutes made with plant stanols really a better alternative? Plant stanols are derived from plant cell membranes. They are found naturally in foods such as nuts, beans, fruits, and vegetables. Past studies have shown that supplements containing these naturally occurring compounds can

lower "bad" LDL cholesterol by up to 14% in people taking 2,000 to 3,000 milligrams (mg) a day. But the problem is that butter-replacement products often don't have enough plant stanols to produce a therapeutic effect.

Improving cholesterol

To see a reduction in your cholesterol levels, you would likely need to consume at least four tablespoons a day, says Kathy McManus, director of the Department of Nutrition at Harvard-affiliated Brigham and Women's Hospital. However, a tablespoon of a butter substitute with plant stanols has about 70 calories. "Doing that math means that in order to have enough of the substitute to see a benefit, you'd have to consume 280 calories' worth. Unless you are underweight, it's probably not a good idea to eat that much," says McManus.

Types of plant stanols

You can purchase plant stanols in pill form. But like other supplements, there is always the question about the quality and quantity of the active ingredients. Some plant stanols come in a chew form, but keep in mind that these products have a big drawback: they contain about 10 grams of added sugar per serving. "It's like candy," says McManus. "So, people need to be aware of that." If you're trying to lower your cholesterol, the best approach is often to focus on tried-and-true strategies, says McManus. These include eating a plant-based diet with more fruits and vegetables and less processed foods, reducing consumption of saturated fat, and working to maintain a healthy weight. If you are looking for a healthier alternative to butter, consider switching to liquid oils, such as olive oil or avocado oil, or use a nut butter as a spread. Some good options are peanut butter and almond butter, says McManus. You can still use traditional butter, but save it for special occasions or for recipes where only true butter flavor will do, she says.

Essential nutrients your body needs for building bone

Eat a well-rounded diet and pay special attention to calcium, vitamin D, and protein.

Many nutrients play a role in bone health, such as calcium, vitamin D, protein, magnesium, phosphorous, and potassium. If you eat a healthy diet (with lots of fruits, vegetables, legumes, nuts, seeds, and lean proteins), you'll get enough of most nutrients needed to keep your bones healthy and functioning well. But some nutrients require extra effort to ensure adequate intake when we're older.

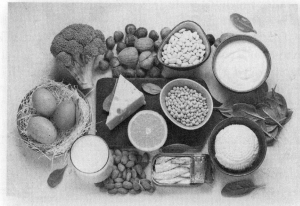

Dairy products, sardines, beans, greens, and nuts contain both calcium and protein.

© bit245 | Getty Images

you'll run out of money. So think of dietary calcium not as building bone, but as preventing calcium from being sucked out of bone," explains Dr. Harold Rosen, an endocrinologist and director of the Osteoporosis Prevention and Treatment Center at Harvard-affiliated Beth Israel Deaconess Medical Center.

Calcium

Calcium is one of the main ingredients of bone, and it's essential for cell, muscle, heart, and nerve function. We don't make calcium on our own—it comes from dietary sources (which are the safest and most effective) or calcium supplements. If there isn't enough calcium in the bloodstream, the body raids the bones for supplies, thinning the bones.

"The parathyroid gland sends a message commanding cells called osteoclasts to chew up bone and spit out calcium. If that's how calcium levels are sustained, it takes a toll on your bones. It's like going to the bank and taking out $100; if you do it every day,

Calcium goals and sources

The Recommended Dietary Allowance (RDA) of calcium for people ages 51 or older is 1,200 milligrams (mg) per day for women, and 1,000 to 1,200 mg per day for men.

Rich sources of dietary calcium include dairy foods (milk, cheese, yogurt), nuts, seeds, beans, soy, certain vegetables (leafy greens, rhubarb, artichoke, squash), fruits, and seafood. "As a rough rule of thumb, I tell patients that a cup of milk, yogurt, calcium-fortified orange juice, almonds, beans, or certain greens [kale, spinach, broccoli] has about 300 milligrams [mg] of calcium. I think that's easy to remember," Dr. Rosen says.

Fortified juices and nut milks have extra calcium. For example, fortified orange juice contains about

300 mg of calcium per cup, compared with 27 mg in regular orange juice. A cup of almond milk has 450 mg of calcium.

If you can't get enough calcium in your diet, take a low-dose calcium supplement to reach your daily RDA goal, but not more. Some studies show that large doses of calcium pills may increase the risk for developing kidney stones and possibly increase the risk of having a heart attack.

Vitamin D

Vitamin D is important for many body systems, especially bones. Vitamin D helps our bodies to absorb calcium (in the gut, which sends it to the bloodstream), and to regulate blood levels of calcium and phosphorus (which are needed to build bone).

Our bodies make vitamin D when sunlight turns a chemical in the skin into vitamin D_3, which the body then transforms into an active form of vitamin D. But be careful about sun exposure; if it's longer than a few minutes, you'll need sunscreen to reduce your risk of skin cancer. It's possible to get some of your vitamin D from food, but few foods contain it. "A 6-ounce portion of salmon has about 1,000 international units [IU] of vitamin D. You can drink vitamin D–fortified milk or orange juice, and certain mushrooms also have vitamin D," Dr. Rosen says. It's easier (and safer than sun exposure) to take a vitamin D_3 supplement. "Healthy older adults who don't have the bone-thinning disease osteoporosis, and those who have the precursor condition to osteoporosis called osteopenia, should take 600 to 800 IU per day. If you have osteoporosis, take 1,500 to 2,000 IU per day," Dr. Rosen advises.

Protein

We call proteins the building blocks of life. They give cells structure; power chemical reactions throughout the body; and build and repair skin, muscles, and bones. In bone, protein makes up a major part of the mass and volume, creating a meshwork of fibers that lay the foundation for growth. "Protein is like scaffolding. Calcium and phosphorous form on it and stiffen up," Dr. Rosen explains.

To support the body's needs, we need to consume healthy sources of protein: dairy products, fish, poultry, legumes, whole grains, nuts, seeds, and some vegetables such as corn, broccoli, and asparagus.

But appetite can decline with aging, and you may find you're cutting back on protein—perhaps eating just a tiny portion of fish or chicken rather than the larger helpings you once enjoyed. "If you're protein-deficient, you can't build muscle, skin, or bones," Dr. Rosen warns. "You need protein for strength and stability."

To figure out how much protein you need, multiply your weight in pounds by 0.36. For example, a 170-pound person would need to eat about 61 grams of protein per day ($170 \times 0.36 = 61.2$). That may sound like a lot, but protein adds up quickly if you eat the right foods. For example, a breakfast of one-and-a-half cups of bran cereal with a cup of skim milk starts you out with 14 grams of protein. A midmorning snack of half a cup of low-fat cottage cheese and some blueberries adds another 12 grams. For lunch, a small spinach salad with half a cup of cooked lentils and 3 ounces of salmon or chicken gives you another 30 grams. That's already 56 grams before dinner! But don't overdo it on protein intake; the jury is still out on whether too much dietary protein is safe for bones.

Two-for-one

You get a two-for-one benefit when you eat proteins that are also calcium-rich. Examples include canned salmon (with the bones) or sardines, beans, dairy products (cheese, yogurt, cottage cheese, milk), leafy greens, and nuts.

And the best way to ensure healthy bones is not only eating right but also maintaining a healthy lifestyle that includes daily weight-bearing exercise (such as brisk walking and weight training), limiting alcohol intake, and not smoking. All of those lifestyle habits are linked to another benefit: warding off chronic disease. Take advantage of these "two-fers" and protect your bones if you aren't already doing it. For more information about protecting bones, check out the Harvard Special Health Report *Osteoporosis* (www.health.harvard.edu/osteo).

More clues about the healthiest carb choices

New evidence links diets that contain more simple, low-quality carbs to a higher risk of heart disease. But the big picture is more complex.

Carbohydrate categories can be bit confusing. Nutrition experts refer to carbs as simple or complex, low-quality or high-quality, or even just "bad" or "good." Carbohydrate-rich foods can also be ranked by how quickly the sugar they contain is absorbed into your bloodstream after you eat it, using a scale known as the glycemic index, or GI (see "Glycemic index and glycemic load, explained"). First developed 40 years ago, the glycemic index was in the news again when *The New England Journal of Medicine* recently published a large international study suggesting that diets with a higher glycemic index and load are associated with a higher risk of cardiovascular disease and death. The link was strongest among people who were overweight or obese.

"Glycemic index is one way to think about carbohydrate quality, but it's not the only way," says Dr. Frank Hu, professor of nutrition and epidemiology at the Harvard T.H. Chan School of Public Health. You can also classify carbs as sugars, starches, and fiber.

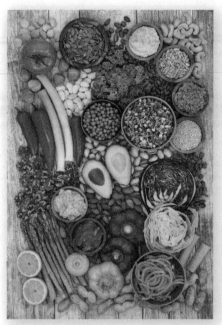

Carb categories

Here's a rundown of these three categories of carbs:

Sugars. Easily digested sugary foods (sodas, candy, and desserts) have a high GI. Eating them causes blood sugar spikes and dips, which over time can make the body less sensitive to insulin, the hormone that regulates blood sugar. The resulting insulin resistance triggers weight gain, inflammation, and other factors that contribute to the artery-clogging plaque that's responsible for most heart disease.

Fiber. Foods full of fiber are digested much more slowly and tend to have a lower GI. Low-GI foods include whole or minimally processed carbohydrate-rich foods, such as whole grains, legumes (beans and peas), nuts, vegetables, and fruits. Here's the easy part: these carbohydrates are also

Glycemic index and glycemic load, explained

Carbohydrate-containing foods have properties that affect how quickly they are digested and how quickly the resulting glucose (sugar) enters the bloodstream. This is quantified by a measure known as the glycemic index (GI). Foods are ranked on a scale of 0 to 100; pure glucose has a value of 100. However, the GI value doesn't account for the quantity of the specific food a person typically eats. A separate measure, the glycemic load, indicates the change in blood glucose level when someone eats a typical serving of the food. It's calculated by multiplying the food's GI by the amount of carbohydrate it contains.

For the highest-quality carb intake, choose foods that have a low or medium glycemic load and limit those with a high glycemic load.

Low glycemic load: bran cereals, apples, oranges, kidney beans, black beans, lentils, cashews, peanuts, carrots.

Medium glycemic load: pearled barley, brown rice, oatmeal, bulgur, rice cakes, whole-grain bread, whole-grain pasta.

High glycemic load: white potatoes, refined breakfast cereals, sugar-sweetened beverages, candy bars, white rice, white-flour pasta.

classified as complex, high-quality, or good carbs.

Starches. Starches are another story. The most commonly consumed form of carbohydrate, starches include cereal grains such as rice, wheat, and corn, and root vegetables such as potatoes. Americans tend to eat mostly highly processed grains, such as white rice and foods made with white flour. These refined starches are quickly broken down into sugar, which is why they have higher GI values.

What is resistant starch?

But some starchy foods—most notably legumes—contain what's known as resistant starch. Resistant starch is similar to fiber in that it cannot be directly absorbed by the body. It has to be broken down by specific gut bacteria. Eating foods high in resistant starch spurs the growth of these health-promoting bacteria. "They produce short-chain fatty acids, which make your body more sensitive to insulin and reduce inflammation," says Dr. Hu. In effect, resistant starch has the opposite effect from sugar and other highly processed carbs in your body.

White potatoes are full of regular starch, which is why they have a high glycemic index. French fries and mashed potatoes are probably the most popular ways to prepare spuds, but potato lovers might want to consider potato salad instead. Why? "If you leave potatoes in the refrigerator for one or two days, the cold temperature transforms some of the starch into resistant starch," says Dr. Hu. Another culinary trick that may slightly lower a food's glycemic impact is to add vinegar or lemon juice, as the acid slows the conversion of starch to sugar in the body.

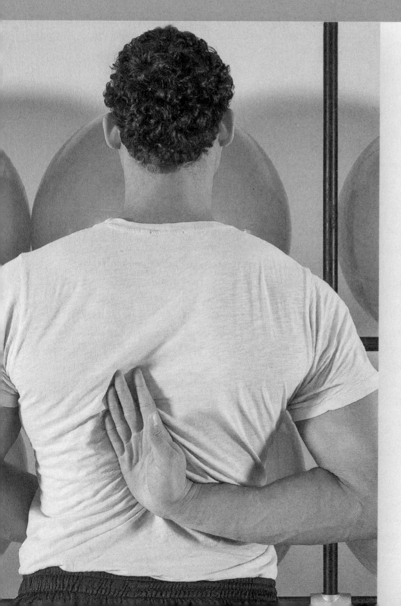

Chapter 6

Pain Management for Arthritis and More

Take Action!
5 Things You Can Do Now

1 **Stretch daily.** Limber muscles can help ease knee pain. (page 131)

2 **Hold a plank.** Stronger core muscles can help back pain. (page 134)

3 **Consider the cost of platelet injections.** They are costly and results are inconsistent. (page 137)

4 **Get a pedicure.** It will help you avoid ingrown toenails. (page 149)

5 **Don't forget your shingles vaccine.** It will lower your risk for this painful condition. (page 150)

Take on chronic pain where it lives

At-home strategies can help you find relief when it hurts.

The good news is that more people are living longer. The bad news is that as a result, more people are also living with chronic pain, which becomes more common with age.

"There are more people over the age of 65 today than under the age of 5. This is a first in our country," says Robert Jamison, PhD, a professor in pain management, anesthesia, and psychology at Harvard Medical School. However, as people age, many of the body's systems start to break down, which can lead to persistent discomfort.

Common causes of chronic pain include anything from osteoarthritis and back pain to migraine headaches and fibromyalgia. In some people who have experienced prior nerve injuries or inflamed joints, the nerve endings keep firing even when the initial problem has resolved, says Jamison. "It's not a psychiatric problem. It's true, it's real, but it's not a sign that something is life-threatening or progressive," he says. But this ongoing pain is something that can significantly affect quality of life.

Chronic pain can be more complex and expensive to treat than many other conditions like diabetes and cancer, says Jamison. This is the case because people experiencing persistent pain often require a lot of doctor visits and medical tests. They may also need to work with multiple health care providers to manage their condition.

"So, for a lot of reasons it's important to manage pain well," Jamison says.

But to truly keep pain under control, you'll need to not only partner with experts, but also develop strategies that you can use on your own at home. Empowering yourself to learn how to manage pain without office visits or procedures is often the most successful way to improve quality of life and decrease chronic pain. "What people can do about it themselves can be just as important as what the doctors do," says Jamison.

At-home options to manage pain

The pandemic has not only magnified the importance of at-home pain management strategies, but also brought forth new options. For example, there

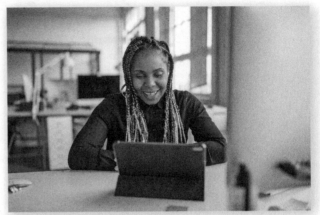

If it's difficult for you to attend group support meetings, an online version may be just as effective in helping you manage pain.

are now numerous telemedicine options, including online support groups sponsored by pain management organizations, Internet-based mental health support programs, and pain management apps.

Using a combination of strategies can help get your pain under control. Here are some you can try.

Increase movement. While it seems like someone who is in pain should rest and avoid movement, this is actually the opposite of what you should do, says Jamison. Increased activity can help relieve chronic pain, so focus on what you can to be as active as possible. Try at-home exercises, such as online yoga classes, or walking. Also test out an activity tracker. It can help you increase your movement over time and to set small achievable goals that won't aggravate your condition.

Try cognitive behavioral therapy (CBT). This psychotherapy practice can help you adopt healthier thought patterns. It's been shown to reduce pain and disability by helping people cope with pain more effectively. CBT offers a way to change your emotional response to pain, starting with the understanding that while you may be hurting, your condition isn't necessarily getting worse.

While therapists often guide people through CBT, you can also try an online CBT program, such as PainTrainer (www.painTrainer.org) or Pain Course (www.health.harvard.edu/pc), says Jamison. It can help you develop strategies to pace yourself as you move toward goals and to solve potential problems that crop up in daily life. For example, how can you manage pain when you have to leave the house to go somewhere?

Join an online support group. The pandemic forced many groups to move to a virtual format, which has proven a good option for some. Online meetings can be as helpful as those conducted in person.

"We did a study looking at a weekly pain group session. We monitored people who participated in either a virtual group or an in-person group and found that both groups did equally well in terms of getting better," says Jamison. But the remote group actually performed better on one measure. "People in the remote group were more compliant and showed up more often," he said. This is likely because people encounter fewer barriers when attending an online meeting at home than they do leaving home to attend a meeting in person. This is particularly true if they care for a child or have other responsibilities. To find a meeting or other resources, visit the American Chronic Pain Association website at www.theacpa.org.

Use support apps. There are a number of apps on the market that can help people manage different aspects of chronic pain. They can help people track certain behaviors, sleep, and mood, and whether their pain has gotten better or worse. Some apps even allow you to connect with your doctor to share information about your pain management efforts.

Mindfulness meditation for pain

Mindfulness meditation can help people manage chronic pain. Here are the basics:

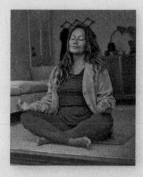

1. In a quiet and comfortable place, sit on a cushion on the floor with your legs crossed, or sit in a chair with your feet flat on the floor. Sit up straight but not stiff. Let your hands rest on the tops of your thighs.
2. Start by bringing your attention to the sensations of your body (sight, sound, taste, touch, scent).
3. Next, bring your awareness to your breathing as you inhale and exhale. Pay particular attention to breathing out.
4. When you become distracted by thoughts and feelings (an appointment you must keep or anger at someone), silently and gently label these as thoughts, let them go, and return your focus to your breath.

Start by setting aside some time to meditate for five to 10 minutes once or twice each day. You can gradually build up to 20 minutes or even an hour. For additional tips, see the Harvard Special Health Report *Pain Relief Without Drugs or Surgery* (www.health.harvard.edu/prds).

"It's amazing how much you can do through an app," says Jamison.

Casing the joints

Is there any protection against osteoarthritis?

If you live long enough, you'll no doubt have days when your joints feel extra stiff, achy, or even painful. The likely reason you feel out of joint, so to speak, is osteoarthritis: it's the most common type of arthritis among older adults. And it can slow down even the most active person.

While osteoarthritis has no cure, there are ways to lower your risk and lessen its impact on your health and quality of life when it comes calling.

Overusing overuse

Osteoarthritis involves damage or breakdown of the joint cartilage between bones. Cartilage is a tissue that acts as a cushion. When it wears away, bones can rub against each other, causing pain, swelling, and stiffness.

The disease usually strikes the knees, hips, neck, spine, and hand (usually the middle joints of the fingers and the ones closest to the nail).

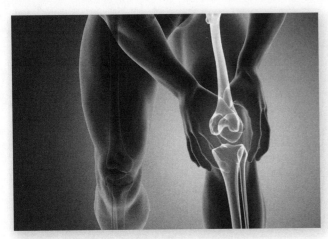

Osteoarthritis often strikes the knees, but can also attack the hips, neck, spine, and hands.

of the rubbery cartilage structures that cushions the shin bone from the thighbone at the knee), a ligament injury, or a joint dislocation.

A range of motions

You are not defenseless against osteoarthritis. Some measures can help you lower your risk and better manage the disease if it appears. The two biggest are losing excess weight and avoiding stress on an injured joint. However, movement is the best medicine.

"It's not clear if specific exercises or activities help ward off or slow the progress of osteoarthritis," says Dr. Shmerling. "The idea is that any type of regular movement can help build the muscles surrounding your joints. Increased muscle strength won't make the joints healthier, but it can help them work better." Some research, though, supports a multi-tier approach to exercise. A study published Feb. 9, 2021, in *JAMA* found less pain and better range of motion in people with hip and knee osteoarthritis who did a combination of aerobics, strength training, and mind-body activities like tai chi and yoga.

During flare-ups, both acetaminophen (Tylenol) and oral or topical over-the-counter nonsteroidal anti-inflammatory drugs can ease pain; the latter can also help with swelling. Occasional use is usually safe (unless your doctor tells you otherwise), but if daily medication is needed, it's best to check with your doctor first.

Also, be mindful that joint pain could be caused by an injury, infection, or a musculoskeletal condition like bursitis or tendinitis. "You should have any ongoing pain checked out by your doctor," says Dr. Shmerling.

Osteoarthritis is often called a "wear and tear" disease, but this is misleading, as it doesn't occur because of overuse. "Your joints don't get worn down like treads on a tire from years of taxing labor or physical stress," says Dr. Robert Shmerling, senior faculty editor at Harvard Health Publishing.

In fact, the opposite may be true. Some studies have found that longtime runners actually have a lower risk of knee osteoarthritis than non-runners.

Here's another way to think about it. Osteoarthritis in the fingers is quite common, so if overusing these joints were the problem, you'd think right-handed people would have more arthritis in their right hand. "But, in general, osteoarthritis affects both hands equally," says Dr. Shmerling.

So, why exactly do some people develop osteoarthritis? There are probably different causes in different people, but at least three factors are known to be important:

Age. The CDC says that approximately 50% of adults ages 65 and older have been diagnosed with osteoarthritis. "You naturally lose some cartilage over time and will probably get some osteoarthritis in one or more of your joints," says Dr. Shmerling. "It's one of the signs of surviving a long time."

Weight. In general, the more extra weight you carry, the greater the risk.

Genes. It tends to run in families. In addition, certain musculoskeletal injuries can damage cartilage and lead to osteoarthritis. Examples include a fracture of a bone near a joint, a tear in a meniscus (one

Contributing conditions

Other conditions also can trigger joint pain and possibly accelerate osteoarthritis. For example:

Hemarthrosis: repeated bleeding into a joint from trauma or a blood clotting disorder like hemophilia.

Gout: a type of arthritis that usually affects the big toe.

Avascular necrosis: death of bone near a joint caused by interruption in blood flow.

Rheumatic disease: joint inflammation from rheumatoid arthritis and psoriatic arthritis.

If standard treatments don't work, the next step is possible surgery. Depending on which joint is affected and the severity of the damage, you may need joint replacement surgery or a procedure to fuse bones together using pins, screws, or rods. "Surgery should be considered a last resort," says Dr. Shmerling. "And it doesn't completely solve the problem in every case. There may still be some pain or stiffness."

The best types of exercise when you have hip or knee pain

Here are joint-friendly moves and machines to keep you active and safe despite joint pain.

Hip or knee pain makes everything harder, especially exercising. How are you supposed to work out when it hurts to bend your joints or put pressure on them?

The answer is to switch to non-weight-bearing exercise that takes the burden off of your hips and knees. "It allows you to move more freely, with less pain, and you wind up feeling better afterward," says Vijay A. Daryanani, a physical therapist and personal trainer with Harvard-affiliated Spaulding Outpatient Center.

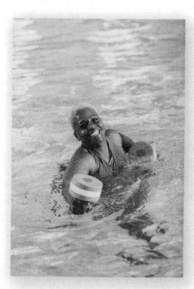

© kali9 | Getty Images

Joint-friendly exercise machines

Several exercise machines are gentle on your joints and provide a great cardio workout while strengthening your muscles, improving endurance, and boosting range of motion.

An elliptical trainer. This machine has pedals that move along an oval-shaped track (either back and forth or up and down), creating a fluid motion that saves you from hitting the ground and putting pressure on your joints. Most elliptical trainers also have handles or poles you move back and forth

IN THE JOURNALS

The most common exercise among people with arthritis

It's hard to exercise when you struggle with the pain and stiffness of arthritis. So how do people with arthritis get moving? Most of them walk, according to a study published online Oct. 8, 2021, by the CDC's *Morbidity and Mortality Weekly Report*. Researchers analyzed the 2019 survey results of 87,000 U.S. adults with arthritis (most of them middle-aged or older) who said they'd been physically active in the past month. About 71% reported that walking was one of their two most frequent activities, even if they had severe joint pain; 13% mentioned gardening;

7% said weight lifting. All of these activities help reduce arthritis pain and fatigue: Brisk walking gets your heart and lungs pumping for an aerobic workout that helps reduce fatigue, inflammation, and excess weight (which contributes to arthritis pain). Weight training reduces pain by strengthening muscles so they can absorb pressure you place on the joints. Gardening helps reduce stress and fatigue. Few survey respondents said they took part in low-impact activities, such as cycling or swimming. However, these activities are great workouts and are particularly easy on your joints.

for an upper-body workout (like a cross-country ski machine). "You need good balance to use an elliptical machine. If it's safe for you to use it, try moving the pedals backward sometimes to challenge your muscles and balance even more," Daryanani suggests.

A stationary bike. A stationary bike (also called an indoor cycling machine) has bicycle pedals and a seat with a back. The machines come in two styles: upright (like a regular bicycle) or recumbent (which has back support). "If you use an upright bike, don't stand up and pedal; that can put extra pressure on your joints," Daryanani says.

A rowing machine. A rowing machine has a seat that slides back and forth on a straight track, and a horizontal bar that you pull toward you. While seated, you place your feet on footpads, pull the bar, and propel yourself backward, simulating boat rowing with little impact on the joints. "The tricky part of using a rowing machine is that it's low to the ground. Make sure you can get down to it and that you'll be able to stand back up," Daryanani advises.

No matter which of these machines you use: "Start out with a few minutes and the lowest amount of resistance, gradually increasing your time. When 15 minutes with no resistance feels easy, add a little resistance to make it harder, and increase it over time," Daryanani advises.

Low-impact exercises

Several low-impact exercises can also provide a good cardio workout and muscle strengthening without stressing your joints.

Pool exercises. These include swimming laps, water aerobics, or walking in waist-deep water. The water keeps you buoyant, takes pressure off your joints, and provides resistance (which helps build muscle and bone strength). Exercising in water is also safer for balance and mobility, as there's no risk of falling.

"You're free to do so much more in water than you would on land. But be cautious and don't necessarily attempt the same kinds of exercise out of the pool," Daryanani says.

Short brisk walks. Taking short walks as opposed to long ones avoids excessive pressure on the joints. "If you can go out for five, 10, or 15 minutes, a few times per day, that adds up," Daryanani says. In terms of aerobic health benefits, three 10-minute walks per

Stretches to relieve hip or knee pain

Standing quadriceps stretch: Stand up straight, feet together, holding the back of a chair. Bend your right knee, grasp your right foot, and pull it behind you, toward your buttocks, until you feel a stretch in the front of your thigh. Hold for 10 to 30 seconds, then repeat with the other leg.

Pretzel stretch: Lie on your back with your left knee bent and the left foot on the floor. Rest your right ankle on your left leg near your left knee. Your right knee should point to the side. Grasp the back of your left thigh with both hands and slowly pull it toward you until you feel a stretch in your right hip and buttock. Hold a few moments, then repeat the exercise with the opposite leg.

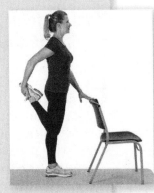

Exercise photos by Michael Carroll

day is the equivalent of one 30-minute walk—and easier on your joints. When walking, wear snug-fitting walking shoes with good support. "And steer clear of tree roots or anything that would make you lose your balance," Daryanani says.

Tai chi. This low-impact martial art is not a cardio workout, but it has many benefits. It involves a series of slow, choreographed movements; you gradually shift your weight from one pose to another as you focus on body sensations and deep breathing. Tai chi has been shown to improve balance, flexibility, range of motion, and reflexes. It's also been shown to reduce falls by up to 60%. "Tai chi will help you function better, especially with hip or knee pain," Daryanani says. "But if shifting into a pose hurts, don't force it."

Making it work

Before starting any of these exercises, get the okay from your doctor or physical therapist. And don't worry about immediately meeting the standard goal of at least 150 minutes per week of moderate-intensity activity; any amount of exercise will help.

"If you're starting at zero and you do a minute, that's progress; and then do a minute and a half, and then two minutes. Keep increasing the time," Daryanani says.

The payoff of exercise is well worth it. "Even small increases in moderate-intensity physical activity provide health benefits. Some of them can happen quickly, such as reduced feelings of anxiety, reduced blood pressure, greater insulin sensitivity, and improvements in sleep," says Dr. I-Min Lee, a senior exercise researcher and a professor of medicine at Harvard Medical School. "And over the long term, you'll get other benefits, such as increased heart and lung fitness, increased muscle strength, and a reduced risk for chronic diseases, such as heart disease, stroke, type 2 diabetes, and several cancers."

Take control of your knee pain

Simple home exercises and stretches can help ease some common types of knee pain.

If you've got sore knees, exercise might seem like the hardest thing you can do—but it's also one of the best.

"Exercise is one of the most important things you can do for knee pain," says Dr. Lauren Elson, an instructor in physical medicine and rehabilitation at Harvard Medical School.

The right combination of strengthening and stretching exercises can relieve pain by helping to improve the way the joint moves and functions.

"The knee is often an innocent bystander between the hip and the foot. Knee pain is often caused by problems occurring above or below," says Dr. Elson.

For example, weak hip muscles may cause more strain on the knee, intensifying your pain.

Strengthening the muscles around the hip joint can help relieve it, says Dr. Elson. In addition, knee pain is sometimes caused or aggravated by tight muscles around the knee, a problem that is often successfully addressed by stretching. If the muscles aren't flexible, the knee joint sometimes won't move properly, says Dr. Elson.

Know when to see your doctor

While many conditions that cause knee pain can be helped by exercise, in some instances it may not be appropriate, says Dr. Lauren Elson, an instructor in physical medicine and rehabilitation at Harvard Medical School. You should stop exercising and see a doctor if you have any of the following symptoms:

▶ fever

▶ pain that is not improving

▶ pain that intensifies with activity

▶ pain that wakes you up in the middle of the night.

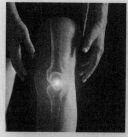

Exercise can help ease knee pain for many people, but there are some exceptions.

What conditions can exercise help?

Knee exercises and stretches can help relieve knee pain caused by many conditions, including these three that commonly affect older adults:

Patellofemoral pain. This condition typically causes a dull, aching pain in the front of the knee that's made worse by daily activities, such as squatting, going up or down stairs, or standing up after sitting for a long period of time. The pain is caused by irritation of the cartilage underneath the kneecap when it does not glide or sit properly. Exercise can help to eliminate problems that lead to this irritation. Stretches can loosen tight muscles on the side of the knee that may be pulling the kneecap out of its groove as it moves. Strengthening weak hip muscles or stretching tight muscles in the front or back of the legs can also reduce discomfort.

Chronic degenerative meniscal tears. When one or both pads of cartilage that cushion each of your knee joints deteriorates or tears, you may feel pain and a sticking or locking sensation. While surgery is sometimes necessary, doctors usually first recommend physical therapy to help build up the muscles around the knee to take the pressure off the joint and reduce discomfort.

Osteoarthritis. If you're over age 50 and you have stiffness, pain, or swelling, it may be osteoarthritis.

Years of wear and tear can break down the cartilage in the knees, leading to chronic joint inflammation. A past injury may also lead to arthritis. While nothing can reverse these physical changes, you can reduce pain by building up the muscles around the knee as well as in the pelvis and core. Strong muscles act like scaffolding,

taking some of the pressure off the joints. Stretching to increase flexibility can help the joint function properly.

Exercises to try

To ease knee pain, you'll want to perform exercises that work a number of different muscles, from the hip abductors to the hamstrings and quadriceps, says Dr. Elson.

Two to add to your routine are the side-leg raise, and the single-leg lift. Do this workout at least two days a week to start and ideally work

Exercises to help control knee pain

SIDE-LEG RAISE

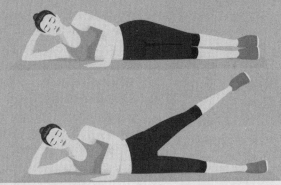

SINGLE-LEG RAISE

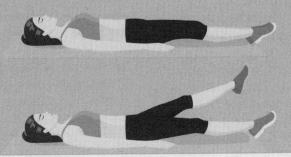

Side-leg raise
Starting position: Lie on your right side, with your legs straight. Bend your right forearm upward and rest your head on your hand.
Movement: Keep your legs straight and slowly lift your left leg up toward the ceiling. Pause, then slowly return to the starting position. Finish all repetitions, then repeat on the left side.
Tips and techniques: Throughout the movement, keep your hips straight and still as if you were lying with your back against a wall. Contract your abdominal muscles and keep your pelvis still (no rocking) throughout. Lift your leg up as high as possible without letting your hip move and while maintaining good form.
Make it easier: Lift your top leg a shorter distance, or lean your back against a wall for support.
Make it harder: Tie resistance tubing around your upper thighs, or increase the number of repetitions.

Single-leg lift
Starting position: Lie on your back with your legs straight. Extend one leg, foot slightly flexed. Rest your hands at your sides on the floor.
Movement: Tighten your thigh muscles and slowly lift the leg in the air until your knees are aligned. Pause, then slowly lower your leg to rest on the floor. Finish all repetitions, then repeat with the other leg.
Tips and techniques: Keep your abdominal muscles contracted. Keep your hips on the floor as you lift one leg. Exhale as you lift.
Make it easier: Lift your leg a shorter distance.
Make it harder: At a slow, controlled pace, try tracing the letter T with your leg in the air. Lift up one leg four inches, move the leg four inches to the left, return to center, move the leg four inches to the right, return to center, then lower your leg to the floor. Finish all repetitions, then repeat with the other leg.

up to every other day. How many exercises you do in each session is your choice. But keep in mind that rushing through exercises can be counterproductive.

"It's more important to have good form than it is to have volume," says Dr. Elson. Start slowly with fewer repetitions to ensure you get your form right. Then add more as it becomes easier.

Stretching

You should also incorporate daily stretching into your routine. Try using a foam roller to work out the kinks in your muscles. The roller targets tight, rigid, and painful areas in both the muscles and the myofascial tissue (a layer of connective tissue around the muscles). This process, called myofascial release, which can also be performed through a hands-on massage, is designed to relax this tissue to reduce pain. It does this by releasing tension in muscles that are pulling abnormally on the knee joint, says Dr. Elson.

Accompanying this article are two stretches to try. Ideally, you should aim to do three or four repetitions of each, holding for 10 to 30 seconds each time.

HAMSTRING STRETCH

QUADRICEPS STRETCH

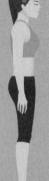

Hamstring stretch
Starting position: Lie on your back with your legs straight and your arms by your side.
Movement: Grasp your right leg with both hands behind the thigh. Extend your leg to lift your right foot toward the ceiling, foot flexed. Straighten the leg as much as possible without locking the knee to feel a stretch along the back of the right thigh. Hold. Return to the starting position and repeat with the left leg.
Tips and techniques: Stretch the leg extended toward the ceiling to the point of mild tension without any pressure behind the knee or any pain. Relax your shoulders down and back into the floor.
Make it easier: Don't lift your leg as high, or use a strap instead of your hands to support your leg.
Make it harder: Pull your leg closer to your chest.

Quadriceps stretch
Starting position: Stand on the floor with your feet spaced shoulder-width apart.
Movement: Bend your right knee and bring the heel toward your right buttock. Reach back with your right hand and take hold of your foot. Hold the stretch, then slowly lower your foot to the floor. Repeat the stretch with your left leg.
Tips and techniques: Stand straight. Keep your bent knee aligned with the hip, not pointing out to the side.
Make it easier: Lie on your stomach to do the same stretch. Place a yoga strap around your foot and hold on to both ends as you get into the starting position. Then use the strap to assist with the stretch.
Make it harder: Doing the stretch on your stomach, lift your knee off the floor slightly, without pulling your foot, to increase the stretch.

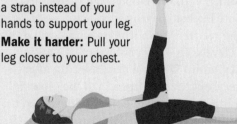

Help for your aching back

At-home strategies can ease many cases of back pain. Others may need a little more assistance from a doctor.

Whether it's sudden intense pain or a long-standing ache, back pain can be debilitating. The question is, what can you do to make it go away?

Dr. Joerg Ermann, a rheumatologist in the Division of Rheumatology, Inflammation, and Immunity at Harvard-affiliated Brigham and Women's Hospital, says that there are several strategies that can help you get back up and moving. Choosing the right ones largely depends on what type of back pain you have. The first question you need to answer, he says, is duration: Are you experiencing a short-term (acute) problem? Or is your pain chronic—lasting for months or even years?

"It's important to distinguish between the two scenarios, because it has a huge impact on what could be driving this pain, and affects its management," says Dr. Ermann.

What to do for acute pain

If you've got what doctors refer to as an acute episode of back pain, it typically comes on suddenly and often goes away within a few days or weeks. This type of back pain is very common. "Almost

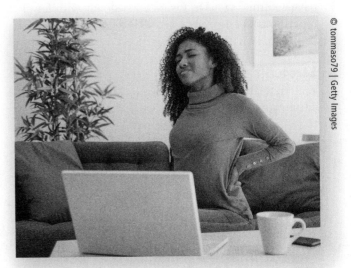

There are numerous strategies that can help lessen both sudden and chronic back pain.

everyone—80% of people—will experience this in their lifetime at some point," says Dr. Ermann. "With most common cases of back pain, we often don't really know why it hurts."

A classic scenario occurs when someone shovels

IN THE JOURNALS

Vitamin D deficiency might affect recovery from knee surgery

Could a vitamin D deficiency be linked to a more painful recovery from knee surgery? A study published online May 5, 2021, by the journal *Menopause* says it's possible.

The study looked at 226 women recruited from 2017 to 2019. Researchers divided women into two groups based on their vitamin D levels before undergoing surgery. One group had normal vitamin D levels (at or above 30 ng/mL); the other group was defined as vitamin D deficient (below 30 ng/mL). The women were tracked to see how well they did after surgery. While there

was no difference found between the groups in how successful the surgery was in improving knee function, there were differences in how much recuperation pain the women experienced. Women with low blood levels of vitamin D were more likely to have moderate to severe pain during recovery than women with normal vitamin D levels. This does not mean that taking additional vitamin D would decrease pain after knee surgery, but the findings add to the growing list of conditions other than bone health related to low vitamin D levels.

snow or does some other unusual physical activity, and—later in the day or on the following day—develops severe back pain. "This is usually due to muscle strain or ligament sprain in the back," says Dr. Ermann.

If this sounds like you, and you're otherwise fit and healthy, you can likely wait a few days to see if the pain starts to go away before you pay a visit to the doctor. In the meantime, there are several pain management strategies that are often helpful.

Medication and heat. Taking an over-the-counter nonsteroidal anti-inflammatory drug, such as ibuprofen or naproxen, can help to reduce pain. Also, try applying heat to the affected area.

Move as much as you are able. While you may be tempted to lie flat on your back until the pain goes away, movement may actually help get you back to normal more quickly. "The general approach these days is that, if at all possible, people experiencing back

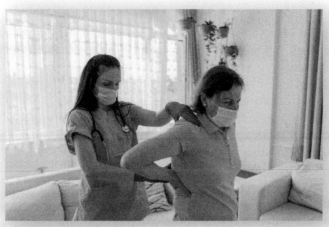

See your doctor immediately for very severe back pain or pain that causes weakness in your legs, or urinary incontinence.

pain should keep moving. We don't treat back pain with immobilization," says Dr. Ermann. The exception to this rule is a fracture or other condition that makes movement inadvisable.

Stay positive. Most episodes of acute back pain resolve on their own within a few days or weeks. "People almost always get back to the status they had before," he says. Other than staying active, no particular strategy has been shown to more quickly resolve pain and stiffness.

See your doctor. There are some instances where back pain warrants immediate medical attention. Signs that you should call your doctor include the following:

- Your pain is debilitating and getting worse. It prevents you from performing your daily

IN THE JOURNALS

A single-session class offers chronic low back pain relief

A single two-hour pain management class may offer months-long relief from chronic low back pain, according to a clinical trial published online Aug. 16, 2021, by *JAMA Network Open*.

The trial involved 263 adults with chronic low back pain that lasted at least six months. Everyone was placed randomly into one of three groups: 87 people took a pain relief skills class (called "empowered relief"), 88 had cognitive behavioral therapy (CBT) for chronic pain, and 88 had back pain education.

Empowered relief consisted of a single-session, two-hour class. It covered areas such as pain neuroscience education and CBT skills like identifying distressing thoughts, cognitive reframing

(shifting your mindset to look at a situation differently), relaxation response, and self-soothing techniques. People received a 20-minute relaxation audio file. The CBT group attended eight two-hour sessions (16 hours total) that also included multiple relaxation audios. The two-hour back health education class included how to recognize warning signs of back pain and advice on nutrition and medication management.

Both empowered relief and CBT were superior to the education class for managing pain. Yet, the single-session empowered relief class was as effective as the eight CBT sessions in reducing pain, improving sleep, and lowering depression and anxiety. The effect also lasted for three months.

- activities.
- You have additional symptoms, such as fever, weakness in the legs, difficulty walking, or urinary incontinence.
- You have an existing disease—for example, you are undergoing cancer treatment or you are on immunosuppressant medications. "Sudden severe back pain in this context may indicate a more serious problem, such as a fracture or infection," says Dr. Ermann.

What to do for chronic back pain

Chronic back pain, defined in the medical literature as pain that lasts three months or longer, typically needs different management strategies than acute back pain does.

"If you are experiencing back pain that has lingered past the three-month mark, is interfering with your life, and requires medications to treat it, it is worthwhile to talk to your doctor about it," says Dr. Ermann. A good starting point might be to mention it at your annual wellness visit. Your doctor might recommend any of the following strategies.

Work with a physical therapist. Getting guidance from a specialist as well as performing regular exercise at home can often help. Core strengthening exercises are especially important, says Dr. Ermann. If the spine is better supported by strong core muscles, it can reduce some of the pressure and pain on your back. "This can be helpful in relieving symptoms," he says. At home, try plank holds (either in a push-up position or using a modified version on your knees). Regular exercise can also help you lose weight, which may alleviate some of the pressure on the back.

Adjust your posture. In some situations, lasting back pain may be aggravated by poor posture, such as slouching. "If you are experiencing pain, look at how you sit at your desk. Relatively simple changes sometimes bring a big benefit," says Dr. Ermann. This might include getting up every few hours to stretch your back.

"I had a patient who started having back pain when working from home. It disappeared when he went back to the office. He realized that at home he was working from his couch. At the office he was sitting at a desk, which improved his posture," he says.

Try, try again. People with chronic back pain may experience pain sensitization, meaning that changes

Is your back pain a sign of an overlooked condition?

Sometimes chronic back pain is caused by conditions that aren't very common. One to consider is axial spondyloarthritis, also known as ankylosing spondylitis. It's a chronic inflammatory condition triggered by a problem with your immune system. It leads to back pain, stiffness, and other symptoms.

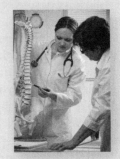

A less common condition that may cause pain is ankylosing spondylitis.

"Axial spondyloarthritis used to be considered a male disease, but that view has changed over the past 10 years. We now have better ways to identify these patients, and have since realized that the disease is as common in women as it is in men," says Dr. Joerg Ermann, a rheumatologist at Brigham and Women's Hospital. Doctors used to think that it was more prevalent in men because males tend to have more severe disease that progresses rapidly, so it's visible on an x-ray, he says.

Signs that you might have axial spondyloarthritis include back pain and stiffness that are worse in the morning and improve with exercise. This condition should also be on your radar if someone else in your family has it, because it has a strong hereditary component.

in the brain cause the body to overreact to pain signals. "Chronic pain may take on a life of its own," Dr. Ermann says. This can be addressed with specific medications, such as certain antidepressants.

"Unfortunately, we cannot really predict which medications will work for an individual, so it often becomes a matter of trial and error to find an appropriate medication or combination of medications that work," he says.

Be patient. "If you are someone who has had chronic back pain for five or 10 years, you can't expect it to go away overnight," says Dr. Ermann. Sometimes it takes time for interventions such as medication or physical therapy to make a difference. Most treatment plans won't work instantly.

Consider alternatives. "Many patients of mine also see a chiropractor," says Dr. Ermann. This doesn't work for everyone, but it is certainly something worth trying. "I personally prefer a more active approach, such as physical therapy, where you empower the muscles and help the back get stronger. Chiropractic medicine is a more passive approach. Nevertheless, I do hear from some patients that they feel better doing it," he says.

Document your progress. Keep a record of all the interventions that you have tried and write down what works and what doesn't. Having a record can be helpful down the road. Also, be certain to keep copies of the reports and the actual digital images. "It's important for a back pain specialist to see the images directly rather than reading a report."

Get a second opinion. Surgery may be necessary for some back problems, particularly those that are causing neurological symptoms, such as numbness or weakness in the extremities. It may also be used to address a tumor or for certain types of fractures. But surgery is not a cure for many back conditions, and it is not uncommon for back pain to persist after surgery. For this reason, if your doctor recommends surgery, consider getting a second opinion, says Dr. Ermann.

Can platelet-rich plasma injections heal your joints?

Research is mixed, but new evidence shows the treatment might fall short for some conditions.

Platelet-rich plasma (PRP) injections are promoted as a way to reduce pain and speed healing for a number of common problems that affect the tendons, muscles, and joints, ranging from arthritis to shoulder pain.

The treatment harvests platelets (tiny blood components that promote clotting and healing) from your own blood. They are then injected back into the injured area along with blood plasma (the liquid part of your blood), with the idea that they will supercharge your body's natural healing process.

"Platelets contain proteins called growth factors that are involved in the natural development of many tissues," says Dr. Jeffrey Katz, a professor of orthopedic surgery at Harvard Medical School. "These factors

---

IN THE JOURNALS

Pool therapy beats physical therapy for chronic low back pain

Aquatic (pool) therapy and physical therapy are two treatments that can reduce pain. But which is better for chronic low back pain? A small randomized trial published online Jan. 3, 2022, by *JAMA Network Open* suggests that buoyancy has the edge. Researchers took a group of 113 people with chronic low back pain, ages 18 to 65, and divided them into two groups. The people in one group had two 60-minute physical therapy sessions per week; the others took part in two 60-minute sessions of pool exercises per week. After 12 weeks, about half of the people in the pool therapy group showed an improvement of two to five points in their pain scores (depending on the scale), compared with only 21% or

fewer in the physical therapy group. And a year later, the pool exercisers still felt better than the land exercisers. Researchers say pool therapy seemed to have a greater influence than physical therapy on pain, function, quality of life, sleep quality, and mental state.

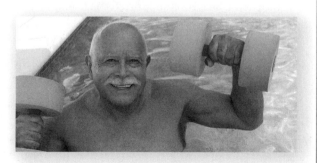

may help reduce the inflammation associated with osteoarthritis and tendinitis."

PRP injections can be done in a 30-minute office procedure and are most commonly used for knee, shoulder, foot, ankle, and elbow problems. Often the underlying conditions are difficult to treat, and a simple injection to provide symptom relief sounds great. But is PRP therapy effective?

"Historically, research into the use of PRP to treat musculoskeletal problems has produced mixed results," says Dr. Katz. Some studies show a benefit; others don't. And now, a series of well-designed clinical trials has found that PRP doesn't appear to work for three conditions that it is often used to treat: knee osteoarthritis, ankle osteoarthritis, and Achilles tendinitis (irritation or inflammation of the tendon that connects your heel to your calf).

New research suggests no benefit

The studies were all published in *JAMA* in the summer and fall of 2021. All three studies came to the same conclusion, says Dr. Katz, whose editorial examining the findings appeared along with the third study in the Nov. 23 issue. Trial participants treated with PRP fared no better than people who received a placebo treatment, he says.

However, that doesn't mean that PRP is completely out of the running. PRP formulations often have different concentrations of platelets and growth factors. It's possible that certain mixtures are more effective than others, which could explain why research results have been inconsistent, says Dr. Katz.

Some professional organizations were already hesitant to endorse PRP injections because of the variable research findings. The American College of Rheumatology and the Osteoarthritis Research Society International, for example, recommended against using PRP for osteoarthritis. The American Academy of Orthopaedic Surgeons supported the use of PRP on a "limited" basis.

Armed with this new evidence, Dr. Katz says he

Weighing the benefits of PRP

If you are considering PRP treatment, there are four questions you should ask.

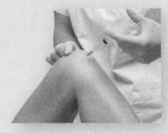

Platelet-rich plasma injections may not be effective for some conditions, including knee and ankle osteoarthritis.

1. Is PRP effective for the condition you want to treat? "The evidence that PRP actually works in osteoarthritis and Achilles tendinitis is not compelling," says Dr. Jeffrey Katz, a professor of orthopedic surgery at Harvard Medical School. PRP appears to be more effective for lateral epicondylitis (tennis elbow). The evidence for other conditions is either limited or conflicting, he says.

2. Is the treatment worth the cost? Most insurance plans don't cover PRP treatment, which can cost $1,000 or more per treatment. Many doctors recommend multiple injections over time, so the cost can add up.

3. What are the risks of treatment? PRP injections are likely safe and don't usually cause side effects, says Dr. Katz. Because it uses your own blood, it's also unlikely to prompt an immune system reaction. Some less common side effects of PRP include skin irritation, bleeding, or infection.

4. Is there a better option? Consider whether another therapy or management strategy might be more effective for your condition.

thinks it's time for doctors to stop using PRP for osteoarthritis and Achilles tendinitis until there is evidence that shows the treatment works. People considering PRP injections for other conditions should do their homework and weigh their options before they move ahead.

The big pain of small-fiber neuropathy

The condition often begins with mild discomfort, but the pain can become debilitating. Here's what you can do about it.

Ever get a sudden tingling or numb feeling in your feet or hands? You often can make it go away with a few good shakes, but if the problem keeps recurring, followed by painful or burning sensations, you may have something called small-fiber neuropathy.

"While not life-threatening, small-fiber neuropathy should always be checked out, as it could be a symptom of something more serious," says Dr. Khosro Farhad, a neuropathy expert at Harvard-affiliated Massachusetts General Hospital.

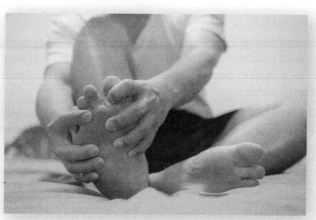

With small-fiber neuropathy, pain and burning sensations usually begin in the feet and hands.

The role of fibers

Small-fiber neuropathy is a type of peripheral neuropathy. Peripheral neuropathy refers to conditions that irritate or damage the nerves that connect our body to the central nervous system—that is, the spinal cord and brain.

These nerves contain both small and large fibers. Small fibers detect pain, heat, and itching sensations in the skin, while large fibers carry the pain signals to the central nervous system and also control muscle movement. In addition to their role in skin sensation, small fibers play a key role in almost all involuntary bodily functions, such as heart rate and blood pressure. They also help regulate body temperature and the proper function of the stomach, intestines, and bladder.

IN THE JOURNALS

Frequent migraines? Eating fatty fish may offer comfort

People who suffer from chronic migraines could find relief by increasing their intake of the omega-3 fatty acids EPA (eicosapentaenoic acid) and DHA (docosahexaenoic acid) found in fatty fish like salmon, herring, sardines, mackerel, and trout. A clinical trial in the July 3, 2021, issue of *The BMJ* looked at 182 people who averaged about 16 headache days per month with attacks lasting more than five hours each. Participants were randomly assigned to one of three diets: One was high in EPA and DHA (1.5 grams total per day) from fish and also high in linoleic acid (an omega-6 fatty acid found in corn and soybean oils and some nuts and seeds). Another diet had high EPA and DHA and low linoleic acid levels. The third was a control diet high in linoleic acid and low in EPA and DHA (only 150 milligrams total per day), a ratio that reflects the average American diet. After 16 weeks, those who consumed the diets high in EPA and DHA had 30% to 40% fewer headache days per month and headache hours per day than people who had a lower intake of these omega-3s. The researchers added that the diets high in EPA and DHA increased blood levels of oxylipin, a byproduct of omega-3s that helps reduce pain and inflammation.

You can experience damage to either type of fiber or both, but small-fiber neuropathy is the more common.

Know the symptoms

Small-fiber neuropathy may initially just cause numbness and tingling, and even itchiness. Symptoms often progresses to an intense burning or stabbing pain. It typically begins in the feet, hands, or both, but it can involve any part of the body. Abnormal signals from small nerve fibers can give skin in the arms and legs a lacy reddish or purplish pattern. Pain tends to be more severe at night or while you are resting.

Small-fiber neuropathy also affects how you feel pain, as you may become more sensitive to pain in general and feel pain you otherwise would not. You also may notice pain concentrated in a small area, like a pinprick.

Less commonly recognized symptoms caused by small-fiber neuropathy include abnormal sweating, dry eyes and mouth, urinary frequency, incontinence, and irregular bowel movements. People with the condition sometimes develop orthostatic hypotension (a sharp drop in blood pressure upon standing), which can cause dizziness or fainting.

Small-fiber neuropathy happens most commonly in people with diabetes. The tingling, numbness, and pain can be the first sign of type 2 diabetes and even pre-diabetes. Other potential causes are

---

ASK THE DOCTOR

by **HOWARD LEWINE, M.D.**

Can dehydration cause headaches?

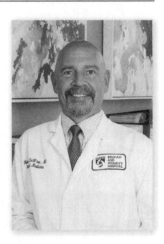

Q *I get occasional headaches. Could it be related to not drinking enough water?*

A Yes, insufficient fluid intake can cause headaches. Some people are much more prone than others to headaches related to dehydration, and people who are more susceptible can avoid the headaches by making sure they drink enough fluids daily. A water-deprivation headache can cause pain throughout the head or be more localized to the front or back. Less often, it is one-sided. The head pain tends to intensify when you bend your head forward or make other head movements. Even walking can make the headache worse.

The exact reason why dehydration causes headaches is unknown. The brain does not have pain receptors. A dehydration headache is possibly triggered by pain receptors in the lining around the brain, called the meninges. When a person is dehydrated, fluid can shift out of the brain, exerting traction on the meninges, which could stimulate the pain receptors. Another possible explanation is the exaggerated response you might feel to any type of pain when you are dehydrated.

A water-deprivation headache should go away within an hour or two after you drink 16 to 32 ounces of water. More prolonged or severe dehydration requires more fluids and lying down for several hours until the pain dissipates. If dehydration is severe and vomiting prevents you from drinking enough to replace the lost fluids, you may need intravenous fluids to relieve the headache. Keep in mind that a migraine attack or any other type of headache can be prolonged if you are not adequately hydrated. Even if you have nausea with a migraine attack, you should try to sip a little fluid every few minutes once your symptoms begin.

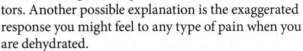

Dehydration can trigger all kinds of head pain.

© Wilson Araújo | Getty Images

Diagnosing the problem

Small-fiber neuropathy is generally underdiagnosed, according to Dr. Khosro Farhad, a neuropathy expert at Harvard-affiliated Massachusetts General Hospital. The problem is that routine neurological exams and tests cannot accurately discriminate between large-fiber and small-fiber neuropathy. "A skin biopsy is a gold standard for diagnosing small-fiber neuropathy; however, this test is not always available," says Dr. Farhad.

vitamin B_6 or B_{12} deficiency, autoimmune disorders like Sjogren's syndrome, an underactive thyroid gland (hypothyroidism), and celiac disease.

Scientists have found that the condition can be associated with mutations in either the SCN9A or SCN10A gene. "These mutations are inherited, which may explain why small-fiber neuropathy tends to run in the family," says Dr. Farhad. Genetic testing can determine if you have these mutations.

Seeking treatment

The best treatment approach is to focus on the root cause. For instance, adopting lifestyle changes like exercising, losing weight, modifying diet, and taking medicines to control blood sugar levels can help prevent and treat small-fiber neuropathy related to

---

IN THE JOURNALS

High-intensity walking may reduce leg pain from artery disease

There are some gains from a bit of pain when it comes to peripheral artery disease (PAD) and walking.

PAD is a circulatory problem in which narrowed arteries reduce blood flow to the limbs and often cause leg pain from walking. Yet, a new study found that a high-intensity walking program that causes some discomfort improves walking performance in people with PAD. The results were reported online April 6, 2021, by *JAMA*.

Researchers recruited 305 people with PAD and divided them randomly into high-intensity or low-intensity exercise groups. A six-minute walking distance measured walking ability. Both exercise groups then followed a program where they were asked to walk up to 50 minutes per day, five days a week, for a year. The high-intensity people walked fast enough during their sessions to cause some short-term moderate to severe pain in their legs during exercise. The low-intensity group always walked at a comfortable pace to avoid any discomfort.

Afterward, when both groups repeated the six-minute walk test, the high-intensity walkers could walk about 38 yards farther than before, while the low-intensity people walked almost seven fewer yards. The participants also underwent treadmill testing at the end of the study. The high-intensity exercisers could walk more than three times as long as the low-intensity group before stopping, primarily because of leg pain. The researchers suggested that higher-intensity walk-

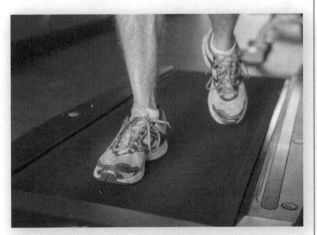

A walking program can improve distance and endurance.

ing might stimulate the formation of new small blood vessels to feed leg muscles deprived of oxygen from arterial blockages higher up.

diabetes, prediabetes, and celiac disease. "However, in about 50% of patients, no cause can be found," says Dr. Farhad.

Symptom relief often requires oral medications, such as duloxetine (Cymbalta), gabapentin (Neurontin), or pregabalin (Lyrica). Unlike drugs that provide immediate relief, these therapies usually take several weeks to produce improvement.

For areas of localized pain, topical skin applications, such as lidocaine patches, gels, or lotions can provide temporary relief. Topical capsaicin is another option, but it can be irritating at first.

Two common shoulder injuries and how to avoid them

These workhorse joints are more vulnerable than you may realize. Protect them now to stay independent.

It doesn't take much to sustain shoulder injuries once we reach our 50s. By then, shoulder muscles and tendons have become weaker, cartilage has worn away, and bones have begun losing density. Two particular categories of shoulder injuries are common among older adults.

Rotator cuff injuries

The rotator cuff—a group of muscles and tendons that stabilize the shoulder and help move your arm—is vulnerable to becoming inflamed or torn.

These injuries often occur when you're lifting a heavy object above your shoulders, such as putting luggage in an overhead bin on a plane or reaching up to trim tree branches. "You're relying a lot on your rotator cuff for motion and strength, but those muscles are very small and not that strong. If you put too much force on them, they can tear," says Dr. Evan O'Donnell, a shoulder surgeon at Harvard-affiliated Massachusetts General Hospital.

Other causes of rotator cuff injury include a bad fall or abnormal areas of bone that pinch tendons as you move your shoulder.

How can you recognize a rotator cuff injury? "Your range of motion will be intact, but you'll feel pain on the outside of the upper arm, especially when using your arm overhead," Dr. O'Donnell says.

He notes that rotator cuff pain is usually worse at night. "That may be because the body releases inflammatory chemicals while you sleep. It could also be

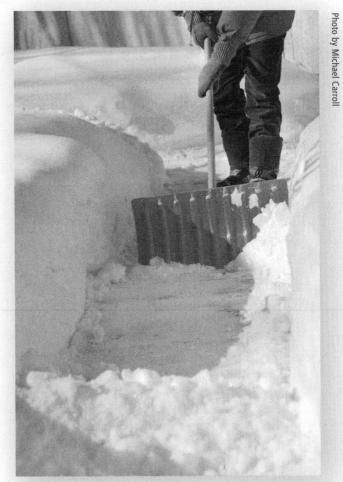

Photo by Michael Carroll

Stretch your shoulders for a few minutes before you put them to work.

because you're sleeping on your shoulder and having a hard time finding a comfortable position," Dr. O'Donnell explains.

Rotator cuff treatment includes corticosteroid injections into the shoulder, anti-inflammatory medications, and physical therapy to stretch and strengthen the shoulder muscles and tendons. "When those therapies aren't enough to manage pain, we can replace the shoulder joint or even take tendons from your back to create a new rotator cuff," Dr. O'Donnell says.

Fractures

The shoulder bones (especially the upper arm bone and collarbone) are two of the bones that are most often fractured (broken) during a fall. These fractures can cause pain, swelling, bruising, a bump at the fracture site, difficulty moving your arm, or grinding sounds as you move your arm.

Many shoulder fractures can be managed without surgery. "The arm is placed in a sling, and you'll have to go through a course of physical therapy to gently stretch and strengthen your shoulder," Dr. O'Donnell says. "The prognosis is excellent. Over three to six months, shoulder pain should decrease and range of motion should increase."

If you suffer a complex fracture, meaning a bone is broken in several places and tissue around the bone is injured, you may need surgery to fix the fracture or replace the shoulder. "It's major surgery and requires physical therapy afterward. But the outcomes are good to excellent. Most people regain their range of motion and are pain-free," Dr. O'Donnell says.

What you can do

The key to warding off shoulder injuries is to keep the joints healthy, strong, and flexible. Many of the

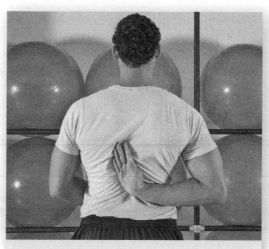

© YinYang | Getty Images

Try this shoulder stretch

Shoulder stretch with internal rotation: Stand up straight with your feet hip-width apart and your hands by your sides. Place the back of your right hand against the small of your back at your waist. Point your fingers up. Slowly slide your right hand farther up your back as high as you can. Stretch to the point of mild tension. Hold for 10 to 20 seconds, then repeat with your other hand.

strategies to do this are the same ones that will reduce fall or fracture risk. Here are some examples.

Weight-bearing activity. Lifting small weights or doing body-weight exercises such as planks or modified push-ups will build both stronger bones and stronger shoulder muscles.

Stretching. A daily stretching routine that includes a warm-up (such as two minutes of marching in place) is important to make muscles long, supple, and better able to react quickly if you lose your balance. Keeping your shoulder muscles and tendons flexible also makes them less likely to tear with activity.

Improving balance. Exercises such as tai chi and yoga require slow, focused movements that challenge and improve balance, reducing fall risk. These practices can also strengthen and stretch shoulder muscles.

Eating a healthy diet. A good diet with colorful vegetables and fruits, legumes, nuts and seeds, some poultry and fish, and some dairy products (like yogurt or cottage cheese) will provide most of the vitamins, minerals, and nutrients to keep your body (including shoulder muscles and bones) healthy.

Getting enough calcium, vitamin D, and protein. These nutrients are especially important for bone health. Women ages 51 or older need 1,200 milligrams (mg) of calcium per day; men 51 or older need 1,000 to 1,200 mg per day, according to the National Academy of Medicine. Adults over 50 need 600 to 800 international units (IU) of vitamin D per day. To calculate daily protein needs in grams, multiply your weight in pounds by 0.36.

The extra mile

These strategies will also help protect your shoulders.

Stretch right before activities. Take a few minutes to stretch before activities requiring shoulder power, like lifting a heavy laundry basket or hanging curtains. "March in place for two minutes to get your blood pumping. Then put your left hand up high on the edge of a wall, and turn your body to the right, so you feel a stretch in your armpit. Then try it on the other side. Now put your left hand lower on the wall, about shoulder height. Turn your body to the right until you feel the stretch in the front of your shoulder, then repeat on the other side," Dr. O'Donnell advises. (Also see "Try this shoulder stretch" on the previous page).

Do an easy shoulder strengthener. "Place your right elbow at your waist, with your forearm in front of you, like you're going to shake hands with someone. Now swing your hand in to your belly, then out as far as you can to your right, then back to your belly, then back to the right. Keep your elbow at your waist the whole time. Do this 10 times, then switch arms. Your shoulder will tire quickly, but you'll be strengthening your rotator cuff muscles," Dr. O'Donnell says.

Reduce fall hazards at home. Eliminating hazards reduces your fall risk. Get rid of floor clutter and throw rugs, make sure hallways are well lit, add grab bars and floor treads to slippery bathrooms, fix broken steps and loose carpeting, and wear shoes with nonslip soles on hard floors.

Avoid lifting heavy objects overhead. If possible, keep those objects at or below your waist. Hug them close (wrap your arms around them), use your legs for power, and stand up straight to reduce strain. Holding heavy objects away from your body and lifting them above your head can tear your rotator cuff.

Are home pain relief gadgets safe for use?

Some make big promises, but may pose big health risks. Here's what to watch for.

Desperate times call for desperate measures. That's how many people feel when they have chronic pain; they'll try anything to get rid of it. For some, the desperate measure is buying a gadget promising to ease aches and pains with the push of a button. If that's your strategy, beware: the move may come with more risks than relief.

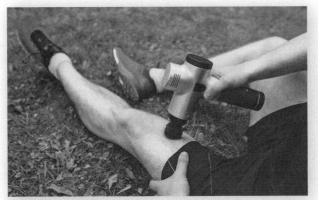

A home massage device might help relieve pain, but talk to your doctor before using it.

These devices often have credible-looking, convincing ads that tout clinical evidence and testimonials from doctors. While there could be something to those claims, don't believe them without doing some digging.

"The problem is there are doctors who will accept money to conduct a small study, and then say a treatment helps, but that's not evidence. The kind of validation that's important is a large study in a well-respected, peer-reviewed medical journal," says Dr. David Binder, a physiatrist and director of innovation at Harvard-affiliated Spaulding Rehabilitation Hospital.

What's out there?

You can find a wide range of pain relief gadgets to use at home. There are devices claiming to interrupt pain signals to the brain with "bio-antennas" embedded in skin patches; squeeze pain away with compression cuffs; or eliminate pain with ultrasound technology, electrical stimulation, heat, lasers, vibration, pressure, light, radiofrequency, infrared rays, or pulsed electromagnetic fields.

What's the risk?

Like any industry, the pain relief industry has some bad actors who prey on vulnerable populations—and that means trouble. Some possible outcomes:

The product doesn't work. No matter how many great testimonials a product receives, it might not work—because it's not right for you or your condition, or simply because it's junk.

You lose a lot of money. Some pain relief gadgets cost hundreds or even thousands of dollars.

Using the product is dangerous. People with particular conditions should avoid some types of devices. For example: "You wouldn't want to put anything with electrical stimulation near a pacemaker. And your doctor needs to weigh in before you use devices that squeeze your legs if you have impaired circulation, swelling of the legs, or a history of blood clots," Dr. Binder says. "If a product uses heat, you could burn yourself if you have nerve damage and can't feel your skin getting hotter."

Using the product keeps you from seeking medical care. "If you buy a pain relief device and skip seeing a doctor about your condition, it might delay an important diagnosis and needed treatment," Dr. Binder points out.

Avoid these

Be suspicious if you see advanced medical technologies in a home pain relief device. For example, Dr. Binder recommends staying away from gadgets that use the following technologies.

Light therapy. Light therapy has many important uses in medicine, but it's not well established for pain relief. "The evidence is weak," Dr. Binder says.

Radiofrequency (RF). For pain relief, doctors sometimes use the heat waves of RF in procedures to dull specific nerves in the spine. "But RF is not a do-it-yourself home treatment," Dr. Binder warns.

Before buying

Talk to your doctor before buying a pain relief gadget. "Print the ad and bring it to an appointment," Dr. Binder advises. "The doctor can assess whether it makes sense, if there's a prescription version of the device that would be safer, or if there's an alternative treatment that would be better."

Another idea: try certain technologies at a physical therapy clinic before buying a home version. One example is transcutaneous electrical nerve stimulation (TENS), which uses tiny electrical shocks on the skin to interrupt pain signals. It doesn't work for everyone.

Also: make sure a high-tech device is FDA-approved (which means it's safe and effective), not just listed or registered with the FDA, which is required of all home health devices. You can look up devices at the FDA database (www.health.harvard.edu/device).

What fills the bill?

A home TENS machine is the only high-tech pain relief device Dr. Binder feels comfortable recommending. "Ask your doctor or physical therapist which voltage is safe for your particular condition," he says.

And don't exclude these low-tech devices, which may also relieve pain:

- a foam roller to stretch out muscles or tight bands of tissue
- massagers such as massage cushions, vests, or handheld devices
- heat or cold packs or skin patches.

You'll find those at any big-box store. They're generally considered safe for use, and they won't break the bank.

Get a helping hand for pain

Hand osteoarthritis can be painful, but there are strategies to help you manage it and maintain function.

Your hands work hard from the moment they pick up your toothbrush in the morning to the time they pull your covers up at night. If you've got osteoarthritis in the joints of your hands, all those daily tasks can become more of a challenge.

Osteoarthritis is a common condition that occurs when the cartilage between the bones begins to break down. Cartilage acts as a smooth padding, cushioning the bones and allowing the joint to move freely. When it deteriorates, the bones may start to rub together, triggering inflammation that causes pain and stiffness.

Osteoarthritis of the hand is not only a common cause of hand pain, but occurs more often in women than in men, says Dr. Barry Simmons, associate professor of orthopedic surgery at Harvard Medical School. The condition also has a strong genetic component. While osteoarthritis in the hands can be debilitating, there are a number of strategies you can use to manage it, he says.

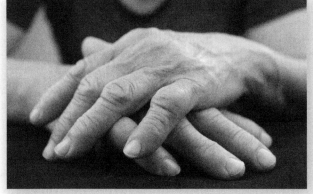

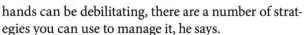
Osteoarthritis can cause stiffness and pain and is often accompanied by swollen joints, bony nodules, and crooked fingers.

The origins of stiffness and pain

Osteoarthritis affecting the hands most commonly occurs in the joints closest to the fingertip, known as the distal interphalangeal joints, says Dr. Simmons. People might notice that the end of their finger looks a little knobby or has started to bend toward the pinky finger. The joint may also feel stiff when you move it.

Other hand joints commonly affected include the proximal interphalangeal joints, which are the joints in the middle of the fingers, and the joint at the base of the thumb, known as the first carpometacarpal joint. Less commonly, the problem occurs in the joint where the finger meets the hand, called the metacarpophalangeal joint, says Dr. Simmons.

While many people are most affected by the pain and stiffness caused by osteoarthritis, some people are also bothered by the physical changes that osteoarthritis may cause. These include the appearance of cysts or bony nodules on the fingers, crooked finger joints, and swelling.

Treating osteoarthritis

The primary goals of osteoarthritis treatment are to relieve pain and improve function, says Dr. Simmons. This may require a combination of approaches, such as the following:

Splinting. Your doctor may recommend immobilizing the joint with a splint. "Splinting is solely for pain relief, but you'll only have pain relief when the splint is on," says Dr. Simmons. Splinting will not correct a joint deformity. The finger will revert back to its former position when the splint is removed.

Ice and heat. Another strategy to soothe sore joints is to use heat or ice. Icing a joint may reduce inflammation and using methods to warm up a joint, such as soaking in warm water, might help ease stiffness.

Medication. Some people effectively manage mild to moderate osteoarthritis pain using topical pain relievers, which come in many forms, including creams, patches, and gels. They are available in both prescription and over-the-counter formulations.

Oral pain medications, particularly non-steroidal anti-inflammatory drugs (NSAIDs) such as ibuprofen (Advil, Motrin) and naproxen (Aleve), can help ease osteoarthritis pain and reduce inflammation. But they will not cure the

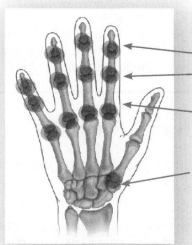

Distal interphalangeal joints

Proximal interphalangeal joints

Metacarpophalangeal joints

First carpometacarpal joint

Osteoarthritis affects four types of joints in the human hand.

underlying problem, says Dr. Simmons.

Injected medications, called corticosteroids, may grant temporary relief. However, many doctors use them sparingly because they may worsen osteoarthritis in the long run, by hastening damage to the bone and cartilage.

Exercise. Building strength and endurance through regular exercise can help reduce hand pain and improve function. Working with a specialist trained in hand therapy can ensure that your efforts are on the right track. A hand therapist will typically help you set goals and design an exercise plan, says Dr. Simmons.

Lifestyle adjustments. A hand therapist may also advise you on ways to change your everyday routines to minimize pain—for instance, by structuring activities to avoid pain flare-ups, or by using tools and assistive devices to ease certain tasks, such as opening jars.

Surgery. Surgery is typically saved as a last resort after other strategies to manage arthritis pain have failed. Options include joint replacement (arthroplasty), which involves removing damaged bone and tissues and replacing them with a prosthetic joint, and joint fusion (arthrodesis) to permanently immobilize the joint.

Typing and tapping despite hand pain

Do stiff hands make it hard to use your smartphone or computer? Try these tips so you can keep using your devices.

Thanks to technology, the world is at your fingertips. All it takes is tapping on a smartphone, typing on a keyboard, or clicking with a mouse. That's not so easy, however, when it irritates underlying conditions, such as tendinitis or arthritis.

"The problem is the repetitive movement of your fingers on a keyboard or reaching and stretching your fingers on a mouse. With a phone, it's the repetitive movement with one hand and sustained grasping with the other hand," explains Eve Kennedy-Spaien, clinical supervisor of the Pain Management, Work Injury, and Integrative Medicine Programs at Harvard-affiliated Spalding Rehabilitation Hospital.

Consider the following strategies when hand pain or stiffness makes computer or smartphone use difficult, and check with your doctor to make sure these tips are right for you.

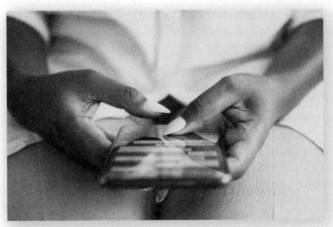

Alternate which hands do the work when using a smartphone or computer.

Distribute the work

Do you have a "hunt and peck" typing style? Do you text only with your thumb? That can lead to overuse injuries. Instead, distribute the work among your fingers and hands. "Alternate which fingers are doing the work," Kennedy-Spaien says. "If you only use a mouse with your right hand, try mousing left-handed. Or switch the hand you use to hold a smartphone."

Take breaks

Using a computer or smartphone is a sedentary activity. It keeps you from being active and restricts blood flow to your hands, which makes them stiffer and harder to move.

To combat it, take scheduled breaks before you feel the need to stop. "By the time your hands are complaining, you've already aggravated them. It takes longer to get the pain and stiffness under control, and you end up needing a longer break," Kennedy-Spaien says. "Take a five-minute break after 45 minutes of activity. Stand up, get a drink of water, or do anything that completely changes your position."

Stretch your wrists and hands

It's important to keep your wrists and hands limber. Stretch them periodically. Start at your wrists, keeping your forearms still and slowly moving your fists in circles. Next, gently open and close your fists, stretching your fingers if you can. "Make sure your fingers are aligned and moving together, and that no finger is going ahead of or lagging behind the others, which can happen when you have arthritis," Kennedy-Spaien advises.

Use heat or cold therapy

Heat and cold therapies have differing uses. Heat is soothing and relaxes muscles. It's helpful before typing or using your phone for an extended period. "It's good for stiffness but not swelling," Kennedy-Spaien says. "Moist heat gets deeper into the tissues and joints. You can get moist heat from warm hand soaks or using microwavable moist heat mittens."

Ice is an anti-inflammatory and a painkiller. "It's best for tendinitis or swollen, hot joints. It helps after you've been using your hands for a long time," Kennedy-Spaien says. Try an ice pack, cold therapy gloves (with gel packs you keep in the freezer), or a hand soak in icy water. Limit therapy sessions to 20 minutes, to avoid hurting your skin.

Avoid awkward hand positions

Holding or moving your hands in unnatural ways can cause pain. For example, maybe you're reaching for the mouse with only your wrist; twisting your wrist as you hold your smartphone; or propping your laptop on your fingers. All of those activities put pressure on the joints and small muscles. "Use your larger muscles—such as your whole arm to move your mouse—and keep weight off of your fingers," suggests Kennedy-Spaien.

Use helpful tools

Go easier on your hands and wrists by using some of the following tools.

"Virtual" assistants or voice-to-text features. Most computers and smartphones have features that allow you to type, text, or carry out commands by simply talking out loud. Don't know how to use them? Search for an instructive video on the Internet or ask a family member for a lesson.

A comfortable mouse. "You should be able to move the mouse without having to grasp it tightly or stretch your fingers out too wide," Kennedy-Spaien notes. Get a mouse that's bigger or smaller to fit you better, or try a vertical mouse that keeps your hand in a handshake position.

A wide-grip stylus. It's easy to hold and saves your fingers from tapping on a smartphone or tablet.

A smartphone holder. "A gooseneck holder enables you to adjust the height and angle," Kennedy-Spaien suggests.

Gel-filled wrist rests. Get them for your keyboard and mouse.

Get a comfy chair. Be sure it has good support and that you sit up straight in it. "The body is a dynamic chain," Kennedy-Spaien says. "When one part isn't in a good position, it affects the rest of the body, including your hands."

5 common foot problems and how to cope with them

Protect your mobility by addressing problems early.

Every day, more than 50 million people in the United States experience some kind of chronic pain, and it often comes from their feet. That's according to a Harvard study published in the February 2022 issue of *Pain*, which also notes how chronic pain limits the ability to work, or socialize, or function in general.

Fortunately, some new approaches along with tried-and-true therapies can reduce foot pain and keep you active. Here are five common foot problems and proven treatments for them.

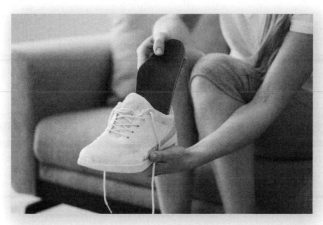

Shoe inserts can help ease the pain of fallen arches and plantar fasciitis.

1. Bunions

A bunion is a deformity at the base of your big toe—a bump formed where two foot bones aren't connecting properly. If it doesn't bother you, there's no need to treat a bunion. If it causes chronic pain, a first step is to wear shoes with roomy toe boxes or a toe sleeve with a cushion so the bunion doesn't rub against the shoe. A toe spacer—a rubber device that sits between the big toe and second toe—can make the toe lie straighter. Surgery to realign the joint is also an option. "We're doing 'keyhole' surgery with thinner tools and incisions that are smaller than ever, just 5 millimeters long. That helps speed recovery," says Dr. Jeremy Smith, a foot and ankle surgeon at Harvard-affiliated Brigham and Women's Hospital and part of Mass General Brigham's Sports Medicine Division.

2. Fallen arches

The arch of your foot can flatten if the main tendon in the foot loses elasticity. That can cause chronic pain in the arch, ankle, and leg when you walk. "Treatments involve supporting the arches with orthotic insoles. And a relatively new approach involves stretching the calf muscles. These muscles can get tight and make the heel bone sit off-center. When the heel bone is off to the side, the foot doesn't sit well in the orthotic," Dr. Smith explains. He recommends stretching the calf muscles a few times per day, and wearing either store-bought or prescription orthotics. "Look for over-the-counter insoles that have a supportive base and a cushion overlay. They're more comfortable than hard plastic orthotics," Dr. Smith says.

3. Hammertoes

A hammertoe looks a little like a claw: a bend in the toe joint makes the tip of the toe angle sharply down.

The bent joint juts upward and hurts when it rubs against the top of your shoe. Dr. Smith says most people can manage this condition without surgery by wearing shoes with roomier toe boxes or silicone toe sleeves that prevent the toe from rubbing against the shoe. When these strategies aren't helping, doctors can stretch the toe with surgery. "We release the soft tissues holding up the toe. Sometimes we need to remove a section of bone, depending on the deformity," Dr. Smith notes. Again, today's smaller surgical instruments require smaller incisions than in the past.

4. Ingrown toenails

An ingrown toenail occurs when a border of the toenail grows into the skin, causing redness, swelling, and lots of pain. It usually occurs in people who can't trim their toenails well anymore because they can't reach or see them. You can prevent it from happening by having a pedicure regularly—yes, even if you are a man. If the ingrown nail isn't infected, soaking it regularly can relieve pain, as can wearing shoes with roomy toe boxes (or sandals). If you can't trim the nail yourself, find a podiatrist to do it. If the toe is red, it may be infected; see your doctor. Treatment may require antibiotic cream and possibly the removal of the nail.

5. Plantar fasciitis

This condition is marked by pronounced heel pain, which can be temporary or long-term. It got its name because doctors used to think the main cause was inflammation (–itis) of the plantar fascia, a thick band of tissue that sits at the bottom of the foot and supports the arch. "It's a misnomer," Dr. Smith says. "The condition usually starts with tiny tears in the plantar fascia where it attaches to the heel bone."

It's typically treated with calf stretching, using heel shoe inserts during the day, and wearing a splint at night to keep the foot at a 90° angle. A corticosteroid injection may offer short-term pain relief. "There's shock-wave therapy, too. It's a fairly new treatment that involves high-frequency 'thumps' to the plantar fascia that may create new blood flow to the area to promote healing," Dr. Smith says. "There are many other treatments out there, but they aren't well supported by evidence."

Who's the right doctor for the job?

"See a podiatrist for ingrown toenails," Dr. Smith says. "For all other conditions, you can see either a podiatrist or a foot and ankle surgeon. We both care for these kinds of problems."

Answers to common questions about shingles

This painful condition is unique in many ways. Our expert explains how it works and how to prevent it.

Shingles is definitely an illness to avoid if you can. Known for its blistering rash, shingles is uncomfortable and sometimes leads to long-lasting complications, including a painful nerve condition called postherpetic neuralgia. While it can affect people of any age, including children, it's

most likely to strike after age 60. Shingles is also somewhat unusual. It's caused by a virus that has often been living inside the body for decades. That means it differs from most viral infections in how you get it and how you can prevent it. We asked Michael Starnbach, a professor of microbiology at Harvard Medical School, to answer some common questions about shingles. Below are his responses.

How do I get the virus that causes shingles?

Shingles is caused by the varicella-zoster virus, which you probably encountered decades ago when you got chickenpox as a child. After your chickenpox infection cleared, the virus stuck around. It took up residence in nerve cell clusters in your spine or at the base of your skull. There it stayed dormant, held in check by your immune system. But it can re-emerge as shingles.

Does everyone who had chickenpox get shingles?

No. Although anyone who has had chickenpox is at

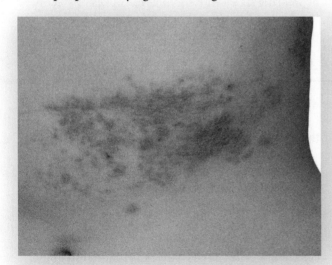

Shingles, which is caused by the varicella-zoster virus, produces a painful rash and may lead to complications.

risk for the condition, only an estimated one in three of those people will actually get shingles. It's not clear why some people get it and others don't. It may have something to do with your immune system. If your immune system is compromised by an illness, surgery, or medication, the virus may be able to shake off its slumber and reactivate. When it does, it typically causes a blistering rash, which often appears as a thick stripe across your ribcage or on the side of your face. It may also bring a painful or burning sensation on the skin, headache, fever, and fatigue.

Is shingles contagious?

Yes and no. If you come in close contact with someone who has shingles, you can't catch shingles. But you can be infected with the varicella-zoster virus and develop chickenpox if you aren't vaccinated against the virus and haven't had chickenpox in the past. If you do develop shingles after you were around someone who had a shingles infection, it came from the virus that was already present inside you, not from the new exposure.

Can a vaccine trigger shingles? My friend got shingles shortly after receiving her COVID-19 vaccine. Is it just a coincidence?

There have been anecdotal Internet reports of shingles following both COVID-19 infection and vaccination for COVID-19. But there isn't sufficient statistical or scientific evidence to show a connection. Just because the two events occur near to each other doesn't mean they are related.

Any medical intervention, even vaccines as safe as the COVID-19 vaccines, can cause health problems in a very small number of individuals. The vaccine manufacturers and U.S. regulatory agencies track these reactions carefully to determine if there is an association between a particular vaccine and an adverse outcome.

Doctors continuously weigh those risks and have uniformly concluded that it is much, much more likely for you to remain healthy if you take the vaccine, despite the super-low risk of an adverse reaction.

Can you get shingles more than once?

Unfortunately, you can. Studies have found that there is approximately a 5% risk of getting a second or a third case of shingles within eight years of your first. This is why doctors recommend that people get

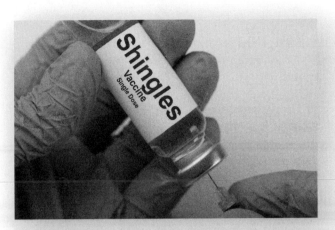

The shingles vaccine, called Shingrix, is 90% effective against shingles and may help prevent complications if you do get it.

the shingles vaccine even if they have already had shingles in the past.

How common are complications from shingles?

A small percentage of people who get shingles experience complications. Approximately 10% to 18% of people develop the nerve pain known as postherpetic neuralgia. About 1% to 4% of people experience other complications that require a hospital stay, such as skin infections or eye-related problems.

Is there a cure for shingles?

No, nothing can cure a shingles attack. However, antiviral medications may help you recover more quickly and reduce your chances of developing complications. These medications, which include acyclovir (Zovirax), famciclovir (Famvir), and valacyclovir (Valtrex), work by blocking the virus's ability to reproduce. When there is less virus present, your immune system has a better chance of getting the reactivation under control.

Be certain to reach out to your doctor quickly if you suspect you have shingles, because these drugs work best if they are started within 72 hours of the start of symptoms.

What is the best way to prevent shingles?

The best way to avoid a painful case of shingles is to get vaccinated. The FDA approved the Shingrix vaccine in October 2017. A few years after Shingrix was approved, an older shingles vaccine called Zostavax was discontinued because it was much less effective.

Shingrix is recommended for adults over age 50 and is given in a series of two injections, six months apart.

Is there anything I can do to help relieve shingles symptoms?

The most bothersome symptoms associated with shingles are typically itching and pain related to the rash. There are a number of strategies that may help. For pain, try

- cool compresses
- an over-the-counter pain reliever, such as ibuprofen (Advil, Motrin) or acetaminophen (Tylenol)
- a topical pain-relieving cream containing capsaicin (such as Zostrix).

If your pain isn't responding to these interventions, your doctor may want to prescribe recommend a topical numbing agent called lidocaine (Xylocaine, others) or use an injected medication in a procedure called an intercostal nerve block.

The best options to help relieve itching are

- soaking in a colloidal oatmeal or starch bath
- applying calamine lotion
- taking an oral or topical antihistamine, such as diphenhydramine (Benadryl). Whenever possible, try to keep your shingles rash clean and covered with sterile bandages to prevent infection.

I already had the Zostavax vaccine. Do I need to get vaccinated with Shingrix?

Yes, it is recommended that you get the Shingrix vaccine even if you already had the older vaccine. The newer vaccine is far more effective. Shingrix is more than 90% effective at preventing a shingles attack. If you are vaccinated and do end up getting shingles, you will likely experience a much milder infection and will be less likely to develop complications.

Does the vaccine have side effects?

Most people who get the shingles vaccine will only experience mild side effects, such as redness or pain at the injection site, fatigue, chills, muscle pain, or stomach upset. While these side effects are temporary, they may be enough to make you feel crummy for a couple of days.

In rare cases, people may experience an allergic reaction to the vaccine. Seek emergency medical attention if you experience hives, swelling in your face or throat, trouble breathing, or dizziness, weakness, or a fast heartbeat.

Are there any lifestyle changes that I can make to prevent shingles?

Keeping yourself and your immune system healthy won't guarantee that you'll never get shingles, but it may reduce your risk. Eating a healthy diet, getting regular exercise, reducing stress, and getting the right amount of sleep at night can keep your immune system functioning well. But keep in mind that immune function naturally tends to decline with age. So, even if you do everything right, you may still get shingles down the line. Getting vaccinated is the best way to reduce your risk.

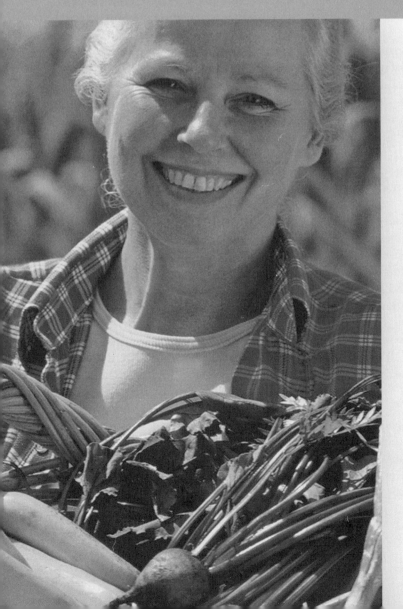

Chapter 7

Cancer Prevention and Early Detection

Take Action!
5 Things You Can Do Now

1 **Skip the soda.** Sugary drinks may increase the risk of colorectal cancer. (page 160)

2 **Examine your nails.** Melanoma can occur there as well as on your skin. (page 164)

3 **Test your home for radon gas.** High levels of this carcinogen may cause lung cancer. (page 166)

4 **Assess your breast cancer risk.** Noncancerous breast diseases may warrant extra vigilance. (page 167)

5 **Add some HIIT workouts.** This kind of exercise might slow prostate cancer growth. (page 171)

Vitamin D and the big C

Research suggests this bone-building nutrient may lower cancer risk, but many older adults still don't get enough.

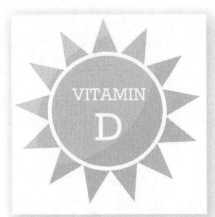

Like school grades, the essential vitamins begin at the front of the alphabet: A, B, and C. Vitamin D? As its letter suggests, many people may view D as one of the lesser ones.

Vitamin D is a fat-soluble vitamin, meaning the body stores what it doesn't use in fatty tissues and the liver. Its main job is to help the body absorb bone-building calcium. But vitamin D could play another significant role in health.

"Vitamin D may reduce chronic inflammation and boost immunity, both of which may lower the risk of some cancers," says Stephanie Smith-Warner, an epidemiologist with Harvard's T.H. Chan School of Public Health.

Finding the link

While research is ongoing, several studies have found a link between blood levels of vitamin D and cancer risk.

For instance, one study published in the February 2019 issue of *The Journal of the National Cancer Institute* looked at the vitamin D levels of 12,000 people. It found that those with inadequate levels, defined as less than 12 nanograms per milliliter (ng/mL), had a greater risk of colorectal cancer compared with those whose levels measured 20 to 25 ng/mL, the lower range of what is considered sufficient for bone health. Additional benefit was seen in people with 30 to 40 ng/mL, levels above what is sufficient. No extra benefit was seen in people with more than 40 ng/mL.

Vitamin D also may help people if they get cancer. A 2020 study called the *Vitamin D and Omega-3 Trial*, or VITAL, found that healthy people who took a daily vitamin D supplement of 2,000 international units (IU) did not have lower rates of cancer overall compared with those who took a placebo. However, among people who later got cancer, those who'd taken the supplements had a 17% lower chance of being diagnosed with metastatic cancer (cancer that spreads from where it began to other parts of the body) or dying from their cancer, compared with those who'd taken a placebo.

While the VITAL study was a randomized trial—meaning it might suggest cause and effect—the earlier study, and similar ones, only show an association, so it's not clear what effect, if any, vitamin D has on cancer prevention and prognosis. Still, it appears there is a higher cancer risk among people with a vitamin D deficiency and amounts higher than the current recommendations may help.

The Dietary Guidelines for Americans 2020–2025 say that adults up to age 70 should get 600 IU daily. Those ages 71 and older should get 800 IU. Yet the guidelines also point out that many people don't get these minimum amounts. The problem may lie in vitamin D's limited sources.

Sunshine and food

The easiest way to get vitamin D is up in the sky. The body manufactures vitamin D when the sun's ultraviolet B (UVB) rays penetrate the skin. But geography, season, time of day, and how much skin is exposed play a big part in how much vitamin D you produce.

However, precautions against skin cancer make many older adults avoid harmful rays through liberal sunscreen application, wide-brimmed hats, and protective clothing. (You still make some vitamin D when wearing sunscreen, as SPF 30 or 50 formulas only block 97% to 98% of UVB rays. You make even more if you apply too little or don't fully cover all exposed skin, but it's still a small amount.)

Few foods are naturally rich in vitamin D. Fatty fish like trout and salmon are the best places to find high amounts of vitamin D. A 3-ounce serving of either offers a robust 570 IU to 645 IU. Perhaps the

Champion D breakfast

A great way to help get your daily vitamin D is with a traditional cereal breakfast. A cup of fortified cereal (preferably whole grain and low sugar) has about 80 IU of vitamin D, depending on the brand. One cup

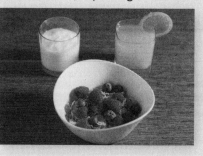

of fortified cow's milk has about 120 IU, while fortified plant-based milks like soy, almond, and oat offer 100 IU to 144 IU. A cup of some fortified orange juice has about 100 IU.

best vitamin D–rich meal is a breakfast featuring cold cereal (see "Champion D breakfast").

Give me a D

Since it can be a challenge to reach your 600 IU to 800 IU via sunlight and diet, you may need a vitamin D supplement, or a multivitamin that contains the RDA for vitamin D. Supplements come in doses of 400 IU, 600 IU, and 1,000 IU or even higher. The National Academy of Medicine considers up to 4,000 IU daily as safe.

A blood test to check your level can help your doctor determine whether you need a supplement and, if so, the appropriate dose. "Focusing on getting at least the minimum daily amount of vitamin D is a good step toward maintaining bone health and may even help prevent cancer development and cancer-related death," says Smith-Warner.

Creating a family medical history

How healthy are your family members? Knowing the answer may help you prevent some chronic diseases.

You've got your father's smile, hazel eyes like your sister, and your grandmother's curly hair. However, while your genes may confer some of your best traits, they can also bring some less-welcome inheritances—namely, a higher risk for certain health conditions.

Your odds for developing heart disease, diabetes, and cancer may be higher than average if these conditions run in your family. By looking for clues in your family's health history, you may be able to identify risks for future illness and perhaps be able to reduce them, says Dr. Jennifer Haas, a professor of medicine at Harvard Medical School. Preventive strategies started early

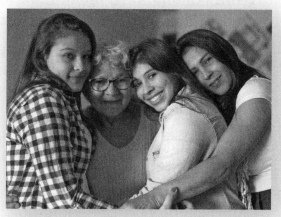

Gathering a family medical history can help you prevent some conditions that have an inherited component.

can reduce your risk.

Gathering important details

When collecting family health information, there are certain items you should prioritize, says Dr. Haas. "It's most important to ask about cancer and chronic diseases," she says. These include diabetes, heart disease, hypertension (high blood pressure), and Alzheimer's disease. These are conditions that have a genetic component, so if others in your family have them, you may be more likely to develop them. Whenever possible, it's also important to get specifics about your relative's condition. For example, if someone in your family had cancer, you'll want to know where in the body the cancer started. "Many types of cancer spread to the liver," says Dr. Haas. But that doesn't mean the person had liver cancer.

Also ask how old they were when they were diagnosed. "It is important to know age of onset. If a condition or cancer started when a family member was young, then an individual may benefit from starting screening or prevention earlier than generally recommended," says Dr. Haas.

Alert your doctor about any illnesses that affect more than one family member and at what ages they were diagnosed, says Dr. Haas.

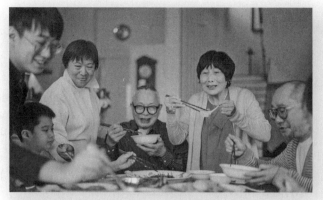

Gatherings provide a good time to talk about your family's medical history.

How to collect the information

When gathering your family medical history, start with immediate family members: your parents, brothers, sisters, and half siblings. From there you can branch out to grandparents, aunts, uncles, cousins, nieces, and nephews. "It is important to realize that it is only blood relatives that share genetic risk, although non-blood-related relatives can share exposures to things like second-hand tobacco smoke, which can also influence risk," says Dr. Haas.

While it's likely fairly easy to identify whom you might want to ask about family history, the challenge often comes in the asking itself. While some family

---

IN THE JOURNALS

Five hours of weekly exercise linked to fewer cancer cases

If you need another reason to get moving, consider this: A study published online Oct. 4, 2021, by the journal *Medicine & Science in Sports & Exercise* suggests that the United States might avoid tens of thousands of cancer cases each year if we all start exercising more. Researchers evaluated the self-reported physical activity of more than half a million U.S. adults, as well as adult cancer cases in every state and the District of Columbia from 2013 to 2016.

Scientists estimated that about 3% of cancer cases per year (about 46,000) could be attributed to inactivity—defined as getting less than 300

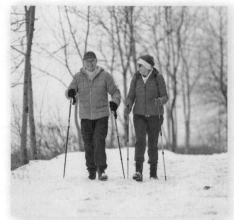

minutes of exercise per week. Rates of cancers of the stomach, uterus, colon, esophagus, breast, and bladder all were lower among more physically active people, particularly those who did at least 300 minutes per week of moderate-intensity activity, such as brisk walking. That works out to about 43 minutes per day.

Because this is an observational study, it doesn't prove that increasing your physical activity will reduce your risk of cancer. But there is strong evidence that this level of activity also is associated with a lower risk of heart disease, stroke, diabetes, dementia—and possibly many common types of cancer.

Tools and tips for gathering your family health history

There are a number of tools and strategies that can help you pull together a comprehensive family medical history. The U.S. Surgeon General created "My Family Portrait," (https://phgkb.cdc.gov/FHH), which is an online resource designed to help you create a family health history. It can become an ongoing library for your family. "The nice thing about it is that people can all orient the information to themselves. So, everyone's tree is different, but they can share information with others," says Dr. Jennifer Haas, a professor of medicine at Harvard Medical School. "This might be helpful if people are hesitant to disclose their information."

Another option is using a medical history binder that family members can contribute to and share. This can be done on paper or electronically using a Google document, says Dr. Haas. These tools may also be used to help you to track who is biologically related and how closely—for example, half siblings versus full siblings, she says.

If you're adopted, have a small family, or don't have access to your biological relatives, there are still ways to get a glimpse into your genetics. "Consider using a DNA testing kit to look for common genetic disease markers or to connect with biological family," says Dr. Haas. However, keep in mind that these decisions can be complicated and should be considered carefully, she says.

members might be open and willing to disclose personal information, others may view a request like this as highly intrusive. Approach the issue with sensitivity, and respect people's differences.

Below are some tips that can help ease the process.

Use gatherings as an opportunity. Family gatherings around the holidays can offer a good opportunity to broach the subject, because everyone is in one place at the same time.

Choose a designee. Assigning a point person to collect the information can be a helpful approach. "Families often have a person who is the 'historian,' which is a good place to start," says Dr. Haas.

Try different methods. People should decide whether the best approach is to speak with the family as a group or individually. Some people may be more honest one-on-one, says Dr. Haas. "Every family is different," she says.

Also, consider whether you should approach people in person, or if it's better to call on the phone or send an email. Your strategy may vary based on the individual. Some people might prefer a face-to-face-conversation, while others would rather talk on the phone or send the information in an email or using an online form.

Be clear. Always explain why you are asking. If people understand that the information may benefit others in the family, they may be more willing to share, says Dr. Haas. It may also help if you explain that you will share health information from others with them, so that they can better assess their own risks.

Protect personal privacy. Ask permission to share someone's health history with other family members. Respect each person's privacy unless you have explicitly discussed sharing the information.

Home screening options for colorectal cancer

Tests are quick and easy, without any prep required. But the tests aren't for everyone.

Among the many things the pandemic has taught us, it's that we can do more from home when it comes to our medical care—whether it's getting a check-up via video or phone call (telemedicine) or sending blood pressure measurements to doctors electronically.

For some people, it's also meant trying an at-home screening test for colorectal cancer. These tests have been approved for years but are often passed over in favor of colonoscopies (see "The gold standard in colorectal cancer screening" on the next page).

Even now, there's still a backlog for colonoscopies because so many people had to cancel their appointments during the pandemic. "We'll never catch up with all the colonoscopies that have to be done. So for people at average risk of colorectal cancer, it's reasonable to use an alternative screening method," notes gastroenterologist Dr. Lawrence S. Friedman, a Harvard

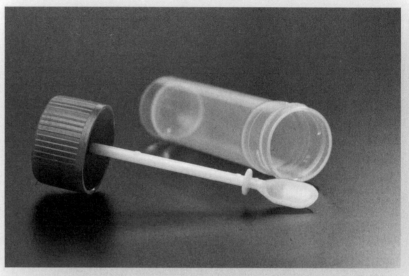

You use a wand like this one to collect a small stool sample for a fecal immunochemical test.

© luchschen | Getty Images

Medical School professor and the Anton R. Fried, M.D., Chair of the Department of Medicine at Newton-Wellesley Hospital.

On the other hand, people who have symptoms

IN THE JOURNALS

New recommendation: Earlier colorectal cancer screening

In a major guideline update, the U.S. Preventive Services Task Force (USPSTF) now endorses screening for colorectal cancer starting at age 45 rather than 50. But the change comes with a caveat: the evidence for benefits from screening at age 45 isn't as strong as it is for ages 50 to 75. The guideline update, published May 18, 2021, in *JAMA*, is the first in five years and brings the USPSTF's advice in line with the American Cancer Society's 2016 call to begin screening at 45.

What if you're older than 75? The USPSTF found no strong evidence of benefit to screening after age 75, especially if earlier tests found no cancer. And a separate study by Harvard researchers, published online May 20, 2021, by *JAMA Oncology*, found that a large group of health care professionals who underwent screening colonoscopy after age 75 were somewhat less likely to develop colorectal cancer or die from it. So if you're 75 or older, and otherwise healthy and free of major chronic illnesses, it's not unreasonable to continue screening.

that could be caused by colorectal cancer, or who are at increased risk for it—because colorectal cancer runs in their family or because they have conditions such as inflammatory bowel disease—should still have regular colonoscopies.

What are the tests?

An at-home screening test is a kit that allows you to collect a stool sample in the privacy of your home. The collection process is quick and easy, and it requires no bowel preparation.

The stool sample is sent to either your doctor's office or a lab. There, it's analyzed for signs of colorectal cancer, such as microscopic amounts of blood (which can come from tumors or precancerous growths called polyps) or DNA from cancer cells.

Three types of at-home screening tests are recommended by the U.S. Preventive Services Task Force:

A guaiac fecal occult blood test (gFOBT) uses chemicals to find blood in the stool. This test must be done once a year.

A fecal immunochemical test (FIT) uses antibodies to detect blood in stool. It must be done once a year.

A multitarget stool DNA (mt-sDNA) test (Cologuard), also known as a FIT-DNA test, can identify DNA from cancer cells in the stool and has a FIT component to look for blood. This test must be done every three years.

Costs and availability

Your doctor typically prescribes an at-home screening test, and Medicare pays for it if you don't have any symptoms of colorectal cancer.

People who don't have a doctor can go online and order a FIT-DNA test (at www.cologuard.com), and the test maker will arrange for a telemedicine visit with a physician who will evaluate you and then can prescribe the test. But you'll probably have to pay for the telemedicine visit.

You can buy some gFOBT or FIT tests online or over the counter for $10 to $25, but these tests may not be as accurate as the kinds prescribed by a

physician. In any case, you should discuss your test results with a doctor.

Test accuracy

At-home screening tests differ in their ability to detect colorectal cancer. "The FIT-DNA is the most sensitive. It finds cancer, when present, about 92% of the time. FIT tests find cancer 80% to 82% of the time," Dr. Friedman says. "The gFOBT test is less sensitive, identifying between 20% and 50% of cancers, and has fallen by the wayside."

Sometimes at-home test results are falsely positive, responding to bleeding from other types of polyps or abnormalities in blood vessels. That can happen about 14% of the time with FIT-DNA tests and about 5% of the time with FIT tests. "But remember that at-home tests suggest you might have colorectal cancer. To diagnose the cancer requires a colonoscopy," Dr. Friedman says.

What happens next?

If you have a positive at-home test result, you'll need to see a gastroenterologist for a follow-up colonoscopy to locate and remove tumors or precancerous polyps. If you have a negative at-home test result,

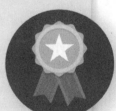

The gold standard in colorectal cancer screening

The most comprehensive colorectal cancer screening test is a colonoscopy—a procedure that enables the doctor to examine the inside of your colon and to snip out suspicious growths.

Before the procedure, you drink liquids that help you clean out your colon so the doctor can see everything. The doctor then passes a long, flexible tube into your colon; the tube carries a tiny video camera and surgical instruments.

The process is lengthy and sometimes unpleasant, but it's worth it. "Colonoscopy is the most sensitive test available for identifying colon cancer; it detects at least 95% of cancers. And when you remove a potentially precancerous polyp, you're preventing a future cancer," explains gastroenterologist and Harvard Medical School professor Dr. Lawrence S. Friedman.

A screening colonoscopy is recommended at age 45, and every 10 years thereafter if no polyps are found (until age 75), or more often if there's an increased risk of colorectal cancer.

you should (as always) continue to watch for potential signs of colon cancer, such as:

- a feeling that the bowel isn't emptying completely
- blood in the stool
- stools that are narrower than usual
- frequently feeling full or bloated
- weight loss with no known reason.

"If you develop any of those symptoms, you may need a colonoscopy for evaluation," Dr. Friedman says. "If you don't have any symptoms, and you're at average risk for colorectal cancer, you'll still need to keep up with at-home testing every one to three years."

Colorectal cancer can be cured if it is caught early with a screening test. But don't put off a screening because you're not sure which one to get. As Dr. Friedman puts it, "The best screening test is the one that gets done."

Can your diet protect against cancer?

Yes, but it's not clear which specific foods are most important.

Evidence has increasingly shown that following a plant-based eating pattern, such as a vegetarian, vegan, Mediterranean, or DASH (Dietary Approaches to Stop Hypertension) diet, helps manage cholesterol and lower the risk for heart disease, the No. 1 cause of death in America. These diets emphasize fruits, vegetables, whole grains, legumes, and low-fat dairy products, with no (or minimal) red meat, processed foods, and alcohol.

But what about cancer, the No. 2 cause of death?

Can this dietary approach also protect you from cancer, or even slow its progression? The short answer is yes, but it's unrealistic to think that one type of diet could reduce cancer risk across the board.

"Linking diet with cancer prevention is like putting together a jigsaw puzzle without all the pieces and the picture on the box," says Theresa Fung, an adjunct professor of nutrition at Harvard's T.H. Chan School of Public Health. "You can develop a sense of what the final image might be, but it remains

---

IN THE JOURNALS

Drinking sugary beverages associated with colon cancer risk

Could sugary drinks be behind the recent increase in early-onset colorectal cancer cases? A study published online May 6, 2021, by the journal *Gut* hints that it might. Researchers examined the dietary patterns of 95,464 nurses who participated in the Nurses' Health Study II from 1991 to 2015. They also asked some 41,000 of the women about their diet as teens (ages 13 to 18). In total, 109 participants went on to develop colorectal cancer before age 50, which is considered early.

The researchers found that adult women who reported drinking two sugar-sweetened drinks a day had more than double the colorectal cancer risk as women who drank less than one sweetened drink per week. The researchers also found for each sweet drink per day that the women drank as teens, they had a 32% higher risk for early-onset colorectal cancer as adults. The researchers speculated that the recent rise in the number of colorectal cancer cases diagnosed before age 50 is connected to an increase in sugary drink consumption—particularly among young adults.

The American Cancer Society now recommends that colorectal cancer screening begin at age 45 instead of age 50, and possibly earlier in people with a family history of the disease. Experts say that these findings should give you another reason to reach for unsweetened options such as water, seltzer, coffee, or tea instead of soda or other sugary beverages.

incomplete and somewhat frustrating."

Why proof is challenging

One of the main reasons for the ambiguity is that diets don't lend themselves to clinical trials, the best types of studies. So, most nutritional research consists of observational studies that show associations but not cause and effect. Take blueberries, for example. Blueberries are high in antioxidants and some research shows a link between eating foods rich in these substances and reduced cancer risk, possibly because antioxidants can dampen inflammation and protect against damage to cell DNA.

But this doesn't mean eating a lot of blueberries will protect you from cancer. "The problem with association studies like this is that you can't say for certain whether blueberries are the cancer fighter, or if it's one of its nutrients, or some other factors," says Fung.

Some studies have shown cruciferous vegetables like broccoli, cauliflower, brussels sprouts, and kale have a cancer-blocking effect similar to fruit. But here scientists have cited the vegetables' high amounts of glucosinolates (sulfur-containing compounds). Still

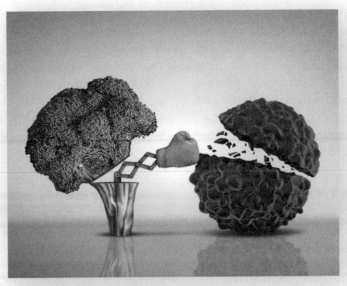

Many fruits and vegetables possess cancer-fighting abilities.

others have touted the phytochemicals in fruits, vegetables, and grains for their ability to protect cells from damage.

A study in the December 2020 issue of *Nutrients* reviewed 54 studies and found a link between eating whole grains and a lower risk of cancers like those of the colon, pancreas, and esophagus. The reason? Scientists believe the high fiber in whole grains dilutes possible carcinogens (substances that cause cancer) and speeds up digestion so smaller amounts can be absorbed by the body.

Then there is the issue of serving sizes. How much is enough? Again, it's up for debate. "Observational studies highlight different ranges but don't provide solid information on specific amounts and servings," says Fung.

Keep eating simple

What does all this mean? Your diet definitely can help with cancer prevention, but Fung says people shouldn't obsess about eating certain foods or specific amounts. Instead, embrace an overall healthy

---

IN THE JOURNALS

Supplements to prevent heart disease and cancer not justified

The U.S. Preventive Services Task Force (USPSTF) recently announced that there was insufficient evidence for using most vitamin and mineral supplements to prevent heart disease and cancer in most healthy adults. In a stronger position, the task force also recommended against using vitamin E or beta carotene to prevent heart disease or cancer, noting that

in high-risk people, like smokers, these supplements could increase the risks of developing lung cancer and of dying from heart disease or stroke. However, people with nutritional deficiencies or requirements may benefit from specific vitamins and supplements and should speak with a doctor. The USPSTF based its suggestions on a review of 78 studies.

diet that includes a variety of fruits and vegetables.

"Follow a Mediterranean or DASH diet or similar plant-based eating plan if you want more structure," she says. "Otherwise, keep it simple."

Focus on consuming various fruits and vegetables every day, along with legumes (beans, peas, peanuts) and whole grains (oatmeal, popcorn, whole-wheat bread, brown rice).

Also, cut down (or cut out entirely) red meat, processed foods, and sugar-sweetened beverages. A recent study in *JNCI Cancer Spectrum* found that consuming these foods was associated with higher risks of various cancers. "If you are eating a lot of unhealthy foods, that probably means you are eating too few healthy ones, and vice versa," says Fung.

Back to the doctor

If you're not up to date on your medical appointments, these are the experts to see and screenings you may need.

If you've skipped doctor visits or health screenings due to the pandemic, it may be time to start catching up—and the sooner you make an appointment, the better. "We've been overwhelmed with people who want to come back," says Dr. Suzanne Salamon, associate chief of gerontology at Harvard-affiliated Beth Israel Deaconess Medical Center.

Need to see your doctor before the first available appointment? It may be possible to get a telehealth visit via video or phone call. Or you can ask to be placed on a waiting list for an in-person appointment, in case a cancellation opens a spot.

Which experts should you see?

If you have chronic medical conditions, you may have been in touch with your doctors during the pandemic. Even if you have no chronic medical conditions, your health needs to be monitored. Start with these three health care professionals.

A primary care doctor. Get a regular check-up, so all aspects of your health can be evaluated.

A dental hygienist. Get your teeth cleaned. You need two cleanings a year, or more if you have gum disease.

An eye doctor. Get a comprehensive dilated eye exam. The American Academy of Ophthalmology recommends this exam every one or two years if you're 65 or older, every one to three years if you're age 55 to 64, and every two to four years if you're 40 to 54—more frequently if you're at increased risk for eye conditions. "As you get older, your risk increases

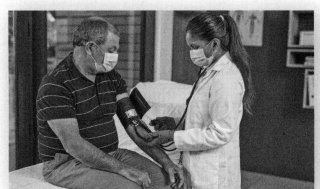

Has your blood pressure changed since your last visit? Your doctor will want to find out.

for glaucoma, which is a common cause of vision loss," Dr. Salamon says.

What to anticipate

If it's been a while, your primary care doctor will have the most questions for you, based on the following aspects of health.

Blood pressure. Has your blood pressure increased in the last year? If so, that could raise your risk for a heart attack or stroke. Has your blood pressure dropped too much? That could increase your fall risk. Your doctor will try to identify what's causing the change and offer treatment to reduce the risks.

Medication changes. Have you started or stopped taking any medications since you last saw your primary care physician? "I'll want to make sure there aren't any potential interactions with your other drugs," Dr. Salamon says.

Weight. Dr. Salamon says she's seen some people who've lost weight since the pandemic started because they've been eating less restaurant food. But she's also seen people who've gained 10 or 15 pounds. "Weight gain is a very strong risk factor for higher blood pressure and diabetes, so we'll talk about why someone gained weight and how to get back into a healthy routine," she says.

Alcohol intake. Be honest if you've been drinking more since your last check-up. Your doctor needs to know, since excessive drinking (more than one drink per day for women and more than one or two drinks per day for men) is associated with an increased risk for many health issues, such as heart problems, stroke, cancer, sleep difficulty, weight gain, depression, and high blood pressure.

Balance and gait. "I'll ask if someone has had any minor falls. Maybe the person needs physical therapy to work on balance, or maybe falls are being caused by medication or an underlying condition," Dr. Salamon points out.

Memory. Have you experienced memory or cognition problems since you last saw your doctor? "I can do a screening and, if necessary, send someone for cognitive testing," Dr. Salamon says. "If I find other neurological problems, I may order an MRI or CT scan to make sure the person hasn't had a stroke and doesn't have a tumor."

Hearing. Hearing loss is associated with isolation, depression, and dementia. Tell your doctor if you've noticed changes in hearing, and ask if you need to see an audiologist for a hearing test.

Mood. "A lot of people have been depressed throughout the pandemic, and it helps to be able to talk about it. You might not need medication. There are pill-free ways to improve mood," Dr. Salamon says.

Exercise. Have you been exercising enough in the past year? Harvard research suggests we need 4,400 to 7,500 steps per day to ward off chronic disease and early death. "Exercising also keeps your legs stronger, making it less likely you'll fall," Dr. Salamon says.

Socialization. "We want to prevent isolation and the health problems it can trigger," Dr. Salamon says. "I'll want to know if someone is in touch with people, especially if they live alone and don't get out of the house. I may recommend taking free classes at senior centers to learn how to use technology for video calls and social media."

Getting blood work

Your doctor will likely order basic blood work if you haven't had any since before the pandemic. "In particular, I'll look at blood sugar levels to check diabetes risk, and creatinine levels to make sure your kidneys are functioning properly," Dr. Salamon says.

Your doctor will also want to see if any new medications are affecting levels of certain minerals in the body called electrolytes. For example, some antidepressants can lower sodium levels, and certain heart medications can raise or lower potassium levels.

Screenings

Your doctor will want to know if you've missed any health screenings. Ask if it's time to screen for

- breast cancer (mammogram)
- cervical cancer (Pap test)
- colorectal cancer (colonoscopy or stool-based test)
- lung cancer (low-dose lung CT for smokers or former heavy smokers)
- osteoporosis (bone density scan)
- prostate cancer (PSA test).

Your need for a screening depends on your age, your risks, and the last time you had the test.

Vaccinations

In-person visits to the doctor's office for routine vaccinations, such as for tetanus or pneumonia, were often postponed during the pandemic. And some people hesitated to get the COVID-19 vaccine, "which is extremely effective and safe, even in people with suppressed immunity," Dr. Salamon says. She also emphasizes the importance of flu and shingles vaccinations. "Shingles is so much more common as you get older, and it can cause pain that doesn't go away," Dr. Salamon notes.

Preparing for the visit

Before the doctor visit, write down questions you have and health changes you've noticed. Bring the notes to your appointment, along with a list of your medications, and some paper and a pen to jot down answers. "And make sure you understand the doctor's instructions before you leave," Dr. Salamon says. "We want to keep you as healthy as possible in between visits."

7 strategies to prevent cancer

Lifestyle changes could prevent more than 40% of malignancies.

Even if you have a family history of cancer, you're not powerless against the disease. Roughly 40% of cancers are preventable through lifestyle changes, says Dr. JoAnn Manson, the Michael and Lee Bell Professor of Women's Health at Harvard Medical School. "Heredity is usually not destiny," she says.

In fact, there are several approaches that can decrease your cancer risk over the course of your lifetime. Some of them are easy, such as getting recommended health screenings. Others may be a little more challenging—for example, maintaining a healthy body weight, squeezing in regular workouts, or changing your diet. But even making small inroads on the strategies below can help protect your health over the long term.

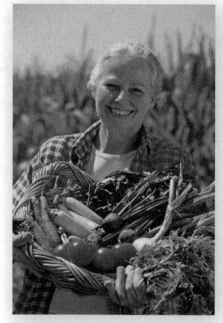

The right diet and other healthy habits can help ward off cancer.

Improve your diet
Reduce your risk for a variety of cancers by eating a diet that is largely plant-based, low in red and processed meats, and low in added sugars, says Dr. Manson. Two examples are the Mediterranean diet and the DASH diet, she says. Both emphasize healthy unsaturated fats, whole grains, fruits and veggies, and nuts and beans, and both are low in processed foods.

Watch what you drink
"Another aspect of diet that people often don't pay much attention to is minimizing alcohol intake," says Dr. Manson. Research has linked alcohol consumption to numerous cancers—particularly in heavy users. But even those who have less than a drink or two daily aren't in the clear. "Recent reports suggest that even modest or moderate alcohol intake is associated with an increased risk of certain cancers, including esophageal cancer, breast cancer, and colorectal cancer," says Dr. Manson. If you enjoy a daily drink, it may be tough to give up. But cutting back on your intake is definitely something to consider. "A drink once or twice a month isn't likely to affect your cancer risk, but more than a couple of drinks per week could," says Dr. Manson.

Get recommended cancer screenings
While some tests, such as mammograms, are

IN THE JOURNALS

Inspect your nails for melanoma

The American Academy of Dermatology (AAD) is encouraging people to examine not only their skin but also their nails for signs of cancer. Melanoma can develop under and around the fingernails and toenails. It often appears on the thumb or big toe of your dominant hand or foot, according to the AAD. Signs of melanoma in and around the nails include a brown or black streak under the nail, a bump or nodule under the nail, darker skin around the nail, a nail that is lifting and pulling away from the nail bed, or a split down the middle of the nail. Melanoma becomes more common as people age and is highly treatable if detected early.

designed to find cancers early when they are most treatable, some screening tests can actually prevent cancer altogether. For example, a colonoscopy can find precancerous polyps and remove them before they do any harm. The same is true of the Pap and HPV (human papillomavirus) tests, which can detect abnormalities before they become cancers in the cervix and vagina.

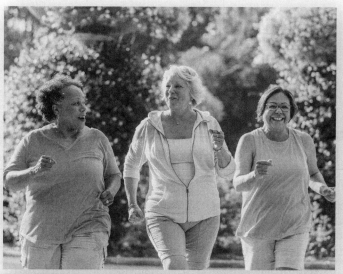

Regular exercise is a tried-and-true cancer prevention strategy that you can use to reduce your risk.

don't respond well to insulin (the hormone that helps your body turn glucose into energy). This malfunction causes your blood sugar and insulin levels to rise, which can promote tumor growth. Obesity also causes chronic inflammation in the body and raises the circulating levels of estrogen and other sex hormones; these changes make certain cancers more likely to occur.

Also make sure you have had a blood test to screen for hepatitis C, which the U.S. Preventive Services Task Force now recommends for all adults ages 18 to 79. Untreated, this viral infection can lead to liver disease and liver cancer.

Maintain a healthy body weight

Obesity is linked to a dozen or more malignancies, from postmenopausal breast cancer to ovarian, endometrial, and kidney cancer. Obesity increases risk through several pathways. It's associated with insulin resistance, a condition where your cells

Exercise regularly

Regular physical activity can reduce cancer risk through several mechanisms, according to Dr. Manson. First, it helps with weight control. Exercise can also moderate levels of sex hormones and inflammation, which may drive certain malignancies. Finally, physical activity is important for stress management. Hormones produced by the body's stress response may increase your vulnerability to cancer. Aim for 150 to 300 minutes of moderate-intensity exercise or 75 to 150 minutes of vigorous exercise each week.

IN THE JOURNALS

Are women being over-diagnosed with thyroid cancer?

Women are four times more likely than men to be diagnosed with thyroid cancer during their lives. But a study published online Aug. 30, 2021, by *JAMA Internal Medicine* found most of the cancers found in women were not the dangerous kind. And autopsy results actually show that men experience these small papillary thyroid tumors at the same rate as women, they are just found less often in men during life, said the study's authors.

In fact, for both men and women, the aggressive and harmful types of thyroid cancer occur equally as often in both sexes. The study authors said it's likely that some women are consequently being overtreated for small papillary thyroid cancers that might never pose any harm to their health. However, when a woman or man has a thyroid nodule, it's still important that it be investigated to be sure it is not one that needs immediate treatment.

Get adequate sleep

Insufficient or poor-quality sleep is associated with obesity and diabetes. Both conditions, in turn, raise your risk for cancer. In addition to this indirect link, some research has found that poor sleep may independently boost cancer risk, says Dr. Manson. Strive for seven or eight hours of good-quality sleep a night. Getting regular exercise can help you sleep more soundly.

Avoid environmental hazards

When possible, cut down on your exposure to potentially harmful chemicals. Some that can raise your cancer risk may be lurking in plastics and in beauty products. Several chemicals in plastics, including bisphenol A and phthalates, are worrisome because there is some evidence that long-term exposure is harmful. Decrease risk by avoiding heating foods in plastic containers in the microwave and avoiding food that is packaged in plastic if another option is available.

Shop carefully for beauty treatments by reading labels to avoid problematic chemicals. Organizations such as the nonprofit Environmental Working Group (www.ewg.org) offer guidance on which chemicals to avoid.

Is there an invisible cancer risk in your home?

A lung cancer threat may be lurking in your home. Radon is a colorless, odorless gas that enters homes from the soil and rocks beneath. Chronic radon exposure is the second leading cause of lung cancer in the United States, next to cigarette smoking. High radon levels (defined as 4 picocuries per liter or higher) are found in one in every 15 homes, according to the American Cancer Society. You can buy a simple test kit at your local hardware store that can tell you if your home is one of them. If testing reveals elevated radon levels, consult an expert who can help you fix the problem by sealing cracks that allow radon to enter or improve ventilation to keep gas levels low.

Also, pare down the number of products you use daily to reduce unneeded exposure. However, keep in mind that while environmental risks may add up over time, the actual cancer risk from these items is minimal. "Don't become preoccupied over what is likely a very small risk compared with the risk of having a really unhealthy diet and being sedentary," says Dr. Manson.

Get vaccinated against cancer

A few vaccines can help protect you from cancer. One is the shot for hepatitis B, a viral liver infection that can cause liver disease and liver cancer. Some people who contract hepatitis B will get sick for a few weeks and then recover. But for others, the infection is persistent, creating long-term health risks. Health care workers are at particular risk of infection. If you have teens or young adults in your life, they should also consider the HPV vaccine, which protects against several cancers caused by the human papillomavirus, including cervical, vaginal, anal, penile, and vulvar cancers, as well as others that affect the head and neck.

If it's not breast cancer, should you worry?

Noncancerous findings on a mammogram are common. Most of the time it's no cause for concern, but some benign breast diseases do increase the risk for cancer.

You found a lump in your breast, and your doctor recommended a biopsy to rule out cancer. Statistically speaking, chances are very good that it's not cancer. Some 80% of breast biopsies are negative. But sometimes what the biopsy reveals is a benign breast disease, such as a cluster of noncancerous cells growing abnormally in the breast. You may wonder what that means and whether it will put you at higher risk for breast cancer down the line.

Most of the time the answer is no. But it depends on what type of benign condition you have. Most noncancerous conditions, such as fluid-filled cysts or fibrocystic breast changes (thickened areas of breast tissue that may be hormonally driven), don't raise breast cancer risk at all. However, other, less common benign breast conditions warrant a little more attention.

"It's important to discuss results of your mammogram with your doctor, even when it shows a finding that's likely benign. Your history and other risk factors need to be taken into account, and you and your physician can decide together what the best follow-up plan is," says Dr. Toni Golen, an obstetrician and

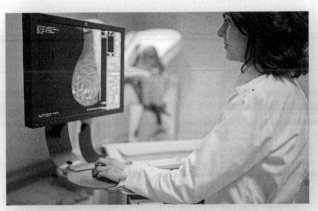

Most breast lumps that show up on a mammogram are not cancerous, but some may require a little extra vigilance.

gynecologist at Harvard-affiliated Beth Israel Deaconess Medical Center and editor in chief of *Harvard Women's Health Watch*.

Proliferative lesions

The benign breast conditions that concern doctors most are areas of growth called proliferative lesions. "Proliferative lesions are an indicator that you are on a

IN THE JOURNALS

Cancer report shows a mixed bag

Women are being diagnosed with cancer at a higher rate than in the past—but death rates for women with the disease are down, says a report published July 8, 2021, in *JNCI: The Journal of the National Cancer Institute*. Researchers came to these conclusions looking at population-based data obtained from national registries and data banks.

They found several noteworthy trends among women when looking at cancer incidence and death over a five-year period (2013 to 2017 for incidence and 2014 to 2018 for mortality): Death rates decreased for 14 of the 20 most common

cancers in women, but increased for five types (uterus, liver, brain/nervous system, pancreas, and soft tissue, including the heart) and remained stable for one type (oral cavity/pharynx).

The death rates for lung cancer and melanoma saw the largest decreases. Breast cancer death rates continued to drop, but at a slower rate than in the past. Overall cancer death rates decreased in every racial and ethnic group from 2014 to 2018. Cancer incidence was slightly lower among Black people than whites; however, cancer death rates were higher among Black people when compared with whites.

pathway to increased breast cancer risk," says Dr. Graham Colditz, an epidemiologist and adjunct professor at the Harvard T.H. Chan School of Public Health.

These lesions may contain cells that grow more rapidly than normal ones, and as these cells divide and multiply, it increases the chance that they will become cancerous, says Dr. Golen. One of the most common types of proliferative lesions is an overgrowth of cells, known as hyperplasia. It can occur in the milk ducts, which transport milk to the nipple, or in milk glands inside the breast.

Hyperplasia is divided into two categories, simple or atypical, says Dr. Golen. Simple hyperplasia is marked by abnormal growth of cells, but the cells themselves look normal under a microscope. It can raise your risk for breast cancer, but is less of a risk factor than atypical hyperplasia. In people with atypical hyperplasia, the growing cells don't look perfectly normal when examined under a microscope, even though they aren't so abnormal as to be considered cancer.

There are a few other types of noncancerous proliferative findings that may increase your breast cancer risk.

Complex fibroadenomas. These are a small subset of the most common type of benign breast tumor, called a fibroadenoma. The vast majority of fibroadenomas don't raise breast cancer risk, but complex fibroadenomas might elevate your risk slightly.

Sclerosing adenosis. This condition is marked by an enlargement of milk-producing sacs in the breast.

Radial scars. These growths are named for their shape, which takes the appearance of a scar. They may slightly elevate your breast cancer risk.

Intraductal papillomas. These small growths inside the milk ducts are most often considered harmless, but may be more of a concern if they contain abnormal cells or if there are numerous growths, typically five or more.

If you do have a benign breast condition that is known to raise your risk of breast cancer, your doctor may want you to undergo more frequent breast screenings using traditional mammography. She may also recommend MRI or ultrasound scans of your breasts. These are typically done in addition to your mammogram.

Depending on your family history and other factors, your doctor may recommend additional preventive strategies as well. says Dr. Golen. However, it's important to note that just because you have one of these conditions doesn't mean you're going to develop breast cancer. Most women with these conditions do not. "Even if you have atypical hyperplasia, the chance of developing breast cancer is relatively small," says Dr. Golen.

IN THE JOURNALS

Adding ultrasound to mammography improves cancer detection rate

A combination of mammography and breast ultrasound might improve breast cancer detection in women being screened for the disease. A study published online Aug. 18, 2021, by *JAMA Network Open* found that the combination of technologies performed better than mammography alone.

Researchers analyzed data from a trial conducted in Japan from July 2007 to March 2011, involving 19,213 women, ages 40 to 49. The trial enrolled asymptomatic women who were randomly divided into two groups. One group was screened using mammography alone; the other group, with a combination of mammography and ultrasound. The cancer detection rate was significantly higher in the combination group than the mammography group. The combined screening also detected more cancers in women with dense breast tissue, which can make it difficult to see cancers on a mammogram.

However, women in the ultrasound-plus-mammography group were also more likely to be called back for additional imaging or a biopsy. The researchers concluded that using mammography and ultrasound together might improve detection of early-stage and invasive breast cancers in younger women regardless of the density of their breast tissue.

Reducing heart risks in the wake of breast cancer treatment

Hormone therapies may increase cardiovascular risks, but making lifestyle changes and being aware of risk factors can help protect you.

Today, the vast majority of women diagnosed with breast cancer survive the disease—91% are still alive five years after their diagnosis. One reason for this is the use of hormone therapies. These drugs can treat—or prevent a recurrence of—estrogen-fueled tumors, which make up a majority (83%) of invasive breast cancers.

Hormonal medications are typically prescribed for five years following treatment to block the effects of estrogen on breast tissue. By hindering the action of this female hormone, these drugs can halt tumor growth. But while hormone therapies bring benefits, they also pose some risks to the heart and blood vessels.

A scientific statement from the American Heart Association (AHA), published online April 26, 2021, by *Circulation: Genomic and Precision Medicine*, outlined some of what's known about the link between hormonal treatment for breast cancer and cardiovascular disease. It stressed the importance of recognizing and reducing risks for women who have been treated with hormone therapies. "Survivors must remain vigilant about cardiovascular disease, which is still the leading cause of death among women who have had breast cancer," says Dr. Kathryn Rexrode, chief of the Division of Women's Health at Harvard-affiliated Brigham and Women's Hospital.

Understanding risks

While several breast cancer treatments can affect cardiovascular health, the AHA statement looked specifically at the role played by hormone therapies. There are two main types of hormones used:

- aromatase inhibitors, which include anastrozole (Armidex), exemestane (Aromasin), and Femara (letrozole)
- selective estrogen receptor modulators (SERMs), which include tamoxifen (Nolvadex), raloxifene (Evista), and toremifene (Fareston).

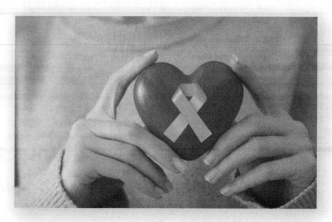

Hormonal breast cancer therapies can raise heart risks. But lifestyle changes can still help prevent problems.

"The specific risks with regard to blood clots, heart attacks, strokes, lipids, high blood pressure, and heart failure depend on the specific hormonal agent prescribed," says Dr. Rexrode. Women treated with aromatase inhibitors, for example, may be more likely to develop plaque buildup in the arteries (also referred to as atherosclerosis), to experience heart failure, or to see an unhealthy rise in the levels of artery-clogging fats in their blood.

"Women treated with SERMs, on the other hand, may be at higher risk for blood clots, hypertension, and pulmonary hypertension," says Dr. Rexrode. Hypertension refers to high blood pressure that affects arteries throughout the body; people with pulmonary hypertension have elevated pressure only in the artery that feeds the lungs.

Reducing your risk

If you've undergone hormonal treatment for breast cancer, you can still make changes to protect the health of your heart and blood vessels over the long term. "The strategies for prevention of cardiovascular disease in women who have had breast cancer and hormonal therapies are similar to recommendations for the general population," says Dr. Rexrode.

Women are advised to follow current guidelines designed to prevent cardiovascular disease. This includes reviewing your risk factors with your doctor and considering treatment if you are at increased risk, says Dr. Rexrode.

The American Heart Association and the American College of Cardiology have developed a risk calculator (www.health.harvard.edu/heartrisk) that allows you to assess your personal risk.

Additional female-specific risk factors aren't always included in these calculations, but they're also worth discussing with your doctor. These include having had an early menopause (before you turned 40) or pre-eclampsia (a potentially life-threatening pregnancy complication marked by high blood pressure and protein in the urine).

Women at elevated risk should closely monitor their blood pressure and get regular cholesterol and blood sugar tests. "In addition, physical activity, a healthy diet, and maintaining a healthy weight can improve both cardiovascular and breast cancer risk," says Dr. Rexrode.

And remember, increased risk doesn't mean you are doomed to experience problems.

Prostate cancer and your diet

Research suggests a heart-healthy diet may offer protection.

Diets that emphasize plant-based foods, like the Mediterranean diet and the DASH diet, help reduce your risk of heart disease by improving factors like cholesterol levels, blood pressure, and weight. But can they also protect against prostate cancer? That disease is second only to skin cancer as the most common cancer among men. "There is no miracle prostate cancer diet," says Dr. Bradley McGregor, an oncologist with Harvard-affiliated Dana-Farber Cancer Institute. "But as we learn more about the role diet plays in disease prevention, there is growing evidence that plant-based diets may lower your risk of prostate cancer and even help slow its spread."

Global impact

The Mediterranean and DASH diets, and other similar plant-heavy diets, revolve around large amounts of whole fruits and vegetables (especially cruciferous vegetables), whole grains, nuts, and olive oil, with fish preferred over red meat.

To understand the possible link between plant-heavy diets and prostate cancer, all you need to do is look at a world map. Prostate cancer death rates are much lower in the Mediterranean and southern European countries that favor this diet than places that don't. Many reasons could explain the difference, such as genetics and lifestyle factors like exercise habits and weight management.

Some research has looked closer at this connection. In a study published March 1, 2021, in *Cancer*, 410 men on active surveillance for localized prostate cancer recorded their daily diets for three years. In those who ate more fruits, vegetables, legumes, grains, and fish, the cancer was less likely to grow to the point of needing treatment.

Other research has focused on individual foods and specific ingredients of plant-based diets. Large prospective studies have found that men with moderate to high intake of fish are less likely to develop prostate cancer or die from it than men who do not eat fish. The protective

© curtoicurto | Getty Images

Foods like tomatoes stand out as special cancer fighters.

Daily cups of joe may serve up anti-cancer benefits

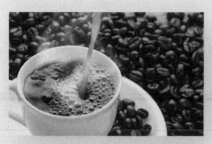

Besides giving a jolt to your day, your morning coffee also may protect you against prostate cancer. An analysis published online Jan. 11, 2021, by *BMJ Open* found that men who drank at least two cups a day had a 9% lower prostate cancer risk than those who drank one cup or none. Coffee may even slow prostate cancer growth. The researchers also examined the coffee-drinking habits of men with advanced cancer. They found that regular coffee drinkers had a 12% to 16% lower risk for progressive and fatal cancer. It's not clear how coffee may help, but scientists point to coffee's high levels of antioxidants as a possible reason. Other research has shown a link between coffee consumption and a lower risk of other cancers, like those of the liver, bowel, and breast.

benefits may come from omega-3 fatty acids, which are known inflammation fighters.

Studies also have shown that carotenoids (compounds that occur naturally in certain plants) have antioxidant properties that may protect the body against unstable molecules that damage DNA and cause cancer cells to form.

Lycopene, found in tomatoes and other red-colored fruits and vegetables, has especially stood out. A study recently published in *Cancer Causes & Control*

IN THE JOURNALS

Exercise may slow prostate cancer growth

Men who follow active surveillance for prostate cancer may improve their outcome by doing high-intensity interval training (HIIT). Researchers had 52 men (average age 63) on active surveillance either do a supervised treadmill HIIT workout three days a week for 12 weeks or follow their usual exercise routine that did not include high-intensity exercise.

With HIIT, you exercise for a short burst at near-maximum effort followed by a brief rest period. You then repeat that pattern a specific number of times. In the trial, the workouts consisted of two minutes of exercise at 85% to 95% of a person's VO2 max (the maximum amount of oxygen the body can use during exercise), then two minutes of recovery at 40% VO2 max. The pattern was repeated five to eight times.

Researchers found that compared with the people doing their usual lower-intensity exercise, those in the HIIT group had lower prostate-specific antigen (PSA) levels, lower PSA velocities (the rate of change in PSA levels

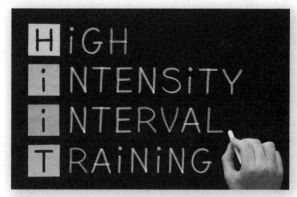

HIIT workouts can benefit men with prostate cancer.

over time), and had slower prostate cancer cell growth. They also had better cardiovascular fitness. The researchers pointed out that men on active surveillance typically have three times the risk of dying from cardiovascular disease than from prostate cancer. The results were published online Aug. 19, 2021, by *JAMA Oncology*.

found that cancer-free men who ate canned and cooked tomatoes five to six times per week had a 28% lower risk of prostate cancer after eight years than those who never consumed the food.

Watch what you eat

When it comes to diet and prostate cancer, it may also be a matter of what you don't eat. Following a plant-based diet means you eat fewer foods high in cholesterol and saturated fat, which scientists have linked to a higher risk of aggressive prostate cancers.

It's important to realize that these studies only show an association. "It's not clear if certain foods or combinations, specific amounts, and other factors like regular exercise and maintaining a healthy weight are the real reasons," says Dr. McGregor. "It also could be a cumulative effect of all of them." Dr. McGregor adds that the dietary recommendations for preventing prostate cancer also apply to managing the cancer if you do develop it.

"The same dietary habits that can lower your risk of prostate cancer can have a similar effect to perhaps slow its spread," says Dr. McGregor. "So, no matter where you are in terms of prostate cancer—from monitoring PSA levels to treating a diagnosis—take the opportunity now to get serious about your diet."

Managing prostate cancer while you wait-and-see

Men who follow active surveillance or watchful waiting for their low-risk prostate cancer still need to stay engaged.

More men are choosing active surveillance or watchful waiting for their low-risk prostate cancer diagnosis. While these two "wait and see" approaches may appear passive, they can provide opportunities for men to get more active about their overall wellness.

"There is a good chance men will live a long time with low-risk prostate cancer, and they should do everything they can to ensure their life is the healthiest and the highest quality it can be," says Dr. Jacob Berchuck, an oncologist with Harvard-affiliated Dana-Farber Cancer Institute.

Know your options

The choice to follow active surveillance or watchful waiting begins after a prostate biopsy, which provides information needed to predict how fast the cancer is growing and the probability of spreading.

Generally, active surveillance is an option for men with low-grade cancer that hasn't spread, who have a PSA level of less than 10 nanograms per milliliter and a Gleason score of 6 or less. (The Gleason system assigns 1-to-5 rankings to the two most common types of cancer cells in a man's biopsied tissue.

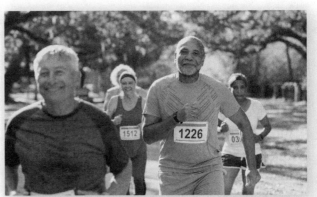

© kali9 | Getty Images

A prostate cancer diagnosis is a chance to get serious about your commitment to health.

The two rankings are added together to get a Gleason score, with 10 being the highest. The higher the number, the greater chance the cancer will quickly grow and spread.)

The reason for choosing active surveillance is to defer immediate surgery or radiation, since low-grade prostate cancer is unlikely to progress. That also means avoiding possible side effects of treatment, such as erectile dysfunction, urinary incontinence, and bowel problems. Men on active surveillance regularly follow up with their doctor for PSA tests, MRI scans, and prostate biopsies. "If there is evidence the cancer has progressed, such as a higher Gleason score or cancer in a greater number of biopsies, then treatment should be considered," says Dr. Berchuck.

In general, PSA is checked every six to 12 months, and MRI is performed every one to two years. Biopsies are done no more than once a year. Watchful waiting is usually reserved for older men with an estimated life expectancy of 10 years or less. Watchful waiting means no special monitoring with PSA or other tests. Decisions about future treatment are postponed until the onset of symptoms, such as difficulty urinating or bone pain. "Men who choose watchful waiting are most interested in their quality of life and wish to avoid the side effects of treatment that probably would not change their life expectancy," says Dr. Berchuck.

Wake-up call

But active surveillance and watchful waiting do not mean you shouldn't do anything while you monitor your cancer. In fact, Dr. Berchuck believes this is a golden opportunity to get proactive about your health. "Men should see their cancer diagnosis as a wake-up call to make lifestyle changes that could not only improve their long-term cancer outcome, but also protect against other serious health issues like heart attacks and strokes," he says. Dr. Berchuck recommends that men consider exploring the following four paths:

Get moving. Do at least 30 minutes of exercise three to five days a week. Intensity matters, too. A study from *European Urology* found that men with prostate cancer who engaged most frequently in vigorous activity had a 30% lower risk of developing advanced cancer and 25% lower risk of developing lethal cancer when compared with men who exercised the least. Men in the study did such activities as running, cycling, swimming, and playing sports like tennis and racquetball.

Get losing. Weight gain is linked with more aggressive cancer. "Even losing five to 10 extra pounds can help lower your risk," says Dr. Berchuck. A healthier weight also keeps blood pressure and cholesterol levels under control.

Get cooking. It's not clear whether specific dietary habits can influence prostate cancer growth. Dr. Berchuck suggests embracing proven healthy diets like the Mediterranean and MIND diets and cutting back on inflammatory foods like red meat, processed foods, and high-sugar foods and drinks. Revisiting your diet is also a chance to beef up your cooking skills and improve eating habits. Take a cooking class, or commit to making a new healthy recipe each week.

Get calm. Many men on active surveillance or watchful waiting may experience stress and anxiety. "Even if men are comfortable following these strategies, there still may be times when they need some emotional support," says Dr. Berchuck. Make time for regular self-care. For instance, reserve 20 minutes each day to listen to music, read, meditate, or just sit still. Also, consider reaching out to prostate cancer support groups.

Radiation for prostate cancer

Here's what you should know about this treatment option.

Men who get diagnosed with prostate cancer have several options to choose from for their next step. Many men with slow-growing, low-risk cancer follow active surveillance, a wait-and-see approach that monitors the cancer for changes.

But if the cancer shows higher risk (a Gleason score of 7 or higher) or has already begun to spread, other treatments are recommended. (A Gleason score classifies prostate tumor cells on a scale from 6 to 10. The higher the number, the more likely the cancer will spread.) There are two options: surgery to remove the prostate (called a prostatectomy) or radiation to destroy the cancer cells.

Studies comparing these two approaches

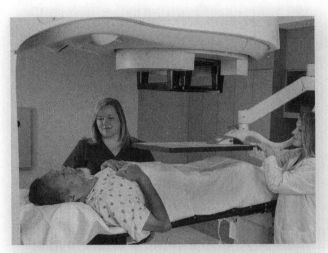
Each radiation treatment for prostate cancer is generally quick and painless.

demonstrate no advantage of one over the other with respect to cancer control. Your path will depend on factors like your current health, the specifics of your cancer, and personal preference. Yet for many men, radiation can be the better option.

"It's much more precise than the traditional radiation used for other kinds of cancer, and research also has found that long-term quality of life is often better, with fewer adverse health effects compared to surgery," says Dr. Anthony D'Amico, a radiation oncologist with Harvard-affiliated Dana-Farber Cancer Institute and Brigham and Women's Hospital.

There are two main ways to deliver radiation to the prostate: external beam radiation and brachytherapy.

External beam radiation

Rays of high-energy radiation are targeted to the site of the cancer on the prostate (and sometimes nearby lymph nodes). External beam radiation effectively destroys cancer cells, but it can also damage healthy tissue. A CT scan determines the prostate gland's exact location to allow for precise focusing and help limit collateral damage to the rectum and bladder. You lie on a table where a device delivers the radiation for five to 10 minutes. In general, treatments are given five days a week for several weeks. There are several types of external beam radiation therapy:

Three-dimensional conformal radiation therapy (3D-CRT). This involves taking three-dimensional pictures of the prostate and surrounding structures before treatment to pinpoint their locations. These images help the radiologist keep radiation away from the bladder and rectum.

Intensity-modulated radiation therapy (IMRT). IMRT is now the most commonly used form of radiation therapy. It is similar to 3D-CRT, but is more precise because it allows doctors to change the radiation intensity within each of several radiation beams, increasing total radiation to the cancerous area while reducing radiation to healthy tissues.

Proton beam therapy. This has the same precision as IMRT but uses protons (subatomic particles with a positive electrical charge) instead of photons (light particles) used in conventional radiation. During proton beam therapy, radiation is released in a narrow

Are you a candidate?

Whether your doctor recommends radiation depends on various factors, including your age, health, and personal preferences. The type of radiation is often dictated by your risk group (low, intermediate, or high) and whether the cancer is localized or has spread.

Sometimes hormone therapy (called androgen suppression therapy, or ADT) is given before radiation or along with it. ADT reduces levels of male hormones, called androgens, which can slow or even stop the cancer's growth. Studies have found this one-two punch leads to higher survival rates than radiation alone among men with localized prostate cancer and a Gleason score of 7 or higher.

If you opt for surgery, your doctor may suggest

radiation afterward, called adjuvant radiation therapy. "You have surgery to remove cancer, and then radiation to eliminate any remaining tumor deposits to keep cancer from returning," says Dr. Anthony D'Amico, a radiation oncologist with Harvard's Dana-Farber Cancer Institute. Cancer that has grown beyond the prostate also may require post-surgery radiation.

After you've had radiation, you'll have a prostate-specific antigen (PSA) test every three to six months for five years and then annually after that to check for recurrence of the cancer. "If your PSA ever rises above 2, then imaging tests are done, and if needed, additional radiation or other appropriate treatment is given," says Dr. D'Amico.

band, thus minimizing damage to surrounding tissue. The downside is that it is more expensive and not available everywhere. "Also, outcomes appear to be equivalent with IMRT in terms of curing the cancer and improving quality of life," says Dr. D'Amico.

Stereotactic body radiation therapy (SBRT). SBRT uses image guidance and computer-controlled robotics to deliver multiple radiation beams to the tumor. Several systems are available, with brand names like CyberKnife, Gamma Knife, and TomoTherapy. Long-term side effects are still being explored.

Hypofractionated radiation therapy. This delivers larger doses with each treatment, requiring fewer sessions—typically, a total of five treatments spaced out over four to five-and-a-half weeks. A man is eligible for this treatment only if he has good urinary flow, doesn't need to urinate often at night, has not had prostate surgery, and doesn't take anticoagulants (blood thinners).

Brachytherapy

Brachytherapy involves placing radioactive pellets, or "seeds"—each about the size of a grain of rice—in or near the prostate tumor. The number of seeds ranges from 50 to 150, depending on the size of the prostate gland.

After the man receives either general or spinal anesthesia, the doctor places an ultrasound probe in the rectum and a catheter in the bladder. The doctor then uses a needle to insert the seeds through the perineum (the area between the scrotum and anus) and guides them into place. The seeds are left there and, over time, emit less and less radiation until they become nonradioactive. Depending on the type of seeds, this may take anywhere from three months to a year.

If cancer returns, a doctor may suggest high-dose-rate brachytherapy. Here, the more powerful seeds are temporarily placed and then removed several days later, with the process repeated for several sessions.

Who needs hormone therapy for prostate cancer?

Here's what you should know about this type of treatment.

The spectrum for treating cancer confined to the prostate gland has a range of options. On one end is watchful waiting (beginning treatment only if symptoms arise) or active surveillance (periodic testing to see if the cancer has progressed). On the other is the surgical removal of the prostate.

Depending on the stage of localized cancer, a man's doctor instead might recommend something in the middle: radiation therapy, which can be delivered alone or combined with hormonal therapy, also known as androgen deprivation therapy (ADT).

"Hormone therapy is a powerful weapon in the fight against prostate cancer because it starves the cancer of the fuel that stimulates its growth and spread," says Dr. Atish D. Choudhury, co-director of the Prostate Cancer Center at Harvard-affiliated Dana-Farber Cancer Institute.

Slowing the growth

Hormone therapy serves to decrease levels of androgens, the male sex hormones. Androgens give men characteristics like facial and body hair, a deep voice, and large muscles. They also help with the prostate's normal growth and function. The most abundant androgens are testosterone and dihydro-testosterone (DHT). The testicles make about 90% to 95% of androgens, while the adrenal glands (located above your kidneys) produce the rest.

Prostate cancer uses signals from androgens to grow and spread. "Androgens—especially testosterone—are fuel for cancer cells," says Dr. Choudhury. "Hormone therapy decreases androgen levels and deprives cancer cells of these signals, causing the cancer to shrink."

Who's a candidate?

Men with biopsy-proven cancer that has not spread outside the gland are offered therapeutic choices based on their age, overall health, and Gleason score (a numerical value that grades prostate tumor cells according to how abnormal they appear compared with normal prostate cells). The usual

A side of effects

Reducing levels of androgens (the male sex hormones) can cause side effects. Some men experience only a few mild symptoms, while others have more bothersome ones. Low libido and erectile dysfunction (ED) are the most familiar. (Taking ED drugs while on hormone therapy may not help.) Other typical problems include fatigue, hot flashes, weight gain, moodiness, and breast enlargement. However, when treatment stops, these problems usually go away. If you take hormone therapy for long periods, or if your cancer is well controlled, your doctor may take you off the treatment for a while to give your body a break from any side effects.

Hormone therapy also can increase total cholesterol, triglyceride levels, and blood sugar levels. Adopting a low-calorie diet and staying active with cardio and weight training can help curb possible weight gain, manage cholesterol and blood sugar levels, reduce sexual side effects, and increase energy. Men can soothe hot flashes by using cold packs and drinking cool water. Relaxation techniques help manage mood swings.

recommendation for intermediate or high-risk localized cancer is surgery or radiation (with or without hormonal therapy).

Hormonal therapy can boost radiation therapy's effectiveness by making the cancer cells "sick" and reducing a tumor's size. The therapy is also used when cancer has spread beyond where it can be successfully treated with surgery or radiation, or if men can't have these treatments for any reason.

Advances in ADT

Previously, the only way to stop cancer-fueling androgens was surgical castration to remove the testicles. Now, many types of drugs can have the same effect without surgery. The most common work by affecting the release of androgens from the testes. Others block the enzyme needed to make androgens or stop growth signals from androgens in the cancer cells. "Your doctor will discuss which one is the best choice for you," says Dr. Choudhury.

These drugs produce similar results, but how they are taken and how often varies based on the therapy's goals and patient preference. In general, injections are given monthly or at three-, four-, or six-month intervals. Prostate-specific antigen (PSA) levels are monitored along the way.

For localized intermediate-risk cancer, men receive the therapy for six months. For localized high-risk cancer, the treatment can last up to two years. For cancer that has spread beyond the prostate, ADT is usually administered indefinitely. Intermittent ADT is another strategy. Therapy is paused once PSA falls below a certain level and then begins again if numbers rise.

Chapter 8

—

Fit and Active

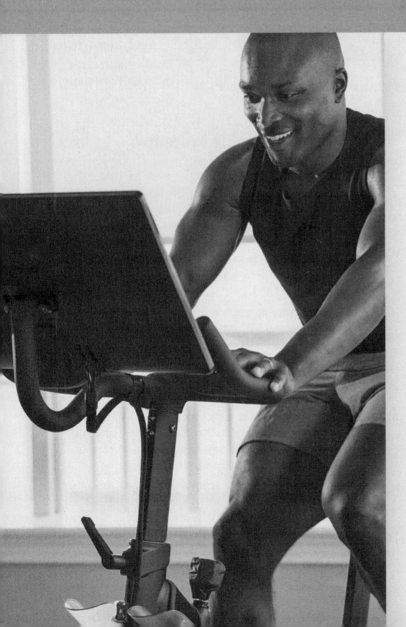

Take Action!
5 Things You Can Do Now

1 **Find fitness buddies.** A workout class or exercise club can provide community support. (page 178)

2 **Check your walking pace.** For most adults, covering about 1.4 miles in 30 minutes counts as moderate-intensity exercise. (page 180)

3 **Invest in new walking shoes.** Use these tips to guide your selection. (page 182)

4 **Pick up a racquet.** Playing racquet sports helps improve your eye-hand coordination. (page 188)

5 **Strengthen your core muscles.** These exercises can be done with grocery bags or a laundry basket. (page 195)

Get SMART about your fitness goals

Take this approach to ensure your strategies are successful.

You're ready to commit to improving your fitness. That's wonderful. But how should you begin? It's not enough to say you simply want to exercise more, get in shape, or be healthier.

"A successful fitness goal should revolve around a specific purpose in your life," says Susan Flashner-Fineman, the Vitalize360 Wellness Coaching Program coach at Harvard-affiliated Hebrew SeniorLife. "What exactly do you wish to accomplish at this time in your life?"

For example, a goal of greater strength or endurance could mean you'll have the stamina to travel again soon. Improved aerobic fitness also may help you lose 10 pounds. Increasing flexibility can mean more mobility and longer independent living. "When you tie your fitness to a specific cause, it gives you the structure and direction needed to plan the right exercise program for you," says Flashner-Fineman.

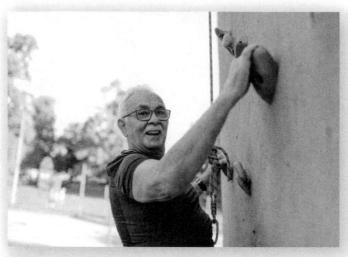

You can reach greater heights in your fitness by creating goals that are detailed and specific.

© RgStudio | Getty Images

Define to conquer

Once you have defined the result of your fitness goal, create a SMART exercise strategy to help achieve it. SMART stands for Specific, Measurable, Achievable, Relevant, and Time-based. Here's a breakdown of each segment:

Specific: Your plan needs to be clear and detailed. If you are too vague, exercise can feel overwhelming. For example, don't say, "I want to exercise most days of the week." Instead, say, "I will do a walk every Monday, Wednesday, and Saturday and do a strength training workout on Tuesdays and Fridays."

Measurable: By measuring your progress each week, you can know if you are indeed improving. For example, consider extending your walking time for two extra minutes each week, with a goal of walking for 40 minutes three times per week at the end of one to two months. Do similar small increments in the intensity of your resistance exercises every couple of weeks.

Achievable: Avoid overly grand expectations. "Base your exercise on what

Build a support system

No exercise strategy is foolproof; there are always setbacks and obstacles along the way. Don't let these derail your efforts. Accept them as part of the process and be ready to implement some counter-maneuvers when they arise. For example:

Some is better than none. Can't do your full workout? Instead of skipping it, just do a mini or abbreviated version.

Monitor your progress. Losing focus? Review your weekly accomplishments to remind yourself how far you've come.

Find fitness buddies. Low morale? Meet like-minded people by joining a workout class, a running or walking club, or an online community.

Use reminders. Not feeling motivated? Keep a visual image related to your goal in constant view: a vacation destination photo, the sign-up form for a 5K race, or your favorite inspirational quotes.

Treat yourself. Don't feel any achievement? Reward yourself whenever you meet a small milestone. For example, when you can do a certain number of push-ups nonstop, buy a new workout shirt.

you realistically can do now, and not when you were younger," says Flashner-Fineman. "If you used to be able to walk five miles and now can only do a mile, that's still a great place to start."

Relevant: Your exercise program should directly benefit or support your fitness goal. If your goal is to improve flexibility and balance, yoga might be a better choice than spin classes.

Time-based: Can you commit to the level of exercise you want right now, or should you begin later? Or maybe you can begin with just 10-minute walks and build up? Also, give yourself a realistic timetable. For instance, if your fitness goal is to compete in a 5K race, you may need more than a month to prepare.

How physical activity keeps your heart in good shape

Findings from the famed Framingham Heart Study address how much exercise you need to stay fit—and how that helps your heart.

The evidence that physical activity staves off heart disease dates back many decades. In fact, that observation was among initial findings published in the late 1960s from the landmark *Framingham Heart Study*, which began in 1948 and is still going strong. Now, two recent studies involving the descendants of the original Framingham volunteers offer insights about how different types of activity affect your fitness and your heart.

"Exercising more and sitting less helps you live a healthier and longer life," says Dr. Hicham Skali, a cardiologist at Harvard-affiliated Brigham and Women's Hospital. These new findings provide further detail about why (and how much) exercise is vital for cardiovascular health, he adds.

The fastest route to fitness

Both studies explored the importance of cardiorespiratory fitness (CRF), which quantifies how well your heart and lungs supply oxygen to your muscles during physical activity.

The first, published Nov. 21, 2021, in the *European Heart Journal*, included 2,070 people

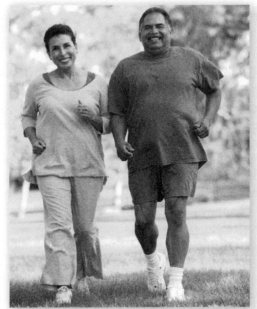

Moderate-to-vigorous exercise boosts fitness and enhances quality of life.

from the Third Generation cohort, many of whom are the grandchildren of the original Framingham participants. All underwent exercise tests on stationary bicycles to measure their CRF; they also wore fitness trackers for one week to measure their activity levels. Researchers then compared the participants' current values to measurements taken eight years earlier.

Not surprisingly, people who did more moderate-to-vigorous exercise, took more steps, and were less sedentary between the two exam periods showed clear improvements in their CRF. This was largely true regardless of a person's age, sex, weight, risk of heart disease, and how active they were at the earlier assessment.

Moderate-to-vigorous exercise (such as brisk walking, jogging, and cycling) was the most efficient way to boost fitness. To reap the same change in fitness level from just one minute of moderate-to-vigorous exercise, a person would have to walk for three minutes or spend about 15 fewer minutes being sedentary (see "Walk, jog, run: How fast?" on the next page).

People whose exercise levels or daily step counts were above the norm had higher-than-average CRF regardless of how much time they were sedentary. This suggests that being more active may partly offset the negative effects of sitting too much. But it's still a good idea to avoid being sedentary for long stretches of time, says Dr. Skali.

Beyond blood vessel benefits

The second study, published Oct. 29, 2021, in *JAMA Network Open*, included 2,962 people in the Framingham Offspring Study. Begun in 1971, this cohort includes a sample of the sons and daughters of the original cohort and their spouses.

Instead of measuring CRF directly (which is costly and requires special equipment), researchers estimated CRF using information such as a person's age, sex, waist circumference, resting heart rate, and physical activity, starting when the participants were middle-aged. But unlike the other study, this one also included relevant measures of the participants' cardiovascular health, notes Dr. Skali. For example, it included tests to check the stiffness of their arteries and to look for early signs of atherosclerosis (plaque buildup inside the arteries).

Over an average follow-up period of 15 years, people with higher CRF at midlife were more likely to have healthier blood vessels that were more flexible with less plaque buildup, compared with people with lower CRF. People who were more fit were also less likely to develop high blood pressure, diabetes, chronic kidney disease, and cardiovascular disease, and were also less likely to die during the follow-up period.

While these findings highlight the value of higher fitness levels in midlife, it's never too late to start exercising, says Dr. Skali. "No matter what age you start exercising, you can improve your cardiovascular health," he says.

Walk, jog, run: How fast?

The CDC defines moderate-intensity walking as a rate of 2.5 to 4 mph. Where you fall within that range depends on your fitness level. If you exercise regularly and are in good shape, moderate intensity might mean 4 mph, or a 15-minute mile. If you're less fit, moderate intensity is closer to the lower end of the range. According to one study, a walking pace of about 100 steps per minute (which translates to 2.7 mph) qualifies as brisk walking for most adults. To reach vigorous-intensity activity, you need to take at least 130 steps per minute (which, at just over 4 mph, qualifies as jogging). Running is often defined as 6 mph or faster.

IN THE JOURNALS

Exercise can add to your sense of purpose—and vice versa

It's well established that regular exercise can improve one's mental outlook. A recent study found the connection also works in the other direction: a sense of purpose makes it more likely you'll stay physically active. Researchers used information from the Health and Retirement Study, an ongoing project involving about 18,000 middle-aged and older adults. As part of the study, participants were asked questions designed to evaluate their sense of purpose in life and how much physical activity they regularly engaged in. The authors defined a sense of purpose as "having goals and aims that give life direction and meaning." The researchers examined data from a specific four-year interval.

No surprise, people who started out leading active lives showed an increase in their sense of purpose four years later. But those who had a strong sense of purpose in the beginning actually increased their physical activity over time. While the results only showed an association, the researchers suggest adopting an exercise routine can provide goals and structure that help offer direction and meaning, especially as people age. On the other end, people who have a strong sense of purpose in life are more motivated to stay physically active. The results were published online April 23, 2021, by the *Journal of Behavioral Medicine*.

3 ways to enhance your walking workouts

Interval and Nordic walking can ramp up your fitness, while mindful walking can alleviate stress.

The beauty of walking for exercise is that it requires no special skills or equipment other than a comfy, supportive pair of shoes. The downside: it can get a little tedious. To break through your boredom, try reinvigorating your walking regimen with some new twists on this popular form of exercise.

"All steps count. But some count a little more than others," says Dr. Edward Phillips, assistant professor of physical medicine and rehabilitation at Harvard Medical School. For example, if you add short bursts of fast walking to your strolls, that elevates your heart rate and improves your cardiorespiratory fitness more than if you simply stayed at a slower pace, he says.

Pick up a pair of Nordic poles to use during your walk, and you'll engage many more muscles and burn more calories. Or you can use walking as an opportunity to practice mindfulness, a mind-calming practice that can help you release stress. Following are suggestions about how and where you might try these techniques.

Interval walking

Dr. Phillips recommends this routine only for more experienced walkers, not beginners. For interval walking, you alternate brief bursts of fast walking with more moderately paced strides. After a five-minute warm-up, walk briskly for 15, 30, or 60

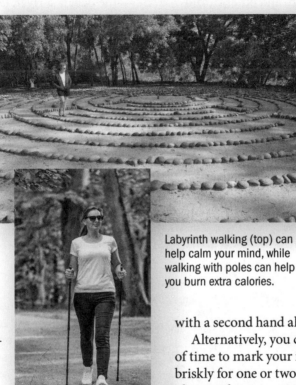

Labyrinth walking (top) can help calm your mind, while walking with poles can help you burn extra calories.

seconds. Then slow down and recover at a normal pace for an equal amount of time (or you may want to double your recovery time).

Start with shorter intervals of rapid walking and gradually lengthen them as you increase your stamina over the following weeks and months. Or you can keep the intervals constant and extend your overall workout time. "A smartwatch programmed to beep at set times comes in handy, but a $10 watch with a second hand also works," says Dr. Phillips.

Alternatively, you can use landmarks instead of time to mark your intervals. For example, walk briskly for one or two city blocks, between two telephone poles, or a quarter of a lap around a local track.

Nordic walking

Nordic walking uses special poles with hand straps that help you engage your upper body. The motion is similar to cross-country skiing, with the poles slanted back behind you as you walk. These workouts may boost your cardiovascular workload and calorie burn up to 25% more than regular walking.

If you'd like to try out the poles, ask around in your neighborhood, because chances are someone has a dusty pair in the garage, says Dr. Phillips. But if you purchase them at an outdoor store, an employee can help you adjust the height and give you a quick primer on how to use them. Most have metal tips (for use on trails) and attachable rubber tips for use on asphalt or concrete.

Mindful walking

If the idea of sitting to meditate doesn't grab you,

perhaps walking meditation—also called mindful walking—is more your speed. The goal is to focus on the present moment without worrying about the past or future. Calming your mind in this way may help ease stress—and excess stress is a well-known contributor to high blood pressure and other cardio-vascular conditions.

Walk in a familiar place, but pay close attention to all the sights, sounds, and smells around you. If you prefer, you can focus on your breathing. As you walk, match your breath to your steps, inhaling smoothly for four steps, then exhaling smoothly for four steps. Do this for a few minutes, then try extending the number of steps per breath, in and out for six paces each breath for several minutes, and then to eight.

See which breath pattern (four, six, or eight) feels most comfortable, and stick with that for a while. Near the end of your walk, switch back to a leisurely stroll and just breathe normally.

If you have the opportunity, try walking close to water—the ocean, a river, lake, or pond—as these locations tend to encourage relaxation, Dr. Phillips suggests. Another option, labyrinth walking, can be especially helpful for evoking a meditative state, he says. A pattern of paths that weave in a circle around a central point (see photo on the previous page), a labyrinth encourages slow, mindful steps. You can find labyrinths in many places, including public parks, houses of worship, and health care facilities such as hospitals and hospices.

Tips for choosing walking shoes

Brisk walking is one of the simplest and best exercises you can do to protect your heart, so put your best foot forward.

A low-impact exercise that you can do almost anywhere, walking is both practical and popular. Another oft-mentioned perk of walking: the only gear you really need is a comfortable pair of shoes. But if you're doing your daily walks in sneakers that are comfy but well-worn, it might be time to invest in a new pair of dedicated walking shoes.

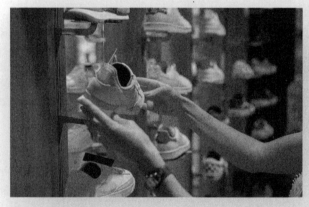

If you walk for exercise on a daily basis, replace your walking shoes at least yearly.

In fact, some experts recommend replacing your walking shoes every 300 to 500 miles. If you walk briskly for 30 minutes a day, five days a week, that translates to a new pair every six to 12 months. Plus, brand-new, well-fitting walking shoes just might put a little more spring in your step and encourage you to walk a bit farther.

Keeping your feet happy

The right shoes may help you avoid common foot and ankle injuries, such as plantar fasciitis (inflammation of the fibrous band of tissue on the bottom of the foot) and Achilles tendinitis (inflammation of the tendon connecting the calf muscle to the heel).

"But if you have any type of existing foot pain or impairment that makes walking uncomfortable, don't rely on a shoe to fix your problems," says Dr. Adam Tenforde, director of the Running Medicine Program at Harvard-affiliated Spaulding Rehabilitation Hospital. Instead, consult a podiatrist or physical therapist to properly address the problem, he advises.

Because feet come in varied shapes and sizes, it's impossible to recommend a specific walking shoe brand or style that would suit everyone. Comfort is the most important factor, and a shoe should feel good as soon as you slip it on. But don't assume that the more support and cushioning a walking shoe has,

© mgstudyo | Getty Images

the better. Some research suggests that thinner, more flexible soles put less stress on the knees, perhaps because they allow your foot to move in a more natural fashion.

If the shoe fits

For the best selection plus expert advice, you're better off going to a specialty running store (many of which also sell walking shoes) instead of a large chain retailer. You can even wear a running shoe for walking because both are designed for forward motion. (But don't wear walking shoes to run, as they aren't made to handle the higher impact.)

Sometimes, employees offer to analyze your feet or your old shoes to see if your foot tends to lean inward (pronation) or outward (supination) as you walk. But Dr. Tenforde isn't convinced this practice is necessary. "Research suggests that for healthy people, matching shoe type to address pronation or supination doesn't prevent more injuries than wearing a neutral shoe," he says.

Here's some additional advice for finding the right pair of walking shoes.

Shop late in the day. Because your feet tend to expand by the end of the day, it's best to try on new shoes when your feet are at their largest.

Choose socks first. The thickness of your socks affects how your shoes fit, so find some you like and take them to the shoe store. Avoid 100% cotton socks, which stay damp if they get wet, setting you up for a blister. Synthetic or

cotton-synthetic blends will wick away moisture.

Give it a bend. Grab the toe and heel of a shoe and pull them toward each other. The shoe should bend easily at the ball of the foot. If it doesn't, look for another style that does. The flexibility offers a greater range of motion and an easier push-off.

Look for a low heel. Stay away from shoes with big bulky heels, which can hinder the natural rolling foot motion of walking and may make you more prone to tripping.

Check for wiggle room. Allow at least one finger's width between your longest toe and the front of your shoe, as your feet may swell more in warm weather and on longer walks.

Take a test walk. To get a feel for the shoe, take

Shoe selection suggestions

When shopping for walking shoes, look for these important features:

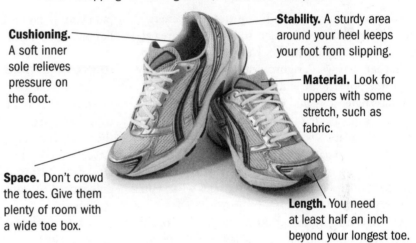

Cushioning. A soft inner sole relieves pressure on the foot.

Stability. A sturdy area around your heel keeps your foot from slipping.

Material. Look for uppers with some stretch, such as fabric.

Space. Don't crowd the toes. Give them plenty of room with a wide toe box.

Length. You need at least half an inch beyond your longest toe.

a few laps around the store. Try on a few different brands, with one on each foot for a side-by-side comparison. If you notice any rubbing, discomfort, or sore spots, try a different pair.

Hike your way to better health

A jaunt through the woods can boost your fitness, your balance, and your mood.

Walking is great exercise, but sometimes you need a break from your usual neighborhood loop or the monotony of the basement treadmill.

Head out for a hike instead. It's similar to walking but can give you a fitness boost along with a dose of novelty and adventure. And not only is hiking great exercise, it doesn't require much equipment.

Reaping physical benefits

Navigating a winding, wooded trail can help your body build endurance, strength, and coordination, says Dr. Edward Phillips, assistant professor of physical medicine and rehabilitation at Harvard Medical School.

Hiking over uneven terrain requires more energy than walking on a level surface, so it burns more calories. If you are hiking uphill, your body has to work even harder, he says. A rigorous hike may offer many of the same physical benefits as interval training, which alternates low- and high-intensity exercise to increase cardiovascular fitness. During a hike, your heart rate goes up as you move up an incline and drops when you head downhill.

Traversing an irregular landscape can also build strength. "You are using different muscles when you climb and descend," says Dr. Phillips.

If you haven't gone for a hike lately, you'll probably feel it in your hips and buttocks when you climb and in your thighs on the way down. "Descending works the muscles in the fronts of your thighs, which need to function like a brake to keep you stable," he says.

Finding your footing on a rutted trail can help you become steadier on your feet. "When you challenge your body, it will adapt. For example, if the terrain

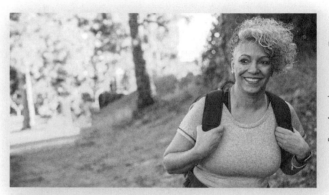

A hike often doesn't feel like exercise, which can help keep you motivated to make it a frequent activity.

puts your balance to the test, it will push your internal balance system to improve," says Dr. Phillips.

Improving mind and mood

Hiking's benefits aren't only physical; they're mental as well. Humans thrive when they are out in a natural setting, says Dr. Phillips. Simply being among the trees may improve a number of health indicators. Research has shown that the Japanese practice of shin-rin-yoku ("forest bathing"), which encourages a slow enjoyment of nature, produces measurable physical changes.

A recent study in the *International Journal of Biometeorology* found that the practice reduced levels of the stress hormone cortisol in the blood. A study in the *European Journal of Applied Physiology* noted its beneficial effects on blood pressure and potentially blood sugar levels.

Being out in nature also exposes you to new sights and experiences. The view from the same trail changes throughout the year as the trees grow or shed their leaves.

"Even when I think I know my way on a familiar path, I see something I've never seen before or haven't noticed, or something that has changed with the seasons," says Dr. Phillips.

The best thing about hiking is that it often doesn't feel like exercise. "Some people who eschew exercise will gladly go for a hike," says Dr. Phillips. And because they enjoy it, they're more likely to stick with

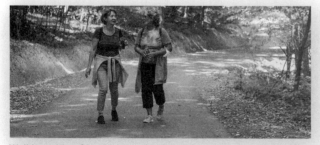

Walking with a friend can make the outing even more enjoyable.

Is it a hike or a walk?

It's not always clear precisely where a walk turns into a hike, says Dr. Edward Phillips, assistant professor of physical medicine and rehabilitation at Harvard Medical School. But there are some clues to help you distinguish between the two, he says.

Your footwear. "One way to tell the difference is to think about your footwear. If you instinctively grab a pair of sneakers, chances are you're going on a walk. If you find yourself anticipating the need for a sturdier shoe to navigate more challenging terrain, you're probably on track for a hike," he says.

The terrain. Most people consider it a walk when you're on a smooth surface, such as a road, a sidewalk, or a trail with few obstacles to navigate. "If the route is more difficult and brings you from lower to higher ground, it's probably a hike," says Dr. Phillips.

The duration. Most walks tend to be quick, typically less than an hour. But a hike will usually last much longer. Being out for more than an hour at a time on a hike isn't unusual.

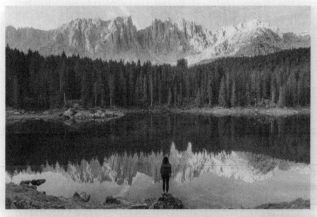

Taking a hike is similar to walking, but provides a change of scenery and potentially some additional health benefits.

it. Some trails even provide their own motivation to keep you going. "If you ever want to hook someone on hiking, go to Acadia National Park in Maine. An hourlong hike there can take you up 400 feet to a peak where you get a panoramic view of the ocean below," says Dr. Phillips.

A destination hike like this allows you to earn a reward, in the form of a sight that you might otherwise not have gotten to see.

How to get started

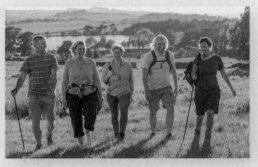

While hiking can be safely adapted to many fitness levels, there are some things you should do to prepare before you head out, says Dr. Edward Phillips, assistant professor of physical medicine and rehabilitation at Harvard Medical School.

Start slowly. If you've never hiked before, don't attempt to trek up a steep mountain. Flat trails provide a great starting place. Look for local rail trails, which are level paths of stone dust or another soft surface. They run along old railway beds where tracks used to be. These are a great place for beginners that still get you out in nature. You can also use a smartphone app or online trail guide to find local routes that suit your ability level.

Bring a buddy. It's safer to hike with a friend, ideally someone who knows the area.

Do your research. Plan your route and know what terrain to expect before you leave. Also, make sure your cellphone will work in the area you choose so you can get emergency help if you need it.

Stop halfway. When you're hiking, only go about half as far as you want to hike. Don't forget, you still need to travel all the way back to your starting place.

Bring the right supplies. Ensure that you have sturdy footwear, and bring a hat and sunscreen to protect yourself from the sun, enough water to stay well-hydrated, insect and tick repellent, and a small first-aid kit.

Be flexible. Don't feel you need to achieve a certain hiking speed or distance goal. Rather, adapt your outing for the conditions you encounter on the trail.

Bolster your balance. If you need a little extra balance support, hiking poles can be a great solution, says Dr. Phillips. They cost around $20 at most outdoor supply stores and can give your arms a mini-workout while you walk.

Exercising safely with hearing or vision impairment

Try these strategies to stay active and protect your health and mobility.

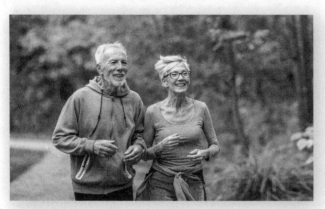

Exercise with a buddy for an extra set of eyes and ears on your daily walk or jog.

Exercising challenges from hearing or vision impairment can start out small. Maybe your glasses slide down while you're jogging, or you can't always hear what a friend is saying as you walk together. As challenges increase, they can make activities so hard or unpleasant that you don't want to do them anymore, or they can put your health and safety at risk. Before it gets to that point, identify difficulties and take steps to resolve them.

Vision impairment

Vision problems can affect your ability to exercise in many ways. For example, you might not be able to see the instructor in an exercise class. And certain eye problems can cause specific challenges.

If you have central vision loss (macular degeneration): "You might have trouble walking on uneven surfaces or navigating obstacles while on a bicycle. And sports such as tennis and golf may no longer be possible," says optometrist Amy Watts, director of the Vision Rehabilitation Service at Harvard-affiliated Mass Eye and Ear.

If you have peripheral (side) vision loss (glaucoma): "You can easily miss steps and curbs while walking or running on uneven surfaces," Watts notes.

ASK THE DOCTORS

by **HOPE RICCIOTTI, M.D., AND TONI GOLEN, M.D.**

Does exercise really boost energy levels?

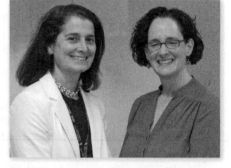

Q *I've been feeling tired lately. My doctor suggested I exercise more. How will this help my energy level? Won't it make me feel more tired?*

A It might sound strange, but it's true that moving more can help give you more energy, through several mechanisms. To begin with, cellular-level changes occur inside your body when you exercise. Exertion spurs your body to produce more mitochondria inside your muscle cells. Mitochondria are known as the powerhouses of cells, because they create fuel out of glucose from the food you eat and oxygen from the air you breathe. Having more of them increases your body's energy supply.

Exercising also boosts oxygen circulation inside your body. This increase in oxygen not only supports the mitochondria's energy production, it allows your body to function better and to use its energy more efficiently. Plus, your body gets a boost from an exercise-induced increase in hormone levels that makes you feel more energized.

In addition to helping your body create and use energy, regular exercise promotes better nighttime sleep. Deep sleep is crucial to your overall health and to feeling well rested and energetic when you wake up in the morning.

"While you're hiking in wooded areas, your side vision might not detect branches until you run into them."

If you're slightly nearsighted or farsighted: Exercising can be uncomfortable with eyeglasses on. Some people take them off to work out. "That's not usually a problem," Watts says. "However, without their glasses, people with particularly poor eyesight have an increased risk of falling."

Hearing impairment

Hearing impairment also has numerous effects on exercise. One is that people with hearing loss can have impaired balance: the ear also contains an important balance center. That makes any movement challenging and increases the risk for falls.

Other problems are related to awareness of your environment. For example:

Missing hazards. "If you're running and crossing the road, you might not hear vehicles around you. Or you might have difficulty identifying the direction of a particular sound, like a siren—you may think it's coming from the left when it's really coming from the right," says Meaghan Reed, director of Clinical Audiology at Mass Eye and Ear.

Missing instructions. "Exercise classrooms with high ceilings and hard floors can increase background noise, which makes it harder to understand an instructor. Loud music can also be a problem," Reed says.

Feeling isolated. You might feel left out if you can't hear other people during activities—even if you're wearing hearing aids. "Hearing aids are optimized for six to eight feet. On a golf course, if you're farther than six or eight feet from others, you might not hear them—especially if it's windy," Reed notes.

Experiencing equipment failure. When you exercise, sweat and moisture can get into a hearing aid and cause it to malfunction.

Simple fixes

A small adjustment could be all it takes to keep you active and exercising.

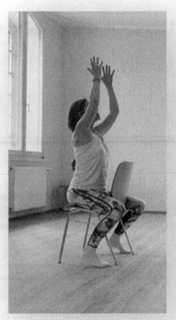

Chair yoga is a good option if you have balance challenges.

If balance is a problem, stick to stationary equipment that allows you to hold on, such as a stationary bicycle or an elliptical trainer. Or try seated exercise, such as chair yoga.

On a walk, take a buddy to act as an extra set of eyes and ears, and walk on smooth pavement, such as paved paths or tracks.

During an exercise class, stand (or sit) in the front of the room and away from loud music. Mention vision or hearing challenges in advance to the instructor, who can check that you're following along during class. "If you have a hard time understanding exercise instructions, ask the teacher to rephrase something rather than just repeat it," Reed says.

Equipment changes

In some cases, you might need to adjust your equipment to keep exercising with hearing or vision impairment.

If you wear eyeglasses during exercise, consider getting either an elastic strap to hold your glasses in place or a pair of prescription sports glasses. "The temples wrap around the ear farther than regular glasses, which prevents the frames from sliding down if you're sweating. The glasses may also come with a strap to help hold them in place. And some sports glasses have lenses that wrap around the eyes to block glare from the sides and protect the eyes from wind and debris," Watts says. She recommends contact lenses as an alternative.

If you wear a hearing aid, consider getting a remote microphone that your exercise buddy or instructor can use; the person's voice will be transmitted to your device. And if sweat is affecting your hearing aid, there are tools that can help. "Get 'dry kits' or electric dehumidifiers to dry out the moisture," Reed says. "That may help prolong the life of the hearing aid."

Whatever the challenge, your clinician will have suggestions to help you keep exercising. It's especially important that you do, since both vision and hearing loss are associated with inactivity and an increased risk for chronic disease.

© SilviaJansen | Getty Images

Activities to sharpen your eye-hand coordination

Racquet sports, swimming, and even playing catch can help.

Think of all the things you do with your eyes and hands at the same time—such as drive a car, cook a meal, pick up an object, or grab a handrail. They're made possible in part by the coordination of the information your eyes take in and the signals your brain sends to your arms and hands. This eye-hand coordination is key to maintaining your independence.

Unfortunately, eye-hand coordination declines as we age. Reflexes, speed, and accuracy dull—possibly because of vision loss, poor health, or changes in brain wiring. "Many people in our society over age 60 who eat a Western diet and don't get enough exercise have tiny, imperceptible 'ministrokes' in their brains. These strokes can disrupt connections in important brain coordination centers. In addition, we all lose some brain cells that produce dopamine, a chemical that helps the brain regulate movement and coordination," explains Dr. Andrew Budson, a neurologist and chief of Cognitive and Behavioral Neurology at VA Boston Healthcare System.

The good news: "You can improve eye-hand coordination by exercising, practicing skills, and treating underlying conditions," Dr. Budson says.

An eye-hand workout

All exercise is good for your brain, and the following may be especially helpful for eye-hand coordination.

Racquet sports. In tennis, racquetball, or pickleball, your eyes watch the ball, and your brain instructs your body to meet up with it. "The speed of the moving ball is challenging. Your brain has to manage that hand and arm not just where you can see it, but also where you can't see it, as the ball flies by and you reach behind you or to the side. It forces your reaction time to be faster," says Jennifer Packard, an

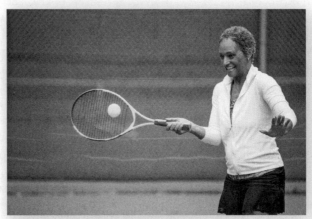

Keeping up with the speed of a moving tennis ball helps sharpen your eye-hand coordination.

occupational therapist at Harvard-affiliated Spaulding Rehabilitation Hospital.

Swimming. In swimming, you often use your arms and hands outside your field of vision, forcing the brain to use its mind's eye. "You visualize in your head what your hands are doing, without watching them," Packard says. "Plus, the sensory input is different in the water, which challenges the brain."

Tai chi. This ancient martial art uses a series of slow, flowing motions and deep breathing. You gradually shift your weight from one pose to another, which improves your reflexes, balance, strength, flexibility, and range of motion. Tai chi reinforces all of these components of movement.

Noncontact boxing. This is a type of exercise program that involves wearing boxing gloves and shadow boxing or hitting soft pads. It's especially challenging for your brain as you quickly aim left with your right hand, or aim right with your left hand. "There is a huge benefit in requiring your brain to cross the midline—an imaginary vertical line drawn from the sky down through your nose to your bellybutton and in between your ankles," Packard says.

Eye-hand activities

You don't have to break a sweat to sharpen your eye-hand coordination; lots of fun activities can help. You could

- play catch with a friend
- bounce a ball against a wall
- play cornhole (a beanbag game)
- take up juggling

- play darts (magnetic darts are a safe choice)
- sew or knit
- paint or draw a picture
- play a video game.

Adapting activities

If any of these activities seem too challenging, you may be able to modify them to make them easier. For example: "If a ball is too small for catch, blow up a balloon and hit it back and forth," Packard suggests. "Play pickleball instead of tennis, since the pickleball court is smaller and you don't have to cover as much ground to hit the ball. Or play Ping-Pong with a pickleball or a light plastic baseball, which may be easier to hit than a Ping-Pong ball."

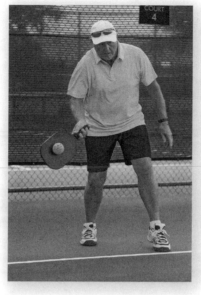

Tennis too hard? Try pickleball.

If you need assistance, occupational therapists can help you modify activities and create programs tailored to your coordination needs. Insurance may cover services only if they're medically necessary; ask your doctor if you qualify.

Whether you're training with a therapist or on your own, make your practice more challenging over time; use a smaller ball or try a more difficult activity. "If you can increase the challenge once a month, that's an impressive feat," Packard points out.

The big benefit: a carryover into your daily activities, such as driving or grocery shopping. "Reduced eye-hand coordination is not something you have to accept," Dr. Budson says. "You can start improving it right now."

Fitness with a function

Add these exercises to your workout routine to improve everyday movements.

Each day you bend, reach, twist, lift, walk, and squat. If you exercise regularly, you may think you address these basic abilities, commonly known as functional fitness.

"Yet, many conventional exercises focus on building individual muscles. While that's important, it doesn't always work on improving how well those muscles move in everyday life," says Dr. Amy Lo, an assistant scientist at Harvard-affiliated Hebrew SeniorLife's Hinda and Arthur Marcus Institute for Aging Research. "If you don't devote enough attention to supporting daily movements, you can have trouble staying active and engaging in even the simplest parts of life."

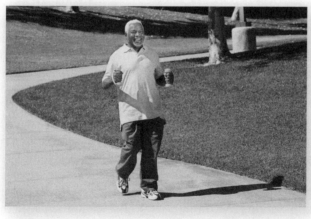

Holding dumbbells while walking makes workouts more challenging.

All day, every day

Functional fitness encompasses not only individual movements, but also how your entire body moves. "The actions required for daily living require multiple muscles, bones, and joints working independently and together in various ways," says Dr. Lo.

To see functional fitness in action, look no further than a grocery store visit. You squat and twist to get in and out of a car, push a cart, reach and bend to pick up items, and lift and carry groceries. "You might take this routine for granted, but if you have problems in just one area, it can make the entire process harder to perform and affect your quality of life," says Dr. Lo.

You can add a few exercises to your daily routine to improve functional fitness. Dr. Lo recommends including the following exercises to your regular workout or performing them on their own.

"They can help strengthen the key muscles needed for optimal functional fitness and let you practice how to better perform daily movements," she says. "Remember that no matter your age or fitness level, there is always something you can do to improve how you move through life."

Walking

Don't underestimate the far-reaching benefits of placing one foot in front of the other. "A regular walking routine not only improves leg strength and endurance, but is a great way to measure your current fitness and note improvements," says Dr. Lo.

It doesn't matter how far or how long you walk. If you are new to walking as fitness, begin with 10 to 20 minutes at home, around your block, or on a treadmill. "You can even break up your walks and do some in the morning and afternoon, or in the evening after dinner," says Dr. Lo.

For more of a challenge, keep track of your time, distance, or steps taken, and try to improve your numbers. Another option is to add several sets of walking lunges during your outing or walk while carrying lightweight dumbbells. To help improve balance and coordination, do a walking routine in your home where you navigate around objects like couches, tables, and chairs.

Sit-to-stand

"This is a great exercise since we execute this movement several times each day, from getting in

How functional are your movements? Do a self-exam

Always pay attention to which daily actions suddenly become more difficult, says Dr. Amy Lo of Harvard-affiliated Hebrew SeniorLife. For example, take note if you don't always make a smooth transition from a seated to standing position or if you have trouble twisting (especially to one side) or moving your arms in specific directions, like outward, across your body, or above your head. "If you notice any limitations, consult a physical therapist or certified personal trainer who specializes in an older clientele," says Dr. Lo. "A professional evaluation and analysis of your movements can identify areas of weakness that may need extra attention with specialized exercises."

and out of bed to rising out of a chair to driving," says Dr. Lo.

Sit on the edge of a chair with your hands crossed over your chest. Keep your feet flat on the floor, shoulder-width apart, and bring your toes underneath your knees. Lean forward slightly and press your heels into the floor as you slowly stand. Pause, and then sit in the same slow and controlled manner. Do this five to 10 times. If you need assistance standing, place your hands on your thighs or the chair's armrests for support.

For a challenge, hold a medicine ball in front of you as you sit and stand, or put a pillow under your feet.

Chair twists and arm raises

Twists and arm raises help with your upper body's range of motion.

For twists, sit tall in a chair with your feet on the floor. Hold a medicine ball or an object of similar weight—like a book or a large filled water bottle—in front of your body, with your arms extended and elbows slightly bent. Twist to the right until the ball or object is over your right hip, or as far as comfortable. Turn your head and neck as you follow its movement. Rotate only your upper body and not your hips or legs. Pause, and then return to the starting position. Repeat the same twist-and-return motion to your left. Do this sequence five to 10 times. You also can perform this exercise while standing.

For arm raises, hold the object with your arms extended in front of you at shoulder height, and then raise your arms overhead. Pause, and then return to the starting position. Repeat about five to 10 times. You also can do the movement without holding anything; just raise your arms and stretch them overhead as high as possible.

Steps to stay safe when you push or pull an object

Follow these instructions to get the job done and avoid injury.

Pushing or pulling heavy objects is often part of everyday activity—such as pulling open a car door or pushing furniture out of the way to vacuum. The keys to maintaining your push-and-pull success are simple: keep your core and leg muscles strong, and use the proper positioning.

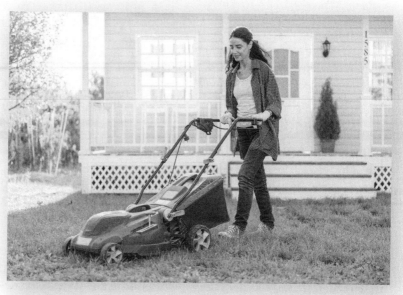

Tighten your abdominals and keep your elbows against your body as you push a heavy object.

Strong core and leg muscles

Your core and leg muscles give you power and stability when pushing or pulling. These muscles include the

- transverse abdominis in your abdomen
- quadriceps in the front of the thighs
- hamstrings in the back of the thighs
- gluteals in the buttocks
- gastrocnemius and soleus in the calves.

If those muscles are weak, you risk back injury when you push or pull a heavy object. "You might overcompensate and arch your back when pulling, or bend forward if you're pushing. That will put stress on your lower back, which can cause spasms, pinched nerves, or bulging or herniated discs," explains Stephanie O'Brien, a physical therapist with Harvard-affiliated Spaulding Rehabilitation Network.

Strengthening ideas

O'Brien says walking is an easy way to keep core and leg muscles strong. "Try to walk 30 minutes once a day or 15 minutes twice a day. You can start with five or 10 minutes and build endurance slowly," she suggests.

O'Brien also recommends performing a muscle-strengthening routine three times per week, such as working out on weight machines in a gym, or using dumbbells and doing body-weight exercises (like modified push-ups or squats) at home. One simple abdominal muscle-strengthening exercise she recommends is called abdominal bracing. "Pull your stomach muscles in, squeeze [contract] them, and hold the squeeze for five seconds. Relax and do it again, 10 to 15 times in a row," O'Brien suggests. You can do this while sitting and reading.

Pushing stance

Make sure you use the right positioning to push a heavy object.

- Stand close to the object you want to push.
- Keep your knees slightly bent, with one leg slightly behind the other so you can push off with it.
- Brace your elbows against your sides.
- Tighten your abdominal muscles.
- Push the object forward.

"Let the power come from your core and legs, and walk forward to move the object," O'Brien advises. "And don't arch your back. Stand up straight, with your shoulders and hips in a straight line."

Pulling stance

If you need to pull an object using two hands, try this method:

- Face the object you're pulling.

- Keep your knees slightly bent and your feet close to the object, hip-width apart.
- Brace your elbows against your sides, and put your hands on the object.
- Tighten your abdominal muscles and take a step backward, pulling the object with you.

"Don't twist or arch your back. Pull with your core and leg muscles," O'Brien says.

If you pull an object using one hand (like a heavy car door), O'Brien recommends standing with one leg slightly behind the other, tightening your abdominal muscles, pulling with your arm, and shifting your weight onto your back leg.

Tips to keep in mind

When you have the choice of pushing or pulling an object—such as pulling versus pushing a cart—go for the pushing option. "Pushing is safer," O'Brien

KNEE LIFT

Stand up straight with your feet together. Hold the back of a chair for support. Tighten your abdominal muscles and exhale as you lift your right knee to hip height. Hold, then lower your foot to the floor. Repeat the move 8-10 times, then repeat the process with your left leg.

says. "People can push about twice as much as they can pull."

If you're generally healthy and the steps to push or pull aren't working, go through the checklist again. "Listen to your body, or think about your posture," O'Brien says. "Have you activated your core muscles? Did you skip a step? If it hurts to move something, don't do it."

Likewise, don't attempt to move an object if you have significant balance issues or you use an assistive walking device (such as a walker). "You don't want to move a heavy object and fall," O'Brien says. "Instead, ask for help."

IN THE JOURNALS

Tai chi offers similar benefits as conventional exercise

Tai chi helps improve balance and coordination, especially among older adults. Now, a study published June 1, 2021, in *Annals of Internal Medicine* has shown that the ancient mind-body practice also offers much the same health benefits as conventional exercise.

Researchers randomly divided 543 obese people, ages 50 and older, into three groups. One practiced tai chi, another worked out with a combination of aerobic and strength training, and the third did not exercise. The tai chi participants followed the common form of slow continuous circular movements known as Yang style. The exercisers did brisk walking and strength-training workouts, such as arm curls and raises, shoulder presses, squats, and heel raises. Both groups did one-hour sessions, three times a week, for 12 weeks.

Afterward, people in both the exercise and tai chi groups had similar reductions in waist size, body weight, and cholesterol levels compared with the control group. It's not clear how tai chi helps, but the researchers noted that the gentle, flowing motions are ideal for people who have trouble staying active and may help them stick with regular exercise.

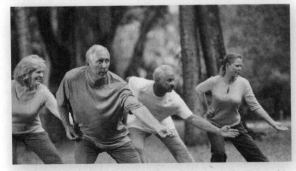

The physical benefits from practicing tai chi go far beyond improving balance and coordination.

Gentle exercises for older, frail people

For older people with heart-related issues, strength and balance exercises may help prevent falls and preserve independence.

Exercise can boost both the duration and quality of your life, especially if you start when you're young and keep at it. But as people age, heart disease or other health problems sometimes derail exercise routines. The resulting loss of muscle and endurance often contributes to frailty, which affects about a quarter of people after age 85 but can also occur at younger ages (see "What is frailty?").

Because frailty often develops gradually, it can be overlooked. "It's usually a family member who notices that the person is looking a little less steady or walking more slowly than usual," says Darlene Harrier, a physical therapist at Harvard-affiliated Beth Israel Deaconess Medical Center.

Realistic options

But if you—or your spouse, partner, or parent—is frail, don't assume there's nothing you can do about it.

For people who've had a heart attack or heart procedure, cardiac rehabilitation might be an option. However, this supervised exercise and lifestyle program involves hourlong sessions several times a week for several months. As such, it probably isn't realistic for people who are frail.

Instead, consider working with a physical therapist, who can provide safe, personalized exercise coaching to help people regain strength and mobility. "Primary care doctors and geriatricians are often happy to refer their patients to physical therapists," says Harrier. They want to keep them as independent as possible and minimize their risk of falling, she adds. During a session, physical therapists can check a person's heart rate, breathing rate, blood pressure,

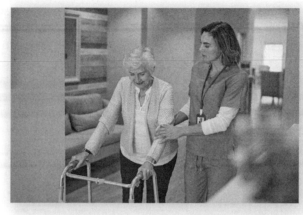

Frail, older people should consult a physical therapist for exercise advice.

and oxygen saturation at rest and then after a short period of exercise. "We want to make sure you're exercising at an appropriate level," says Harrier.

Heart disease and frailty

Expert guidance and monitoring is particularly important for people with cardiovascular problems. Coronary artery disease may limit

What is frailty?

Clinicians use the term "frail" to describe people ages 65 and older with age-related physical decline that leaves them vulnerable to injuries and other health problems. Although we usually think of frail people as being thin, people who are overweight or obese also can be frail. In fact, overweight frail people may be even weaker than their slimmer counterparts because their muscle has been replaced with fat, and they have extra weight to move around.

According to one widely accepted definition, you are considered frail if you meet three of the following criteria:

▶ You have lost 10 or more pounds in the past year without trying.

▶ You have trouble standing without assistance or have a weak grip.

▶ You walk slowly; it takes you more than six or seven seconds to walk 15 feet.

▶ You feel exhausted often and can't get going three or more days most weeks.

▶ You aren't very active; household chores and activities you once did for fun feel too challenging.

© Ridofranz | Getty Images

exercise capacity, leading to chest pain or short-ness of breath even at low levels of effort among those who are frail. Other cardiac conditions such as a narrowed heart valve or a heart rhythm disor-der can leave people more vulnerable to dizziness or fainting, which increases the risk of falling. And falls are especially dangerous for people taking anti-clotting medications (which are prescribed for many heart problems) because these drugs increase the risk of bleeding.

Gentle exercise examples

Walking—even at a slow pace and with a cane or a walker, if needed—can help build stamina. Sim-ple strength exercises can be done while sitting in a chair or even lying in bed so you don't have to get up off the floor afterward, says Harrier.

Two leg-strengthening exercises she recommends are clamshells and bridges. Clamshells are done lying on your side with your knees bent and rais-ing and lowering only your top knee while keeping your feet together. For a bridge, lie on your back with your knees bent, then lift and hold your buttocks off the ground. You can also do mini-crunches on your back to engage your core muscles—just reach up to your bent knees with your fingertips. To build arm strength, make fists and do punches, both straight ahead and over your head, while seated in a chair.

If balance is a challenge, here's an exercise to try. Stand with your back in a corner, with the back of a chair facing you so you're supported on all sides. Practice standing with your feet close together, then one in front of another, and if possible, on one foot at a time.

Cycling: A low-impact exercise that helps the heart

From small, under-desk cycles to high-tech stationary bikes, there's a pedaling machine to suit all fitness levels.

They say you never for-get how to ride a bike. So even if you haven't ridden one in decades, you might be pleasantly surprised to find it easy to take up cycling later in life. More good news: Recent research suggests this popular exercise may help people live longer (see "Cycling linked to lower risk of death from heart disease" on the next page).

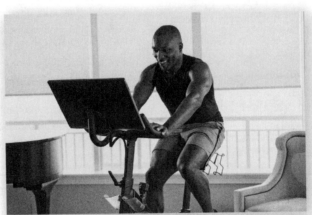

Some stationary bikes feature touchscreens to play live or recorded fitness classes.

© kali9 | Getty Images

and Women's Hospital. Because cycling causes less wear and tear on your joints, many people find they can continue to ride long after they've had to stop jogging, he adds.

When it's too dark, cold, rainy, or snowy to cycle safely outside, using an indoor cycling machine is a convenient way to stay fit. These machines are also ideal for people with physical limitations (such as mobility or balance issues) that make it difficult to ride a traditional bike. There's a variation to accommodate nearly everyone, from peo-ple with low fitness levels or limited mobility to those who want a challenging, heart-pumping workout.

Riding a bike outdoors offers other rewards as well, including fresh air and varied scenery. But there are also some downsides, including traffic and inclem-ent weather. "Cycling can be a great way to stay fit and strong, especially if there's a bike path or a road with less traffic where you can ride," says Dr. Brendan Everett, a cardiologist at Harvard-affiliated Brigham

During the pandemic, many people have avoided gyms and fitness centers, opting instead to buy home machines. Here's a rundown of a few options.

Under-desk cycling machines. These small, portable machines can be tucked under your desk or placed in front of any chair. Easy to use with low resistance levels, they're good for people who are older or who have a limited range of motion due to an injury, arthritis, or another health condition. No-frills models start around $40, or you can pay more for features such as a monitor that tracks your speed and time.

Stationary recumbent cycles. These machines allow you to pedal in a semi-reclined position, which puts less strain on your back, hips, and knee joints. The seat is wider, lower, and more comfortable than a traditional bike. But you still exercise the same muscles (thighs, calves, and buttocks) and raise your heart rate. Basic models start around $250, but high-tech, fancier versions with many added features can run as much as $1,800.

Stationary upright bikes. These machines more closely resemble a traditional bike, with the pedals positioned under your body. Upright bikes also work your core muscles—especially if you switch between standing and sitting while pedaling.

For a full-body workout, you can choose a dual-action stationary bike, with handlebars that move back and forth so you exercise your arms while you pedal. Prices are similar to the recumbent bikes or higher. The more expensive models include touchscreen

Cycling linked to lower risk of death from heart disease

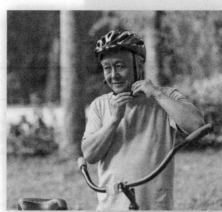

People who ride bicycles regularly may have a lower risk of heart disease.

Regular cycling outdoors may help people with diabetes—a strong predictor of cardiovascular disease—lower their odds of premature death from any cause, including heart disease, a recent study finds. Published online July 19, 2021, by *JAMA Internal Medicine*, the study included more than 7,400 people from 10 Western European countries who were part of a large observational study that began in 1992. On average, the participants were 56 years old and had diabetes for nearly eight years. After an average follow-up of 15 years, about 1,700 people had died; 800 of these were heart-related deaths. After adjusting for confounding factors, researchers found that cycling between one and five hours per week was linked to a 20% to 30% lower risk of death from all causes compared with no cycling.

displays so you can watch live or recorded classes led by fitness instructors; most also require a monthly fee for this service.

Easy exercises to shore up your core

Adding a few simple moves to your daily routine can help you strengthen your midsection.

Many people think that core exercises mainly target your belly, but there's much more to your core. It also includes the muscles in your back, sides, pelvis, hips, and buttocks. "Think of your core as all the muscles that help stabilize your trunk so your limbs can move," says Eric L'Italien, a physical therapist and certified strength and conditioning coach with the Harvard-affiliated Spaulding Rehabilitation Network.

A strong core helps support cardiovascular health by helping you stay active. First, many physical activities and sports depend on a stable, flexible core, including cycling, golf, tennis and other racquet sports, and swimming. Second, core exercises (if done regularly) may also help prevent low back pain, which affects four in five Americans at some point in their lives. Back pain is one of the most common reasons people see a doctor—and a major reason people don't exercise.

Easier options

However, some popular core exercises done on the floor, such as planks and crunches, may be too challenging for older people and those who aren't very physically active. (Planks involve holding the "up" part of a push-up, while crunches are variations of sit-ups.) But there are other ways to improve your core strength that don't require you to get down on the ground. "Any movement that requires you to control and stabilize your trunk while moving your legs or arms will train your core," says L'Italien.

Check with your doctor before starting a

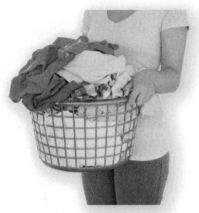

You can use a laundry basket for walk-and-carry exercises to strengthen your core muscles.

program of core exercise if you've had hip or back surgery or pain, or if you have heart disease or another chronic health condition. Two easy exercises, the chair stand and the standing side leg lift (see photos), are good options for people who are just getting started with core training.

Carry that weight

To strengthen your entire core, L'Italien also recommends walk-and-carry exercises (also referred to as loaded carries), in which you hold a weight or another heavy object in one or both hands while you walk for short distances. "I like these exercises because they train your core really well and they also simulate real-life activities, such as carrying groceries or a laundry basket," he says. In fact, you can use those or similar items instead of dumbbells during the exercises.

Choosing the correct weight is important, says L'Italien. It should be heavy enough that you feel like you need to stabilize your abs to stay steady, but not so heavy that you feel any discomfort. Make sure your spine—including your neck—stays straight and you don't slouch or lean forward, backward, or to one side.

For each of the three examples below, walk for 30 to 60 seconds, remembering to breathe and keep the tension in your abs as you move. Put down the weight and rest for at least 30 seconds. Repeat the walk once or twice more.

Laundry basket carry. Stand up straight and hold a either a dumbbell or a full or partly filled laundry basket in front of your body, keeping your elbows and upper arms close to your body.

Farmer's carry. For this carry (so named because it mimics a farmer carrying buckets of milk), you hold either a dumbbell or a bag of groceries in each hand, with your arms

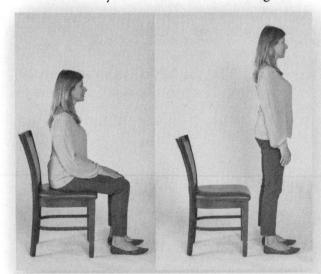

Chair stand

Sit in a chair with your feet hip-width apart, with your hands on your thighs. Tighten your belly muscles and buttocks. Slowly stand up, then sit down with control. Repeat 7 to 9 times.

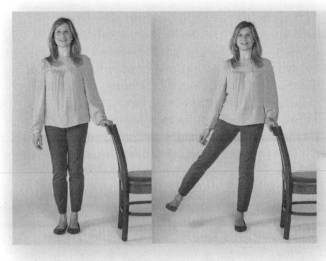

Standing side leg lift

Stand next to a chair, holding the back with your left hand. Keep your weight balanced on both feet. Slowly lift your right leg to the side until your foot is about six inches off the floor. Hold and return to starting position. Repeat 7 to 9 times, then repeat with the left leg.

down by your sides.

Suitcase carry. This is done like the farmer's carry, except you hold a weight or bag in only one hand while your other hand is free. Having all the weight on one side forces your core muscles to work a little harder so that you don't lean. Do two to three walks with the weight on each side.

For more information and many more core exercises, see the Harvard Health Publishing Special Health Report *Gentle Core Exercises* (www.health.harvard.edu/GC).

Keep exercise-related injuries from derailing your workouts

You can prevent many common injuries by incorporating these seven simple strategies into your routine.

Whether it's knee pain, a sore elbow, or a pulled muscle, exercise-related injuries are common in people of all ages. They can derail your fitness efforts, sometimes setting you back for weeks or months.

Often these injuries are preventable, says Dr. Beth Frates, clinical assistant professor of physical medicine and rehabilitation at Harvard Medical School. Below she offers some tips that can help you stay healthy and keep you moving toward your fitness goals.

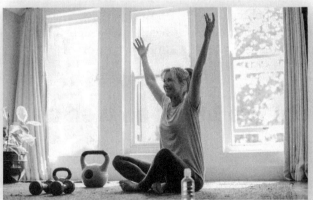

Safety first is rule No. 1 for starting any exercise program so you can stay with it for the long haul.

Select a low-impact activity. While no activity completely eliminates the risk of injury, it's less likely you'll get hurt doing a low-impact exercise that puts less strain on your joints. Walking, swimming, or indoor cycling are all good low-impact options, says Dr. Frates. The highest risk of injury comes from contact sports, such as football, ice hockey, basketball, or soccer. But injuries are also common in high-impact, non-contact sports, such as running.

Choose the right shoes. Blisters, foot pain, and joint injuries can sometimes stem from wearing the wrong type of footwear. It's also easy to run into trouble if your footwear doesn't fit properly. Try to match your shoes to your activity. If you're going running, for example, choose sneakers that have extra cushioning and support. If you're heading out for a hike, put on sturdy footwear that provides good traction and keeps your feet stable. Ankle sprains can result from poor form, missteps, footwear that doesn't support the ankle, or exercising on uneven surfaces, says Dr. Frates. If you're having foot pain, see your doctor. He or she may recommend custom orthotics or shoe inserts.

Start low, go slow. Start any new exercise program gradually. If you're strength training, begin with a small amount of weight and add more as you get stronger. The same goes for a cardiovascular workout. "Add time, then add frequency, and then increase intensity slowly," says Dr. Frates. Too much, too soon can do more harm than good.

Loosen up. Don't jump right off the couch and into a high-intensity workout, says Dr. Frates. Give your body time to adjust by performing a short 5-minute warm up. "Going from being sedentary to vigorous activity is the time you are at greatest risk not just for injury, but also for heart attack," she says. At the end of an exercise session, also take five minutes to slowly cool down, she says.

Mix it up. Injuries can arise if you do the same activity all the time. For example, someone who plays golf six days a week may be more prone to a type of tendinitis (inflammation or irritation of the tendons) called medial epicondylitis—popularly known as golfer's elbow. The same is true of other activities, such as running and tennis, which often trigger repetitive strain injuries. Tennis players commonly develop another type of tendinitis called lateral epicondylitis (tennis elbow), and runners are prone to iliotibial band syndrome, which causes pain on the outside of the knee, says Dr. Frates.

Instead, try a cross-training approach, she says. Play tennis, but also walk, swim, or do yoga. This will not only protect against repetitive strain injuries, but also benefit different parts of the body, which can help your overall fitness. "Working on all four types of exercise—aerobic, strength training, balance training, and flexibility—will help keep your body in good shape," says Dr. Frates.

Check your form. Using an exercise machine or weights incorrectly can lead to muscle or joint problems. Keeping your body in the proper position when you're on a machine or doing strength training can keep you injury-free. If you are starting a new activity at your local gym, check in with an on-site trainer to make sure you are using the equipment properly, says Dr. Frates. Also watch for proper form and body alignment in a mirror.

Drink up. Staying well hydrated during exercise can keep you from experiencing dehydration-induced dizziness or unsteadiness that can trigger a fall. "Exercising when you are not well nourished is also not advised, as you will be weak and find it harder to keep your balance, which may lead to injury," says Dr. Frates. Protecting your overall health puts you in a better position to reap the benefits of your workout.

Exercise may heal the heart as well as prevent future problems

A daily walk and twice-weekly strength training can help to reverse heart stiffness and improve cardiovascular health.

When it comes to heart health, a lot of the focus is rightly on prevention. Eat right and exercise, and you'll have a healthier heart when you get older. But what if you're already older and your heart is showing signs of trouble? Is exercise going to do anything to help you?

As it turns out, the answer may be yes.

"Because physical activity has physiological benefits for the heart, it can not only help prevent, but also reverse some of the earlier damage to the heart and blood vessels," says Dr. JoAnn Manson, the Michael and Lee Bell Professor of Women's Health at Harvard

Medical School.

One study, published Sept. 21, 2021, in the journal *Circulation*, showed that a yearlong exercise program helped improve heart health in people who had heart-related changes that put them at increased risk for heart failure.

People in the study had a condition called left ventricular hypertrophy, which is a thickening of the left chamber of the heart. This condition makes it harder for it to pump blood efficiently. They also had elevated levels of cardiac biomarkers—certain chemicals in the blood that indicate heart injury or increased risk of heart failure. People with these conditions often go on to develop a specific type of heart failure, called heart failure with preserved ejection fraction. The study's authors set out to see

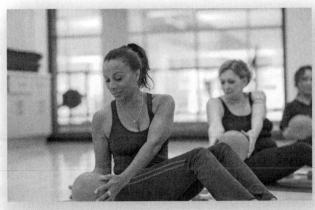

Regular exercise not only helps maintain a healthy heart, it may also help heal a damaged one.

© FatCamera | Getty Images

if exercise could help improve heart health in this situation.

The researchers enrolled 46 people between the ages of 45 and 64 and randomly assigned them to either a year of high-intensity exercise training or to a control group, whose members did yoga, balance training, and light resistance exercises.

Those in the exercise group got individualized exercise plans based on their fitness levels, worked with a personal trainer, and used heart rate monitors. They walked, swam, or cycled at least three times a week for 30 to 60 minutes. They used a strategy called interval training, which involves alternating between short periods of vigorous exercise and lower-intensity

---

© adamkaz | Getty Images

IN THE JOURNALS

Leisure time exercise better than work-related physical activity

Although exercise guidelines encourage all types of physical activity, a recent study suggests that while leisure-time activity promotes cardiovascular health, job-related activity does not.

The study included more than 104,000 men and women ages 20 to 100 living in Copenhagen who rated their leisure and work-related physical activity as low, moderate, high, or very high.

After an average follow-up of 10 years, researchers found that the more leisure-time activity people reported, the lower their risk of experiencing a heart attack or stroke. In contrast, the people who got most of their physical activity on the job were more

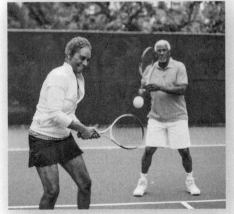

likely to experience those cardiovascular problems. These findings held after researchers adjusted for factors such as lifestyle habits, health conditions (such as high blood pressure and high cholesterol), and socioeconomic status that could sway the results.

One possible explanation: compared with leisure exercise, work activity doesn't raise a person's heart rate enough to improve fitness. The study was published April 9, 2021, in the *European Heart Journal*.

periods throughout a workout, and which has been shown to lead to larger improvements in cardiovascular fitness compared with other types of exercise. The exercisers also did strength training once or twice per week.

All of the participants underwent heart imaging and tests designed to assess the flexibility of their heart muscle at the start of the trial and again at the end of the training program. After a year, the researchers found that the hearts of the people who participated in the exercise program had become less rigid and were more efficient at pumping blood than those of the control group members. The researchers said that this led them to believe that

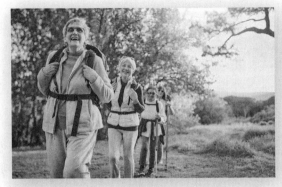

Walking is a great form of exercise to help keep your heart in shape.

exercise training could help protect against heart failure, but they added that a year wasn't enough time to assess long-term outcomes and more study is needed.

Exercise and the heart

It's not surprising that the researchers found improvements, given all the heart-related benefits of exercise, such as reducing blood pressure, says Dr. Manson.

"If you are already healthy, exercise can keep you that way. But exercise can also help you lose weight, decrease damaging inflammation inside your body, reduce insulin resistance, and improve your blood flow," she says. "All of those things could help reduce cardiac stiffness."

Research has also shown that sitting around for long periods of the day and a lack of regular physical activity can take a toll on heart health. A sedentary lifestyle can lead to weight gain, a higher risk of hypertension, diabetes, and high cholesterol. These conditions, in turn, increase the risk of atherosclerosis, heart attack, stroke, heart failure, and even atrial fibrillation (a type of irregular heartbeat), says Dr. Manson. They are all interrelated.

"Physical activity is probably as close as we've come to a magic bullet for good health," she says. "It can favorably influence multiple biological pathways and risk factors very early in the process to prevent development of diabetes, obesity, and atherosclerosis. As a result, you will have a much lower risk of heart attack and stroke."

Even at the molecular level there are many benefits to regular exercise, she says. It improves the ability of the cells to respond to insulin and can enhance the function of

It's not too late to get your heart into shape

No matter when you start exercising or what condition you're in when you start, know that it can improve your health, even if you already have heart problems.

"Cardiac rehabilitation is extremely beneficial in reducing cardiovascular death in people who have had heart attacks or heart failure," says Dr. JoAnn Manson, the Michael and Lee Bell Professor of Women's Health at Harvard Medical School. And remember, even if you have a family history of cardiovascular disease, that doesn't necessarily mean you will end up going down the same road.

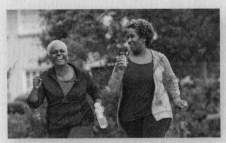

Exercise can benefit your heart no matter when you start.

"The point that I often make is that heredity isn't destiny. Many people do have a family history of heart disease and certain medical conditions. They think they're predestined to develop these problems, too. But one of the most important things you can do in terms of modifying your risk and taking control of your health is to be physically active," says Dr. Manson.

Ultimately, there are two things that people should remember when it comes to exercise: "It's never too late to start, and it's also never too early to start," says Dr. Manson.

blood vessels—for example, by improving their ability to dilate. Physical activity also reduces inflammation within the blood vessels, the body, and tissues.

What type and how much?

A heart-healthy exercise program is one that includes both cardiovascular exercise and strength training, says Dr. Manson. If you've had a heart attack or are at high risk for cardiovascular problems, it's best to run your exercise program by your doctor before you get started.

"Walking is typically a great option for most people, regardless of their health history," says Dr. Manson. She points to a study, published online Sept. 3, 2021, by *JAMA Network Open*, that found that people who took 7,000 or more steps a day were less likely to die prematurely than those who came in under that 7,000-step mark.

Researchers asked 2,110 participants ages 38 to 50 to wear a tracking device for seven consecutive days. They were divided into low, moderate, and high step groups and then followed for an average of almost 11 years. In that time, 72 people died. The researchers found that people who took fewer steps—less than 7,000 a day—were more likely to die during the follow-up period than those who were in the moderate (7,000 to 9,999) or high (10,000 or more) daily step ranges. Walking intensity didn't seem to affect death rates.

In general, people should aim to do at least 30 minutes a day of walking, which adds up to 150 minutes of moderate to vigorous activity each week. However, if you're at increased risk of cardiovascular disease due to risk factors such as hypertension, you should aim for more—closer to 45 minutes over the course of the day, says Dr. Manson. If you are trying to lose weight, try to fit in 45 to 60 minutes a day.

"It definitely doesn't have to be done at the same time. Break it into 10- to 15-minute bouts of exercise several times a day," she says.

Strength training twice a week is also recommended.

Also try to minimize the amount of sitting around you're doing during the day. Sitting for nine to 10 hours a day has been linked to increased heart risks, says Dr. Manson. If you work at a computer, get up and walk around at regular intervals (such as every 30 to 60 minutes), invest in a standing desk, or walk when you are on the phone.

"You can still be active even when you have a desk job," says Dr. Manson. Regular exercise can offset many of the risks of sitting. "You can mitigate some of that risk by being physically active at other times of the day," she says.

How low can you go?

What's the shortest amount of time you can exercise and gain benefits?

Everyone wants to do more in less time. This is especially true when it comes to exercise. Why work out for an hour if you can get the same benefit in half the time?

That's the attraction of short-duration high-intensity interval training (HIIT), which research has found produces similar—and possibly better—health outcomes than longer, lower-intensity exercise. HIIT consists of quick spurts of draining physical effort, followed by rest, repeated multiple times. HIIT workouts usually last from 15 to 30 minutes, compared with up to an hour of traditional lower-intensity exercises.

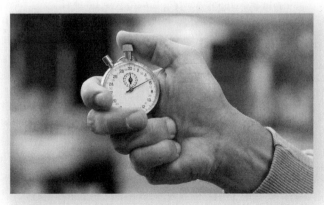

Time efficiency and intensity are key to getting the most from shorter high-intensity interval training.

But now, science has explored whether you can shrink that 15- to 30-minute time frame even more without sacrificing gains. In other words, how low can you go? It turns out possibly quite low.

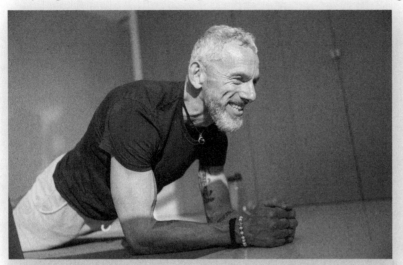

Five by five

Want to try low-volume HIIT training? Here is an all-around routine to begin with that uses familiar exercises. Perform 10 to 12 reps for each of the five exercises. Go from one to the next with only a 10-second break in between. Once you have completed all five exercises, repeat the sequence for five minutes.

Angle push-ups. Do them against a countertop or wall, so your body is positioned at a 45° angle. You can also do push-ups on the floor, regular or from the knees.

Chair squats. These replicate the motion of standing from a seated position. Stand in front of chair like you are going to sit. Lower down into a squat until you barely touch the seat, and then come back up.

Floor dips. Sit on the floor with bent knees. Place your hands behind you with the fingers pointing toward your body. Lift your hips off the floor. Now, slowly bend your elbows, lower your body close to the floor, and slowly push back up.

Lunges. Stand with your feet shoulder-width apart. Step forward with one leg and bend it until your knee is aligned over the front of your foot. The trailing knee should drop toward the floor. Hold for a few seconds, and then return to the starting position. Repeat with the opposite leg forward to complete one rep. Stand next to a wall for support if needed.

Plank pose. Lie face down with your forearms resting on the floor. Raise up your body, so it forms a straight line from your head and neck to your feet. Hold for 15 to 30 seconds. You can also hold the plank from a full push-up position, or on your forearms with your knees on the ground.

Short and sweet

A review published online March 24, 2021, by *The Journal of Physiology* looked at various trials involving HIIT workouts lasting less than 15 minutes, which the authors called low-volume HIIT.

They found that, compared with both regular HIIT training and moderate-intensity aerobic exercise, these shorter-duration HIIT workouts can produce equal or even greater improvements in various measures of health, like cardiorespiratory fitness, glucose control, and blood pressure.

Another study, in the October 2020 *Diabetes Care,* showed that as little as four minutes of low-volume HIIT, three times a week for 12 weeks, could lower blood sugar levels, reduce fat in the liver, and improve cardiorespiratory fitness in people with diabetes. These results were comparable to those from 45 minutes of moderate-intensity cardio exercise.

All the right moves

But are these shorter HIIT workouts really the best moves? While the idea of a five- to 10-minute workout may sound appealing, HIIT workouts have their challenges, especially for older adults.

"Intensity is the key with any variation of HIIT," says physical therapist Vijay Daryanani with Harvard's Spaulding Rehabilitation Network. "A sufficient level of exertion needs to be met for the exercises to be effective."

Also, "high intensity" can be difficult to judge. You want to work out hard enough to get the heart pumping to the point where you're close to exhaustion, but without risking injury or overdoing it, which can be dangerous for some older adults. (It's always best to check with your doctor first before fully engaging in a new routine like HIIT.)

Low-volume HIIT also requires keen attention to form and execution. "Since you work out for such a brief period, you have to ensure you maximize the moves for efficiency and safety," says Daryanani. He suggests first seeing a trainer to learn proper technique before doing any HIIT-based routine. A trainer can also help create a sequence of exercises to fit your needs and limitations.

Give yourself time

Still, approached the right way, low-volume HIIT that lasts five to 10 minutes can be a valuable tool for your workouts. While it's possible to make low-volume HIIT your primary exercise, Daryanani says it's better as a complement to your regular routine.

"Use it whenever you don't have the time for a regular workout to ensure you get in some kind of movement, or if you need a spark to jump-start your motivation, or just to shake things up."

If you do a low-volume HIIT session four days a week, then divide the routines: focus on your upper body one day and your lower body the next. If you do an HIIT workout once or twice a week, do an all-body routine each time. (See "Five by five" on the previous page for a sample workout.)

Perhaps the greatest appeal of low-volume HIIT is the reminder that doing something is always better than nothing. "A five- or 10-minute workout shows you are committed to your health, no matter how much time you have," says Daryanani.

High-intensity exercise and your heart

Brief bursts of strenuous exercise may be safe for some—but not all—older adults.

The fitness trend known as high-intensity interval training (HIIT) is still going strong, both at gyms and in online workout classes. HIIT features short bursts of high-intensity exercise (usually lasting one to four minutes) interspersed with periods of lower-intensity activity or rest. But is it a good idea for everyone? Not necessarily.

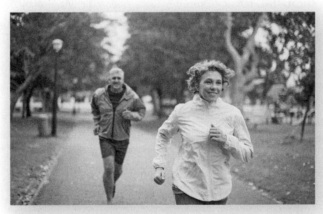

Adding stints of high-intensity exercise to a workout may improve some heart-related risk factors.

an exercise stress test to make sure people don't have symptoms such as chest pain, which might make strenuous exercise dangerous. Outside of such settings, HIIT may be unsafe for people who have or are at risk for heart disease.

One of the largest randomized controlled trials of HIIT, recently published in *BMJ Open*, suggests that healthy people in their 70s can do these workouts with little risk. But in terms of longevity, moderate-intensity exercise seems to be just as good.

"HIIT is a great regimen for people who are young and healthy. If you're older or have heart disease, check with your doctor before trying it," says Dr. I-Min Lee, a professor of medicine at Harvard Medical School and an expert on the role of physical activity in preventing disease.

Increasingly, cardiac rehabilitation programs (which help people recover from heart attacks and related conditions) are using tailored versions of HIIT. But these closely monitored sessions start with

A faster route to fitness

The main advantage to HIIT is that you can boost your cardiovascular fitness faster by working harder instead of longer. Some small, short-term studies hint that HIIT workouts can produce equal or greater improvements in blood pressure and blood sugar compared with moderate-intensity exercise. But because the duration and intensity of the interventions in these studies varied (as did the age and fitness levels of the participants), it's hard to generalize about the benefits, says Dr. Lee.

The *BMJ Open* study included 1,567 healthy, active Norwegians with an average age of 73. About half (the control group) were assigned to do 30 minutes of exercise most days. The rest got the same instructions, but half were assigned to replace two of the week's exercise sessions with HIIT workouts. The other half swapped in moderate-intensity continuous training twice weekly (see "A tale of two workouts").

Similar survival rates

During the five-year follow-up, just three people in the study had adverse events (injuries from slipping while exercising outdoors). There were no survival differences among the three groups, although there were slightly fewer deaths in the HIIT group. One possible explanation for the similarity in outcomes:

People in the control group exercised more than expected (including doing some high-intensity exercise), and only about half of those in the HIIT group actually did regular high-intensity workouts. Also, the people who agreed to participate in the study were more active than the general population, and they had a death rate that was about half of that expected in the general population of the same age.

The take-home message: If you get your doctor's okay, go ahead and try adding some high-intensity sessions into your workouts, whether that's jogging, cycling, swimming, or other aerobic exercise. But if that extra effort and sweat sound unpleasant, don't be concerned that you're missing out. "If doing HIIT fits in with your lifestyle, go for it. But the most important thing is to find an activity you enjoy and to keep doing it," says Dr. Lee.

A tale of two workouts

Researchers compared two workout strategies in healthy adults ages 70 to 77 during a five-year study in Norway (see main text for more details and results). The moderate-intensity continuous training workout involved exercising for 50 minutes. Participants aimed for a target heart rate of 70% of their estimated maximum heart rate. The "4×4" HIIT workout, which lasted 43 minutes, followed this pattern:

1. 10-minute warm-up (brisk walking or jogging) at 60% of maximum heart rate

2. Four minutes of high-intensity exercise at 85% to 95% of maximum heart rate

3. Three minutes of lower-intensity exercise (jogging or brisk walking) at 60% of maximum heart rate

4. Repeat steps 2 and 3 three times, for a total of 4 cycles

5. Five-minute cool-down.

Note: To get a rough idea of your maximum heart rate, subtract your age from 220. For 60%, multiply by 0.6; for 85%, multiply by 0.85, and so forth. As an example, the estimated maximum heart rate for a 75-year-old would be 220 – 75 = 145; 60% of that would be 145 × 0.6 = 87.

Master the stairs

Stair climbing is one of the best workouts to help with balance, endurance, and fall prevention.

Your ability to climb a flight of stairs is one of the great markers of health. It's often used to gauge your mobility and stamina, fitness level after an injury, and whether it's safe to resume sex after a heart attack.

But stair climbing can offer much more. "Stair climbing is an excellent form of overall exercise for older adults because it challenges multiple muscle groups at once, such as your quadriceps, glutes, and calves, as well as improves cardiovascular strength and endurance," says Michelle Munley, a physical therapist with Harvard's Spaulding Outpatient Center Peabody. "If you can safely and effectively navigate up and down stairs, you can stay more active in life."

Going up and down

There are different places where you can practice stair climbing, from gym stair machines to stairs in stairways and stadiums to basic household stairs. The type of stair doesn't necessarily matter, but keep in mind that not all steps are created equal in terms of height, depth,

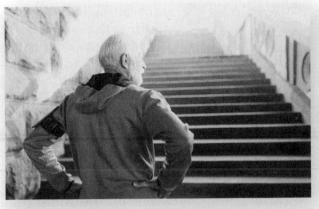

Improving how well you navigate stairs helps you stay active and safe.

and surfaces. Also, stairs that don't have rails are more challenging and potentially more dangerous. "Choose stairs in a comfortable environment using steps you feel safe negotiating," says Munley.

Also, going down stairs is just as important as going up. When you walk up the stairs, your glutes and quadriceps muscles perform concentric, or shortening, contractions. By contrast, when you walk down, the muscles perform the opposite—an eccentric, or lengthening, contraction. "Both movements are needed to provide optimal muscle strength and function," says Munley.

Stairways that are heaven

Consult your doctor before initiating a stair-climbing program, especially if you've had heart trouble, orthopedic conditions, or balance or mobility problems. Also, get comfortable with the stair-climbing movement by practicing step-ups (see "Taking small steps" on the next page).

When you are ready, here are three sample

IN THE JOURNALS

Another benefit of exercise: Eye comfort

In addition to many other health benefits, vigorous exercise may potentially help with dry, itchy eyes by boosting tear production and quality, a new study suggests.

The study included 52 adults, whom investigators categorized as either "athletes" or "nonathletes." Participants in the athlete group exercised at least five times a week, while non-athletes exercised no more than once a week.

All the participants engaged in a treadmill-based exercise session. The researchers performed eye exams just before and five minutes

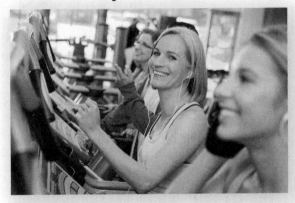

Move more to boost eye moisture.

after the sessions, measuring tear production and how long tear film on the eye remained stable before beginning to dry. While all participants experienced boosts in both tear amounts and quality after exercise, those in the athlete group showed greater benefits.

Healthy tear film not only keeps the eyes moist, but also protects them against irritants such as dust or dirt and dry spots that can lead to itching, stinging, or burning. The findings, published in the January 2022 issue of *Experimental Eye Research*, suggest that better physical fitness and longer periods of exercise might be important ways to enhance eye moisture.

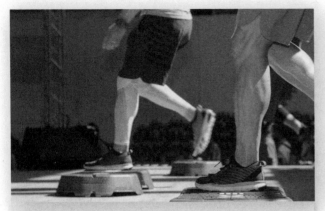

Taking small steps

Before you begin stair climbing, first practice with step-up exercises. Here, you step up and down using only one step, either on a real stairstep or using a piece of equipment called a step-up platform. (These platforms are broader and deeper than typical steps for easier use, and you can adjust the height. They are common in most gyms but can be purchased online or at sporting goods stores.)

"The motion of step-ups mimics the stair climbing movement, but with less effort, and can help people build up their strength and endurance before moving up to regular stair climbing," says physical therapist Michelle Munley with Harvard's Spaulding Outpatient Center Peabody. "And some people who are uneasy about climbing a full flight can feel more confident seeing only one step instead of 12."

workouts you can try that use a gym stair-climbing machine or outdoor or household steps with rails.

Steady climbing. Set a stair-climbing machine to a comfortable resistance level and speed, and climb for five to 10 minutes. Lower or increase the speed as needed. Over time, try to increase your minutes, resistance level, or both.

Intervals. Begin the stair machine at a comfortable speed as a warm-up. Increase your speed or resistance to reach a moderate-intensity level (about 5 to 7 on a 10-point exertion scale) and climb for one to two minutes. Then reduce the intensity to a comfortable level again and climb for two minutes, or long enough to bring down your heart rate. Continue alternating between the two speeds for 10 to 20 minutes.

Outside or in your home. Choose a comfortable stairway that includes a rail for balance. Set a timer on your watch or phone and walk up and down one or two flights at a steady pace for five to 10 minutes. As you improve, try to increase your time, climb without using a rail, or climb more flights at one time.

When stair climbing, always maintain good posture. Place your entire foot flat on the step. Don't climb using your toes, which can overtax your calves. Hold rails or machine handles as needed for support and balance, but avoid pulling yourself forward. As you progress, you can climb stairs without holding on, or challenge yourself using steps without rails, like stadium stairs.

A stair-climbing machine only allows you to walk in an upward motion. So Munley suggests complementing your stair-climbing workout with leg press machine exercises, which mimic the leg action of walking down stairs. "Stair climbing can be a demanding and intense exercise, so always begin slowly, never rush yourself, and take breaks when needed," says Munley.

Rowing or paddling after age 60

If you're new to these sports, or if you're returning to the water after time in dry dock, you'll want to know the risks.

There's something quite satisfying about dipping an oar or paddle into the water and pulling your craft along the surface. It's hard work that produces tangible results (moving from here to there). And when you add the calming element of nature and the camaraderie of working with others, rowing or paddling winds up being a great physical workout with many health benefits. Still, it comes with some risks to consider.

Types of activities

A variety of water sports involve either rowing or paddling. Rowing can be done with one or two oars. You can row in a long boat called a shell that accommodates two, four, or eight people; you operate just one oar in that setup. Or you can operate two oars in a smaller boat called a scull that accommodates one, two, or four people.

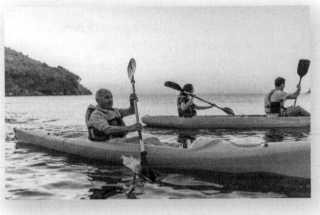

Paddling in a kayak or a canoe is a fun and effective way to strengthen your core muscles.

Paddling refers to water sports that use paddles. Single paddles, which have a flat blade at one end, are used in canoeing, dragon boat racing (with 10 or 20 people in a long canoe-like boat adorned with a dragon head and tail), and paddleboarding (standing or kneeling solo on a paddleboard, which looks like a wide surfboard).

A double paddle, which has a blade at both ends, is used in kayaking. Types of kayaks range from wide, flat recreational kayaks to long, skinny, streamlined kayaks called "surf skis" (a new trend among kayakers).

Benefits

Rowing and paddling have many health benefits.

They work your heart and lungs. Aerobic exercise helps build endurance and promotes cardiovascular health, mobility, better mood, and sharp cognition.

They use lots of muscle groups. "The activities are good for strength and coordination. Rowing mainly uses the legs and back, while paddling uses the core muscles to generate power for propulsion. Paddleboarding works the muscles in the buttocks and the sides of the trunk, and improves standing balance," explains Denise Frost, a long-time sculler, physical therapist, and director of Movement Health at Harvard-affiliated Spaulding Rehabilitation Hospital.

They promote socializing. Spending time with others counters isolation and loneliness, which are associated with chronic disease and premature death.

They help manage stress. Exercising and spending time in nature wards off chronic stress—a contributor to chronic inflammation, chronic disease, and premature death.

Risks after 60

While you might have jumped into a boat years ago, you need to use more caution now and consider the physical risks of rowing or paddling. "These sports have a repetitive component. Paddling can stress the shoulder tendons. Rowing can lead to low back strains," Frost says. "Neither sport is a good idea if you already have tendinitis at the shoulder, elbow, or wrist; a diagnosed back problem such as a disc injury or spinal stenosis; or a previous back surgery."

The sports might also be risky if you're not a good swimmer, haven't exercised in a long time, or have a heart or lung condition. Check with your doctor before getting involved in either sport.

Getting started

If you're interested in paddling or rowing, Frost says paddling might be the smarter way to go, since it can be as easy or demanding as you make it. Rowing, however, has a longer learning curve and is more physically demanding than paddling, so you'll need to be in good shape to try it. You should also wear

Rowing strengthens the leg and back muscles. It's more physically demanding than paddling.

sunblock and sunglasses; stay hydrated; and (during summer) restrict your participation in the activity to early mornings or late afternoons, to avoid getting overheated.

If you want to try paddling, Frost recommends renting the type of boat (such as a canoe or kayak) that interests you and taking a lesson to see if you like it. For dragon boat racing or rowing, Frost says it would be best to join a local club that offers introductory courses and could place you in a boat with similarly experienced teammates.

And even though paddling and rowing may look easy, remember that it takes time to learn a new skill and develop coordination. "You may feel strain and stiffness in many parts of your body as it adapts to new demands and forces," Frost says. "So start slowly, with shorter sessions, and build up your tolerance."

Tune in to better video workouts

Whether you are new to online exercise or want to make it part of your regular routine, here are 10 tips to follow.

One bright spot of the pandemic has been the growing availability of video exercises. Even now, many fitness centers still routinely offer livestreamed classes, and video workouts are more readily available online.

"Online workouts are ideal, as you can do them at your leisure and stop and repeat as needed," says Dr. Edward Phillips, assistant professor of physical medicine and rehabilitation at Harvard Medical School. "They also are a great option if you aren't ready to return to the gym, or want a new way to exercise."

If you decide to log on, make sure to follow these basic tips to ensure you get the most from your online experience.

1. Find the right workout. There are many types of exercises available online, so you are likely to find some that fit your fitness level, interests, and goals. Some have a specific focus, like low-impact cardio, resistance band routines, body-weight training, or balance training (tai chi and yoga). Many of these programs are free. YouTube (www.youtube.com) is

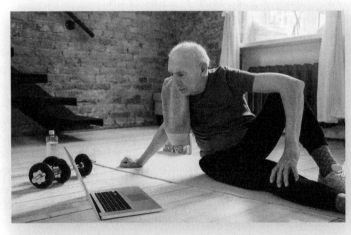

Basic equipment and a proper exercise space are essential for successful video workouts.

© blackday | Getty Images

an excellent resource. To begin, search using terms like "older adult fitness channels" or "senior fitness videos." Or look for a specific style of workout like "standing exercises for older adults" or "seated exercises for older adults."

2. Work your whole body. Routines should work all the major muscle groups, especially the core, back, and legs. But mix in some routines that focus on functional fitness, which support activities of daily living. Examples include getting up from a chair, raising your arms overhead, and squatting.

3. Find qualified instructors. Top instructors have certifications from organizations like the Athletics and Fitness Association of America (AFAA), the American College of Sports Medicine (ACSM), and the National Academy of Sports Medicine (NASM). Look for titles like Certified Group Fitness Instructor, Certified Personal Trainer, and Certified Exercise Expert for Aging Adults.

4. Create a workout space. Set up adequate floor space with no obstacles so you can move freely. Make sure the TV or computer is situated close enough to follow the workout as you move around. Position a portable fan nearby, if you need one to keep you cool, and keep a water bottle and towel handy.

5. Get essential equipment. Invest in basics like dumbbells or kettlebells in various weights, resistance bands, exercise balls, and yoga mats, or arrange for alternatives like gallon water jugs for weights and rolled towels for stretching.

6. Follow a proper sequence. A complete workout video includes all the necessary elements in the right order—a warm-up to slowly raise your heart rate and activate the muscles; the main workout routine; a cool-down to slow the heart; and an ending stretching routine.

7. Look for modifications. If the workout has several difficulty levels, it should be clear how to modify them to make something more manageable.

8. Maintain good form. Ensure the video clearly demonstrates the proper form for each exercise—and then follow it. Working out in front of a large mirror can help you maintain correct form.

9. Monitor movements. Take note if a video includes both standing and floor exercises. "Avoid videos with excessive changes from standing to lying down, as making quick transitions may increase your risk of falling," says Dr. Phillips.

10. Enlist a workout buddy. Online exercises don't have to be solo adventures. Make a workout date with someone; that can help keep you both motivated.

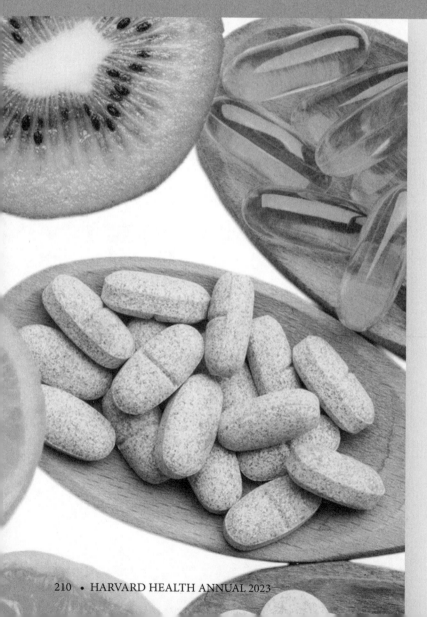

Chapter 9
—
Women's Health

Take Action!
5 Things You Can Do Now

1 **Weigh the pros and cons of a coronary artery calcium scan.** It may help your doctor better assess your heart risk. (page 215)

2 **Make some space.** Establishing boundaries may help ease a stressful relationship. (page 217)

3 **Be skeptical of "natural" hormone treatments.** They may carry risks. (page 222)

4 **Drink more water.** It helps flush out bacteria in the urinary tract and ward off infection. (page 231)

5 **Choose low-sodium foods.** Cutting your salt intake can reduce water retention. (page 236)

Women's heart symptoms not so different after all

New medical advice reflects evolving knowledge about cardiovascular disease in women.

For years, women have been warned to stay alert to "atypical" symptoms of heart attack that are different from what men experience.

But new guidelines co-authored by a Harvard cardiologist flip that advice on its head. It turns out that chest pain—the trademark symptom of heart attack—isn't as different between women and men as doctors believed and is indeed the most common sign of heart attack in both sexes.

The caveat? Women having heart attacks are more likely to report additional symptoms, such as shortness of breath, nausea, or fatigue, among others.

"For many years, clinicians believed there was a real difference in how men and women experienced chest pain," says Dr. Deepak L. Bhatt, executive director of Interventional Cardiovascular Programs at Harvard-affiliated Brigham and Women's Hospital and a professor of medicine at Harvard Medical School. "It's been the conventional wisdom, but it turns out it's not true. It probably turned out to be a hurtful thing."

"For a long time, we said women's symptoms are atypical, which promoted the concept that men are typical," agrees Dr. Emily Lau, a cardiologist at Massachusetts General Hospital who specializes in women's cardiovascular health. "As a community, we're trying to change the language surrounding how we think about women's heart disease and health." (For details, see "Do these 3 things if you're having chest pain" on the next page.)

Heart failure revelations

The new guidance on evaluating patients with chest pain, co-authored by Dr. Bhatt and published Nov.

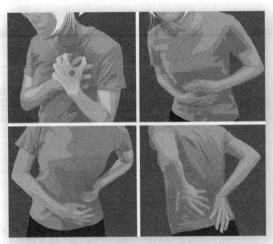

Mention chest pain to your doctor first, even if you're also experiencing other symptoms.

30, 2021, in *Circulation*, is part of a broader shift in the medical community's understanding of key differences in how women and men experience cardiovascular disease.

Another recent Harvard-led insight surrounds heart failure, which strikes one in five people overall. Women are more likely to have a specific type, called heart failure with preserved ejection fraction (HFpEF, also known as diastolic heart failure). This means the heart is stiff and unable to pump well.

Recent research by Dr. Jennifer En-Sian Ho, a cardiologist specializing in advanced heart failure and transplantation at Harvard-affiliated Beth Israel Deaconess Medical Center, suggests that, compared with obese men, women with obesity face higher odds of developing HFpEF. Additionally, women with HFpEF have a tougher time exercising because their hearts have a harder time keeping up with the body's needs, according to recent research by Dr. Ho, Dr. Lau, and colleagues.

Unfortunately, science hasn't yet caught up on effective treatments for this female-dominated heart failure type. Many more medications are available for the type most common in men, known as heart failure with reduced ejection fraction. "It's a major knowledge gap in the field, where we simply know less about how to effectively treat women with heart failure in general," says Dr. Ho.

Reproductive history and heart risk

Ironically, even as research continues to clarify sex-specific differences in heart disease, women's overall awareness of its seriousness is plummeting. A 2019 survey by the American Heart Association found that only 44% of women correctly identified

© Jong-eun Kim | Getty Images

heart disease as the top killer of women, compared with 65% in 2009.

"It's shocking that less than half of women know this fact," says Dr. Lau.

While scientists are still teasing out why our cardiovascular risks and symptoms may vary from men's, it's become clear in recent years that our reproductive history is integral to evaluating our heart health. Dr. Lau says cardiovascular risks may depend on factors such as

- diabetes or high blood pressure during pregnancy
- age and symptoms of menopause
- past infertility.

"Make sure your doctor is asking you questions about your reproductive history," Dr. Lau says. "No one's thinking about how something that happened during pregnancy 20 years ago might affect heart risk, but it may be incredibly important."

Do these 3 things if you're having chest pain

Most patients who go to the emergency room with chest pain are women, especially those over 65. But women are less likely to get timely care, in part because they might mention other symptoms— such as nausea, fatigue, or shortness of breath—first, or dismiss them as something less serious and delay going to the ER, says Dr. Deepak L. Bhatt, executive director of Interventional Cardiovascular Programs at Harvard-affiliated Brigham and Women's Hospital.

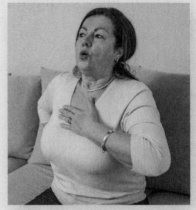

Don't drive yourself to the hospital if chest pain strikes.

Dr. Bhatt recommends anyone experiencing chest pain to follow three key steps:

Call 911. Even if you're not convinced you're having a heart attack, call an ambulance. "We're never angry if someone shows up in the ER and they're not having a heart attack," he says. "Treating it quickly really does matter."

Mention chest pain first. Don't just add it to the list of other symptoms you may be having, and don't minimize what you're feeling.

Be aware of the nuances of chest pain. Some experience chest pain as actual pain, but others may feel pressure, squeezing, or discomfort. "It's important to realize people perceive chest pain in different ways," he says.

IN THE JOURNALS

Regular solo dining may be linked to a higher risk of heart disease

Could eating alone be a heart disease risk factor? A Korean study published November 1, 2021, in the journal *Menopause*, found that older women who often ate more than two meals by themselves each day were more likely to have symptomatic heart disease than those who regularly shared a table with others. To come to this conclusion, researchers looked at data from a 2016 Korean nutritional survey, studying 590 women ages 65 and older. They divided women into two groups: the frequent solo diners, and those who ate more than two meals a day with others. They found that the women who ate by themselves more often not only had less nutritional knowledge, but also ate less nutritious meals. They were also more likely to be widowed and to have lower income levels. These factors might explain why they were at elevated risk for heart disease. The researchers suggested that doctors might consider whether women who often eat alone might be good candidates for cardiovascular screening and nutrition education.

Want a healthier heart? Seriously consider skipping the drinks

The World Heart Federation says that even moderate alcohol consumption harms your cardiovascular health.

Red wine actually isn't good for your heart. Really.

For the past 30 years, health experts have touted red wine (in moderation) as a heart-healthy beverage. But a January 2022 policy brief from the World Heart Federation (WHF) aims to set the record straight. No type of alcohol—including wine—is a friend to your heart.

"Alcohol seems to have adverse effects on nearly every form of heart disease," says Dr. JoAnn Manson, the Michael and Lee Bell Professor of Women's Health at Harvard Medical School. It increases the risk of

- hypertension
- heart failure
- stroke
- cardiomyopathy (a disease of the heart muscle)
- aortic aneurysm (a dangerous bulge in the wall of the aorta)
- atrial fibrillation (an irregular heart rhythm).

It may also play a role in coronary artery disease, says Dr. Manson. But the evidence for this is less clear.

"People should clearly understand that alcohol is linked to several heart-related risks," she says. "The message they may have heard that alcohol is good for the heart has been debunked; it's a myth."

Changing advice

You may wonder, what changed? Why did experts say that alcohol was good for the heart if that's not the case?

One reason for the shift is that researchers now know that there were some procedural flaws in past research, says Dr. Manson. Past studies often compared people who drank alcohol against a mixed group of nondrinkers. Although some of the people in the nondrinking group never drank alcohol, some had stopped drinking because they were recovering from alcohol use disorders and had been

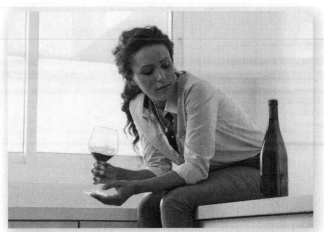

Alcohol consumption can sneak up on you. It's too easy to progress from light to moderate to heavy drinking. The key is to be mindful about your intake.

heavy drinkers for years before they quit. Others had given up alcohol because of health problems, such as heart disease or diabetes, or because they were taking medications that interacted with alcohol, says Dr. Manson.

"When studies excluded former drinkers and people with underlying health problems, they didn't show the same alcohol-related cardiovascular benefits," says Dr. Manson.

In addition, the WHF noted that much of the past research on alcohol and heart health consisted of observational studies—not the more reliable randomized controlled trials. When randomized trials were conducted, they failed to find a heart benefit from drinking alcohol. Also, some of the most favorable effects of alcohol had been found in studies paid for by the alcohol industry, which raised the potential of bias.

Women at higher risk

Although more men than women die from alcohol-related causes (including accidents and liver disease), women may be more susceptible than men to several health problems caused by alcohol, says Dr. Manson.

"Women metabolize alcohol more slowly than men and, generally, can tolerate only about half as much alcohol as men before experiencing adverse effects," she says.

In addition to raising the risk for heart-related problems and liver disease, alcohol use has also been linked to a higher risk of certain cancers, including those of the mouth, throat, esophagus, and liver. In addition, drinking even small amounts of alcohol can raise the risk of breast cancer, says Dr. Manson.

Alcohol also increases the risk of atrial fibrillation, which is more dangerous in women than in men. "Women are more likely than men to have a stroke if they have atrial

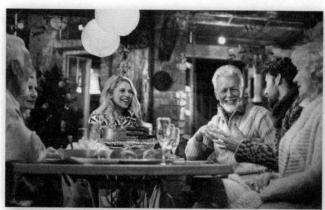

© gilaxia | Getty Images

fibrillation, and women who have a stroke are more likely to have a fatal stroke," says Dr. Manson.

To drink or not to drink?

With this in mind, it may be time to rethink your drinking habits.

"I don't think that everyone who is drinking, even in moderation, needs to stop drinking urgently," says Dr. Manson. But if you do drink regularly, it might be a good idea to cut back. Also, if you're drinking expressly because you've been told it protects your heart, you should stop.

"I'm often amazed to hear people say, 'I didn't used to drink until I heard it was good for my health, so I try to have at least one drink a day,'" says Dr. Manson.

Don't panic if you think you might be drinking too much. People who drink in moderation, especially while dining, don't need to stop drinking immediately. But taking a hard look at your drinking style, in consultation with your doctor, is a good first step.

You should be particularly cautious with alcohol if you have hypertension or other risk factors for heart disease, atrial fibrillation, or heart failure, or if you're at a high risk for cancer. This includes women who have already had breast cancer or who have a strong family history of breast cancer, she says.

It's also time to retire the notion that there is a "safe" type of alcohol, she says.

"People are always interested in whether some types of alcohol are better than others—is red wine or white wine or any wine better than other forms of alcohol?" says Dr. Manson. The answer is that no type of alcohol is good for your heart or your health.

"The difference with wine is that it is often consumed with meals," she says. When you have alcohol with food, your system is likely to absorb it more slowly. You are also more likely to drink in moderation while eating than if you're out at a bar where drinking is the main attraction. "I think there are certain types of alcohol that people might be more likely to consume in excess, which is particularly deleterious," says Dr. Manson.

Alcohol and your heart by the numbers

The World Heart Federation included some statistics about alcohol and health in its January 2022 policy brief, "The Impact of Alcohol Consumption on Cardiovascular Health: Myths and Measures." Here are some of the highlights:

▶ Globally, alcohol use contributed to 2.4 million deaths in 2019—4.3% of all deaths.

▶ Some 230 diseases are linked to alcohol use.

▶ Alcohol, even in small amounts, is linked to a higher risk of breast cancer. It's also a risk factor for cancers of the mouth, throat, and liver, among others.

▶ People who drink moderately are about 14% more likely to have a stroke compared with those who don't drink at all, and also 15% more likely to suffer a fatal aortic aneurysm.

▶ Alcohol use is linked to narrowing of the carotid arteries and the coronary arteries, which may lead to stroke or heart attack.

How to cut back on your drinking

While the World Heart Federation says there's no safe amount of alcohol for your heart, moderate use is typically defined as no more than one drink per day for women.

One drink equals
- 12 ounces of beer
- 5 ounces of wine
- 1.5 ounces of hard alcohol, such as vodka or whiskey.

A woman is considered a heavy drinker if she has eight or more drinks per week, or a binge drinker if she has more than four drinks in one sitting. If you'd like to cut back on your drinking, the U.S. Substance Abuse and Mental Health Services Administration offers some tips that can help:

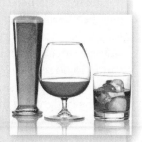

- Set a limit on the number of drinks you will consume each day and week, and track your intake.
- Drink slowly, no more than one drink per hour.
- Avoid situations that make you want to drink.
- Enlist a friend for support in sticking to your alcohol plan.
- Talk to your doctor if you are having trouble managing your alcohol use. She or he may be able to help you find resources in your area that can help.

Do you need a coronary calcium scan?

This heart test is designed to look for dangerous plaque in the arteries, but it may be helpful only for certain people.

When it comes to monitoring the health of your heart, there are numerous tests your doctor might recommend. One on the list is a coronary artery calcium (CAC) scan, which uses a special type of x-ray to look for signs of plaque in your arteries. This arterial plaque often contains calcium, which is how the scan got its name.

Doctors want to identify people with a lot of this arterial plaque because it raises the risk of heart-related problems. Plaque can create a blockage that cuts off blood flow, causing a heart attack or other problems.

While a CAC scan can be a valuable tool in detecting people at higher risk of heart problems from plaque buildup, this test isn't right for everyone, says Dr. Ariane CoCo Fraiche, a cardiologist at Harvard-affiliated Beth Israel Deaconess Medical Center. It's typically most useful for people who don't yet have symptoms of heart disease, but do have some risk factors. If your doctor is on the fence about how aggressively to treat you based on these risk factors, a CAC scan may help her or him determine the most appropriate treatment plan.

"The goal of the CAC score is to go beyond just traditional clinical risk factors to identify patients who are most likely to derive benefit from preventive therapies such as cholesterol-lowering medications," says Dr. Fraiche. "A CAC score may add helpful information to promote shared decision making in these situations."

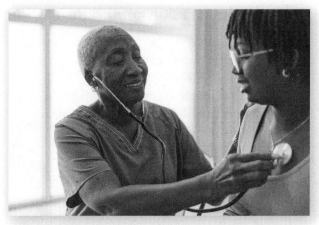

A test that measures arterial plaque may help your doctor determine the best strategies to reduce your heart risk.

The test can also encourage patients to take their own health more seriously, she says. "If a patient is hesitant to start a medication or make lifestyle changes, an abnormal CAC score may provide motivation to do so," says Dr. Fraiche. On the other hand, if the calcium scan shows that the arteries are clear, everyone might feel more comfortable taking a more conservative approach to treatment.

Weighing the pros and cons

In some instances, however, a CAC scan will add little to the equation. "A CAC score is less useful when a patient is at very low or high risk for heart disease because the score will not change management recommendations or may lead to unnecessary testing," she says.

This might be the case for a 62-year-old woman with a family history of early coronary artery disease who already has concerning symptoms. "I would pursue other testing, such as a stress test or assessment of coronary anatomy, rather than a CAC scan," says Dr. Fraiche.

The test would also not be useful in a 57-year-old woman with diabetes and high cholesterol, but no symptoms of heart disease, she says. "For this patient, guidelines would call for a statin to improve cardiovascular risk, so the test would be less likely to provide added value to her traditional risk factors," she says.

If your doctor recommends a CAC scan, there are some pros and cons to consider, says Dr. Fraiche. On the positive side, these scans are readily available and easy to perform.

Among the cons are

- radiation exposure, (although it's a relatively low level)
- cost (you may face out-of-pocket expenses depending on your insurance).

Keep in mind that your doctor may see something on your scan that may lead to additional tests, either for heart-related issues or something unrelated but concerning. Both scenarios may lead to additional hassles and costs, sometimes unnecessarily.

Understanding your results

If you do undergo a CAC scan, you should review your results with your doctor, who can help you understand how the findings relate to your personal risk factors. Typically, scans are graded on a scale as follows:

- 0 (no plaque)
- 1 to 99 (mild disease)
- 100 to 399 (moderate disease)
- 400 or higher (severe disease).

Unless your calcium score is 0, your physician may want to talk about lifestyle modifications and medication to reduce cardiovascular risk, says Dr. Fraiche. However, an abnormal score does not necessarily mean that you need more heart testing, as long as you don't have symptoms. "Rather, it can be used to guide preventive therapies," she says.

Your score is just one of several factors to consider. One thing to bear in mind is that in women, a lower score may still carry additional risk. A woman can have the same score as a man, but have a higher risk

Study sheds additional light on who should get CAC scans

A study published in October 2021 in *JAMA Cardiology* may help doctors decide who will benefit most from coronary artery calcium (CAC) scans.

"This study is getting a lot of attention because it highlights limitations of CAC scores," says Dr. Ariane CoCo Fraiche, a cardiologist at Harvard-affiliated Beth Israel Deaconess Medical Center.

The study looked at more than 20,000 people who had symptoms related to arterial blockages. A large number of them got a score of 0 on a CAC scan despite the fact that they already had plaque-related obstructions in their arteries. This was particularly

true in people under age 40. More than half (58%) scored 0 on a CAC scan, compared with 5% of people ages 70 and older.

This study showed that CAC scanning is not necessarily an accurate gauge of risk in younger people and in those with symptoms of artery obstruction, notes Dr. Fraiche. CAC scores can lead to inappropriately reassuring results in this population since calcium may not get deposited into potentially dangerous plaques. "If I am worried about coronary artery disease in any patient with concerning symptoms, I would consider a different diagnostic test," says Dr. Fraiche.

due to sex differences in atherosclerotic plaque, says Dr. Fraiche. "The distribution of the calcium may also influence risk," she says.

Ultimately, measuring calcium in the coronary arteries can be a very helpful tool for certain patients who have an intermediate or uncertain risk for heart disease. "If you are concerned about your risk of heart disease or weighing pros and cons of preventive therapies, I recommend talking to your physician about the potential role of a calcium score," says Dr. Fraiche.

Fostering healthy relationships

Stressful interpersonal connections may lead to health problems, such as heart disease.

If the pandemic has taught us anything, it's the importance of social ties and human connections. Not only do they improve your emotional well-being, but they can bring physical benefits. "Having nurturing relationships is protective of mental health and overall brain health," says Dr. Jennifer Gatchel, an assistant professor of psychiatry at Harvard Medical School.

However, while positive relationships can boost health, the opposite is often true when it comes to problematic relationships. Chronic emotional stress may put you at higher risk for a number of health problems.

A study published March 2, 2021, in the *Journal of the American Heart Association*, for example, found that women who reported having high levels of social strain were more likely to have a heart attack or die of cardiovascular disease during nearly 15 years of follow-up than women who did not.

To determine this, researchers asked women how many people in their life irritated them, were too demanding of them, excluded them, or tried to "coerce" them in their daily life. Based on their answers, the women were categorized as having low, medium, or high social strain. Those who scored in the high category were 9% more likely to develop cardiovascular disease than women who scored in the low category.

Another study, published by the *Journal of*

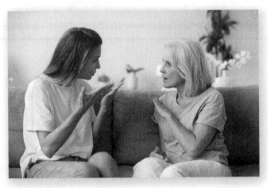

Relationship stress can lead to potential health problems, but there are strategies that can help, such as establishing boundaries.

Epidemiology & Community Health, found that women who reported high levels of social stress had lower bone density six years later. The authors speculated that stress may harm bone health because stress raises blood cortisol levels, which may be linked to bone thinning. Troubled ties with others may also lead to other physical or mental health problems.

Defining a difficult relationship

A stress-inducing relationship can be one with a partner, a family member, a friend, or a professional colleague. People may find themselves at odds with others for many reasons. The pandemic and political polarization that has occurred in recent years may be exacerbating factors for some, says Dr. Gatchel. Relationship stress is often particularly challenging for people who are in a role as caretaker for a child, ailing adult relative, or partner. "Caring for a spouse or a loved one can lead to increased stress, which puts you at risk for depression or physical health problems if the you don't feel supported," says Dr. Gatchel.

Identifying a toxic trend

While your relationships with others may seem like they are outside of your control, there are things you can do to take them in a more positive direction, Dr. Gatchel says. The first step is identifying a problematic dynamic. A trying relationship typically comes with some warning signs, she says. These include

- feeling burned out or depleted after interactions
- having negative thoughts about the relationship
- feeling like the relationship is imbalanced—that one person gives or takes more than the other
- feeling that you are not valued or respected by the other person.

Look at the patterns of the relationship over time. Has it been more take than give? Is it stressful? "If you recognize those signs in yourself, it's a red flag to take a closer look," she says.

Making a change for the better

If you do determine that a relationship is detrimental, that doesn't mean you necessarily have to cut ties with the person, but you will need to make some changes.

Establish boundaries. If there is a person in your life who is difficult, setting boundaries can help put the relationship back on track. You can be there for someone and still establish limits, so that the relationship isn't so taxing. While burnout is common in caregiver relationships, it's a feature of other relationships as well. For example, it may stem from a friendship with someone who is in constant need of emotional support, which may feel draining.

Solve the issue by setting clear limits. If the friend calls with a problem, establish a time to discuss it, rather than always jumping the second she calls. "You can express concern; say, 'I'm sorry to hear that, and about what you are going through. I can't talk right now, but can I give you a call tonight or this weekend to talk about it,'" says Dr. Gatchel.

Tips for healthier relationships

Do your part to help form healthy relationships with others by practicing some good habits, says Dr. Jennifer Gatchel, an assistant professor of psychiatry at Harvard Medical School.

Be an empathetic listener. Practice paying close attention when someone is speaking to you, and take the time to understand what the person is saying. "This can often be done by reflecting back some of their statements to them, to reinforce that you have gotten the point and that they are being heard," says Dr. Gatchel.

Share the spotlight. When someone is talking to you about a problem, keep the focus on them; avoid turning it into a discussion about an issue that you might be facing.

Stay calm. If you can, keep calm during discussions to ensure that they are constructive rather than destructive. If you aren't able to stay calm in the moment, step back and ask to revisit the conversation later when you are in a better place.

HALT. Remember the acronym HALT. When you are upset about something, first ask yourself if you are hungry, angry, lonely, or tired. If so, "halt" in order to first address those needs, and then revisit the problem.

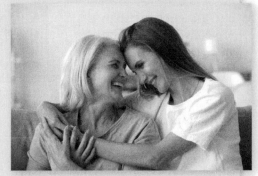

Setting some guidelines for interactions with friends and family can be beneficial.

Interact in person. Sometimes a stressful relationship can be made worse by social media. People may have more aggressive confrontations online than they do in person. "I would say in general, limit social media exposure," says Dr. Gatchel. Reducing time online encourages direct communication, either in person, by phone, or on video, which can often be far less contentious than words spoken from behind a keyboard, such as in text messages.

Emphasize the positive. "Research increasingly supports associations between intentional practices of gratitude and positive mental health, which can extend to improved relationships," says Dr. Gatchel. Such practices can include getting into the habit of writing down two or three specific things that you are grateful for each day. "These things can include anything, including a positive interaction with a friend or partner," she says. "If so, don't be shy about sharing it or making a point of expressing this appreciation to the person."

© fizkes | Getty Images

If you have differences with someone, setting boundaries can also make certain that you aren't forced outside of your comfort zone. This might occur if a friend calls and asks you for a favor you don't feel comfortable performing. "You would have to evaluate if you feel safe and comfortable with that. If not, be clear that you want to help them, but you'll need to do that in another way," says Dr. Gatchel.

Prioritize your own well-being. Establishing boundaries with a child, grandchild, spouse, or other family member can be more challenging than it is with a friend. In these instances, it may be more about designating space for yourself to recharge and reset. This is something that many people have been unable to do during the pandemic.

"People were being asked to do more than they ever would and had to maintain a marathon pace for a really long time," says Dr. Gatchel. To get needed breaks, hire child care or enlist help from a professional, a friend, or a family member.

Don't underestimate your need to recharge. "There is only so much nonstop care that you can provide," says Dr. Gatchel. It's okay to ask for support. It's like what flight attendants say before takeoff: put the oxygen mask on yourself before you then help someone else, says Dr. Gatchel.

Protect your health. You should also take steps to mitigate the stress you are experiencing as a result of unhealthy interactions with others.

Practice self-care. Make time for physical activity, mindfulness relaxation practices, and activities that you enjoy. Sometimes activities that tap into the senses, such as gardening, coloring, painting, or even something as simple as sorting beads can help you relax, says Dr. Gatchel. Also, be certain to make time for good friends who are a source of support for you. And pay attention to your physical needs.

Try to get the right amount of sleep. "Sleep is central to mood, as well as your anxiety and energy level," says Dr. Gatchel. The same is true of a healthy diet and getting enough physical activity.

Achieve some distance. Sometimes when a relationship is no longer positive, taking a step back can help. For example, if you have a friend who doesn't make you feel valued or who is critical or negative, you might want to continue the friendship, but take a closer look to see if it should occupy less of your time. "Friendships change, relationships change,

circumstances change," says Dr. Gatchel. "Investing less in some relationships is normal even if you're not clear why you're having negative feelings toward that person."

Open the lines of communication. Depending on the relationship, you can sometimes address problems directly. "Just be open with them about it," says Dr. Gatchel. The relationship at its core might not be problematic, but there could be a particular topic that puts you at odds. If you continue to disagree, setting boundaries about what you can and cannot discuss is one way to address these conflicts.

When you are talking to someone about a tense subject, be certain to use positive communication strategies. "Use 'I' statements," says Dr. Gatchel. "For instance, 'I've noticed that when we have this discussion, things seem to get heated.' And avoid using 'you' statements that might sound more accusatory, such as 'You always want to argue about this.'"

Ultimately, these strategies can help put many relationships in a better place and protect you from health-harming strain.

Menopause and brain fog: What's the link?

Research ties severity of certain menopause symptoms to cognitive performance.

Reaching for the right word. Wondering why you walked into a room. Forgetting appointments. These signs of "brain fog" might be common at midlife, but our accumulation of birthdays doesn't necessarily tell the whole story.

With midlife comes menopause, and new research suggests cognitive blips may be linked to how severely we experience menopause symptoms—especially depression and sexual problems such as painful sex, low desire, or trouble with arousal.

"Brain fog is one of the lesser-known symptoms of menopause, but it's so common," says Dr. Heather Hirsch, head of the Menopause and Midlife Clinic at Harvard-affiliated Brigham and Women's Hospital.

"We're talking about it more now, but the majority of women don't associate brain fog with menopause the way they do hot flashes."

Stages and symptoms

Indeed, the new study drives home that hot flashes—while considered a menopause hallmark—are far from the only menopause symptom that can dramatically influence daily life, says Dr. Hadine Joffe, executive director of the Connors Center for Women's Health and Gender Biology at Brigham and Women's Hospital and a professor of psychiatry at Harvard Medical School. "People think of brain fog more as a result of chronological aging than of hormone-related aging," she says. "Either way, it can have a

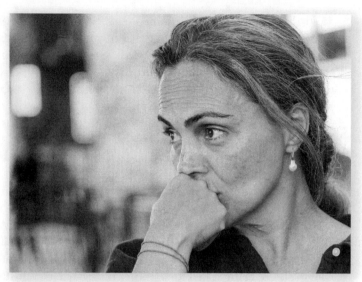

Trying to multitask can make brain fog worse.

IN THE JOURNALS

Risk factors for benign breast conditions identified

Noncancerous breast changes appear to be more common in women with a family history of breast cancer. That's one of several factors linked to benign breast problems, according to a study published online June 25, 2021, by *JAMA Network Open*.

The study looked at 61,617 women, ages 40 to 69, who underwent screening mammograms in Sweden. Of this group, 5,341 women were found to have benign breast conditions during the average 35-year follow-up period. The researchers found the following factors were linked to an increased risk of certain benign breast problems:

A family history of breast cancer. Premenopausal women with a family history of the disease were twice as likely to develop a type of noncancerous abnormal cell growth called epithelial proliferation with atypia (EPA). This condition can raise breast cancer risk. They also were more likely to have several benign breast conditions that don't generally raise cancer risk.

Postmenopausal hormone therapy. Women who used hormones after menopause had higher rates of EPA, in addition to two other benign conditions that don't raise cancer risk, compared with women who did not use hormones. The authors pointed out that more research is needed to determine the impact of taking hormones. The study also linked several factors to lower rates of benign breast conditions:

Obesity. Noncancerous breast conditions were less likely to develop in women who were obese than in women of normal weight, with the exception of epithelial proliferation (EP), another type of abnormal cell growth, similar to EPA but without atypical cells. It can also raise the risk for breast cancer (but less so than EPA).

Not giving birth. Premenopausal women who had not given birth were less likely to develop EP compared with women who'd borne three or more children. However, they were more likely to develop fluid-filled cysts.

Use of oral contraceptives. Women who took birth control pills were less likely to develop a type of breast growth called fibroadenoma with atypia, fibrocystic changes, and cysts compared with those who did not take the pills.

comprehensive effect on well-being."

Published online Jan. 12, 2022, by the journal *Menopause*, the research focused on 404 women in India ages 40 to 65 who weren't using hormone therapy. The researchers divided the women into groups based on their stage of menopause to compare how often and how severely they experienced various symptoms. The researchers also examined how the severity of menopause symptoms related to cognitive performance in areas such as memory, attention, and language skills.

Late-postmenopausal participants, whose periods had ceased more than five years before, scored highest for depression and sexual dysfunction, while anxiety and hot flashes were most often reported among those who entered menopause fewer than five years earlier.

Estrogen drop to blame?

After adjusting the results for factors such as age, marital status, and education level, researchers learned that severe depression and greater sexual dysfunction stood out as the only symptoms significantly linked with cognitive performance. No link was found between hot flashes and brain performance, though earlier research has shown inconsistent results.

The study had several limitations. While it shows an association between severity of menopause symptoms and cognitive problems, it can't prove a cause-and-effect relationship. We also don't know which came first—depression and sexual problems, or brain fog. "We just see they happened around the same time," Dr. Hirsch says.

Why might this occur? With estrogen receptors in virtually every organ, our bodies are highly sensitive to hormone fluctuations, Dr. Hirsch explains. This means estrogen loss can announce itself in how our brain works. Ultimately, however, "we don't know why this happens," says Dr. Joffe, "because many things are happening across the menopause transition along with the drop in estrogen."

But this brain fog probably won't last. The long-term SWAN (Study of Women's Health Across the Nation) trial, to which Dr. Joffe and other Harvard researchers contribute, suggests perimenopausal women temporarily have trouble learning new information. "It does get better with time as women get past menopause," Dr. Joffe says.

Tackling brain fog

Dr. Joffe and Dr. Hirsch offer these strategies to compensate for brain fog.

Stay calm. Panicking about thinking and memory issues can actually make them worse. "Awareness is valuable, but go easy on yourself," Dr. Joffe says. "Menopause is an intense time of life, and midlife changes on the brain and body come and go."

Challenge yourself. Take a different route to familiar destinations like the grocery store and walk down aisles in a different pattern when you get there. "You want to create new memories and new processes rather than always going by habit and routine," Dr. Joffe says.

Get moving. Regular exercise benefits your brain along with the rest of your body, with research indicating it improves cognition.

Focus. "How many of us go into a room and say, 'Why am I in here?' It's because we thought of three other things along the way," Dr. Joffe says. "Slow down, and prioritize the one thing at hand."

Write it down. Sticky notes, lists, and other reminders pay huge dividends when you're feeling frazzled.

Sleep more. This can be a tall order during menopause, since the fall in estrogen levels has also been linked to insomnia. Cut back on caffeine, and skip caffeinated drinks after lunch.

Treat underlying conditions. Tackle depression or mood issues with cognitive behavioral therapy, medication, or a combination.

The truth about nutrient deficiencies

Some women do need a boost. Find out if you're one of them.

Strolling past drugstore shelves teeming with dietary supplements might make you wonder: Am I getting enough nutrients? The $35-billion-per-year supplement industry feeds this curiosity with splashy labels and claims, hoping to fuel the belief that we all need to fill a few dietary gaps.

The good news? Most supplements aren't necessary. It's also time to think bigger—as in maximizing the mix of foods on your plate.

"People tend to ask about different supplements, but we want them to focus on an overall balanced eating pattern," says Emily Blake, a registered dietitian at Harvard-affiliated Brigham and Women's Hospital.

"Quick fixes are often promoted as a gateway to health, when more sustainable changes are what's going to move the needle."

Ones to watch

Few of us face nutrient deficiencies unless we intentionally avoid entire food groups or otherwise drastically limit our diet, says Teresa Fung, an adjunct professor of nutrition at the Harvard T.H. Chan School of Public Health. If anything, "we're a country of excess consumption," she says. While food insecurity is a significant problem in the United States, if you are eating several meals each day, and

---

ASK THE DOCTORS

by **HOPE RICCIOTTI, M.D., AND TONI GOLEN, M.D.**

Are bioidentical hormones superior to hormone medications?

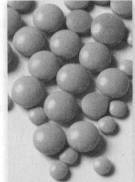

Q *I recently heard a friend say she was taking bioidentical hormones to treat menopausal symptoms. What are they, and are they better than taking traditional hormone therapy medication?*

A The North American Menopause Society and other organizations have warned that there are risks related to using bioidenticals, which are defined by the Endocrine Society as "compounds that have the same chemical and molecular structure as hormones that are produced in the human body." Bioidenticals are often prepared at compounding pharmacies and sometimes used as alternatives to synthetic hormones like Premarin (conjugated equine estrogens) and Prempro (conjugated equine estrogens plus medroxyprogesterone acetate).

Bioidentical hormones are often billed as "natural," but they may bring risks.

While advertisers may claim that these bioidentical hormones are "natural" alternatives to hormone medications, the truth is that the two are often very similar—but bioidenticals may come with less quality assurance. Many FDA-approved hormone therapies also meet the description of a bioidentical (although they're not usually advertised this way). In some cases, they are actually made using the same ingredients as bioidentical hormones. There's little evidence that bioidenticals are superior to FDA-approved hormone medications, and in fact, bioidenticals may be riskier, because they aren't scrutinized or tested by the FDA to verify dose and purity.

© art-4-art | Getty Images

a variety of different types of food, it is unlikely that you are deficient in calories or nutrients.

That said, women are indeed vulnerable to coming up short for a handful of vitamins and minerals due to age, hormone changes, or other factors. Here are nutrients that are most likely to be deficient.

Vitamin D. Vitamin D deficiency is especially common as we get older, since few foods are naturally rich in it. Getting enough sunlight for our skin to convert to vitamin D may be easier in the summer months, but we need to balance that benefit against skin cancer concerns. Signs of deficiency include fatigue, bone pain, mood changes, muscle aches, and weakness.

Foods high in vitamin D include fortified cow's milk and cereals, soy milk, mushrooms, canned tuna, shrimp, and salmon. Daily recommended intake is 600 IU for adults up to age 70 and 800 IU for those 71 and older; a daily 1,000-IU vitamin D supplement provides ample coverage.

Iron. Red blood cells, which carry oxygen throughout the body, rely on adequate

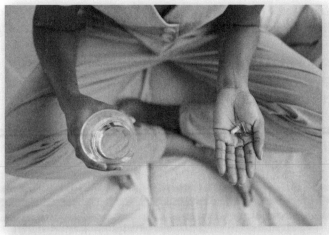

Few of us face nutrient deficiencies. Tests are needed to pinpoint if you have one.

iron stores. But pregnancy or heavy menstrual periods can take a toll, potentially leaving us lacking. So can increasingly popular plant-based diets, since animal products provide higher amounts of iron, and our bodies absorb iron more easily from animal sources.

If you're low on iron, you may feel cold, tired, or short of breath. You

Who needs a multivitamin?

Big containers, bright colors, and even candy-like gummies: Who can resist the ease and appeal of multivitamins? It may feel like a nutrition insurance policy to pop a daily pill or down a specialized formula containing a combination of vitamins, minerals, and other nutrients.

But if you're generally healthy and eat a varied diet, there's just no need, says Teresa Fung, an adjunct professor of nutrition at the Harvard T.H. Chan School of Public Health. "A vitamin pill does not contain all the beneficial stuff in food," Fung says. "It's not a shortcut."

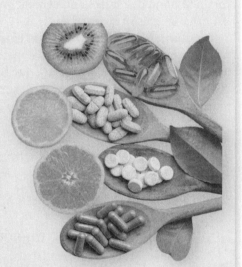

The following factors, however, make it more likely someone will benefit from taking multivitamins:

Age. With advanced age may come trouble chewing and swallowing or a drop in desire to eat adequate meals.

Pregnancy. Since many pregnancies are unplanned, women of childbearing age should consider a daily multivitamin containing the B vitamin folate, also called folic acid, which—if taken early in pregnancy—can lower the risk of brain and spinal cord defects in the developing embryo.

Digestive challenges. Some conditions, such as celiac disease, ulcerative colitis, and cystic fibrosis, can interfere with normal digestion. So can gastric bypass, a weight-loss surgery that removes parts of the digestive tract.

Certain medications. Proton-pump inhibitors for acid reflux and heartburn can prevent us from properly absorbing vitamin B_{12}. Some Parkinson's disease medications also inhibit B vitamin absorption, and diuretics, taken to lower blood pressure, can deplete your stores of magnesium, potassium, and calcium.

may have headaches more frequently. Meat and seafood typically offer plenty of iron, and plant-based sources include beans, lentils, grains, spinach, and fortified cereals. Women over 50 need 8 milligrams (mg) of iron per day; younger women, 18 mg daily.

Vitamin B$_{12}$**.** B$_{12}$ is crucial to healthy nerve signaling and red blood cell production, but we get progressively less efficient at absorbing it as we age. Vegans and vegetarians are also at higher risk of deficiency, since plants don't contain the vitamin.

Signs of a B$_{12}$ shortfall include fatigue from anemia; numbness in hands, legs, and feet; or trouble with balance and walking. Memory can also suffer. Vitamin B$_{12}$ is readily found in fish, chicken, milk, and yogurt. If you prefer plant-based options, try fortified nondairy milks and cereals. Adults need 2.4 micrograms of B$_{12}$ each day.

Calcium. Most of us know that calcium keeps bones strong; it also helps control muscle and nerve function and regulate our heartbeat. As estrogen drops, our ability to absorb calcium diminishes, and those on vegan diets can compound the risk by avoiding dairy products.

Calcium-rich foods include cow's milk, fortified soy or almond milks, yogurt, cheese, fortified cereals, and dark green vegetables like kale and broccoli. Most adults need 1,000 mg each day, but women over 50 need 1,200 mg.

To test or not to test?

Don't count on symptoms—or their absence—to clue you in to a possible nutritional deficit. Most deficiencies are subtle, with few glaring signs, Blake says. And it's not something you can diagnose on your own.

"The term 'deficiency' is really a medical term," says Fung. "Even if you enter your diet into an app that shows its nutrient composition, it will not tell you if you have a deficiency. That requires medical testing."

Additionally, our bodies store small amounts of extra vitamins and minerals that would tide us over several weeks of poor eating, meaning our levels would have to be extremely low before a problem even shows up. A vitamin D deficiency,

---

ASK THE DOCTORS

by **HOPE RICCIOTTI, M.D., AND TONI GOLEN, M.D.**

How can I reduce lasting menopausal symptoms?

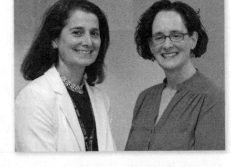

Q *I had my last menstrual period four years ago, but I'm still having hot flashes and night sweats. Is this normal, and is there anything other than hormones that might alleviate my symptoms?*

A Unfortunately, while menopausal symptoms are short-lived for many women, others can have symptoms for years after their menstrual cycles have stopped. These may include heart palpitations, vaginal dryness, night sweats, hot flashes, sleep disruptions, and mood disorders, such as depression and anxiety.

There are some nonhormonal approaches that might help. Some of the best options for hot flashes and night sweats are those that help keep you cool. These include dressing in layers, so you can quickly remove clothing to adjust your body temperature; keeping a small fan nearby that can be flipped on as needed; using cool-water compresses on your skin; keeping your bedroom at a lower temperature at night; and wearing light clothing to bed (ideally made of fabrics designed to wick away moisture).

In addition, try to get regular exercise. It's been shown to reduce menopausal symptoms overall, and it may help to improve your sleep quality. Also, be sure to speak with your doctor. She or he may be able to offer you some additional treatment options and can also rule out other conditions that might be causing the problems you are experiencing.

for instance, might only announce itself in a broken bone.

Calcium levels can't be accurately gauged from a blood test, Fung says. Typically, however, blood tests can reveal whether you're lacking in key nutrients, including vitamin D, iron, or B_{12}. While there's "no need to test for every deficiency under the sun," Fung advises asking your doctor if she or he feels your risk factors warrant a closer look. "If you're concerned or even curious, it's absolutely worth a conversation with your doctor," says Blake.

Vitamin D and fish oil may prevent autoimmune disease

More than 24 million Americans cope with autoimmune disorders such as rheumatoid arthritis, psoriasis, or thyroid disease. But so far, scientists haven't identified potential ways to prevent these burdensome conditions, which disproportionately affect women.

Now, however, a Harvard study suggests that vitamin D and fish oil supplements may offer adults over 50 protection against developing autoimmune disorders. All these conditions—which number more than 80—occur when the immune system mistakenly attacks healthy cells, tissues, or organs. Their symptoms vary, but may include pain, fatigue, skin problems, and other chronic problems.

"We were surprised that a signal for a benefit could emerge for such a broad and varied group of diseases," says Dr. JoAnn Manson, chief of the Division of Preventive Medicine at Harvard-affiliated Brigham and Women's Hospital, who led the main Vitamin D and Omega-3 Trial (VITAL) and co-authored the new report, published Jan. 26, 2022, in *The BMJ*. "Because there are no known ways to prevent autoimmune diseases—whether lifestyle, diet, or medications—these results were exciting."

Longer use, stronger findings

The randomized controlled trial—considered the gold standard of research—included 25,871 racially diverse older adults over age 50, who were split into four groups. People in one group took 2,000 IU of vitamin D_3 each day; those in another took 1,000 milligrams of fish oil (containing marine-based omega-3 fatty acids); those in a third group took both; and the rest took two placebos. None knew which group they were in.

The vitamin D dose used in the trial is more than twice the recommended daily intake of 600 IU (or 800 IU for people 71 and older). During a five-year follow-up period, participants told researchers whether they'd been diagnosed with any autoimmune diseases, and diagnoses were confirmed through medical records.

Compared with placebo, vitamin D supplementation was associated with a 22% reduced risk of autoimmune disease overall. The improvement was greater (39%) after the first two years of treatment. Fish oil by itself showed less robust results, but still showed fewer participants with confirmed autoimmune diagnoses compared with placebo.

"The results suggest that the risk reductions strengthened with longer treatment," Dr. Manson says.

Inflammation-fighting effects

How might vitamin D and fish oil thwart autoimmune disease? Researchers expected the duo might show preventive effects because of their ability to regulate the immune system and tamp down inflammation, which drives autoimmune disorders. The results carry important implications for women, who are at least four times as likely as men to be diagnosed with an autoimmune disorder. But it's too soon to make a public health recommendation that everyone take vitamin D or fish oil supplements in hopes of preventing autoimmune disease, Dr. Manson says. More research should also focus on the effects of these supplements in people at higher risk and in younger adults, as autoimmune conditions often develop earlier in adulthood.

"But those with a strong family history, or who have been told they may have early signs of an autoimmune disorder, may want to talk with their health care providers about whether to begin taking these supplements," says Dr. Manson.

FDA wants women to understand the risks and benefits related to breast implants

The agency approved a series of new requirements to help improve safety.

When a woman decides to get breast implants, she's signing on for a long-term relationship. Implants bring many benefits, both physical and psychological, whether a woman is choosing them for cosmetic reasons or for breast reconstruction in the wake of cancer surgery. But they also bring risks.

"A woman who decides to have breast implants should know that they may not last forever," says Dr. Andrea Pusic, the Joseph E. Murray Professor of Surgery at Harvard Medical School. "That means that she may need a future surgery or have longer-term complications. Surgery is a serious decision, and devices aren't perfect."

The FDA recently moved to help make certain that women considering breast implants have a clear picture of what implants involve before moving ahead with surgery. The agency announced a series of changes in October 2021, including these:

- establishing new labeling requirements for breast implant manufacturers, including a boxed warning
- allowing the sale of breast implants only to facilities that agree to provide patients with a comprehensive checklist outlining potential risks and benefits related to breast implants
- updating screening recommendations designed to detect leaks in silicone breast implants
- releasing updated information on breast implant post-approval studies to better inform patients.

The changes are good news for women, says Dr.

IN THE JOURNALS

Laser therapy for vaginal symptoms comes up short

A small study, published online in July 2021 by the journal *Menopause*, suggested that vaginal laser therapy could help treat vaginal symptoms caused by menopause. However, a second, much larger study has determined that the intervention comes up short. This study, published Oct. 12, 2021, in *JAMA*, found that fractional carbon dioxide laser treatments were no better than a sham treatment in improving vaginal symptoms brought on by menopause.

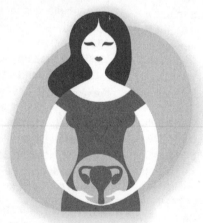

Vaginal laser treatment didn't help menopausal symptoms in a recent study.

The 12-month trial involved 85 postmenopausal women who were experiencing vaginal symptoms, such as dryness, itching and burning. Half of them underwent three laser treatments spaced four to eight weeks apart. The others received a sham treatment.

Researchers assessed the women's symptoms at the start and end of the trial and found no significant difference between the groups with regard to symptom severity or quality of life. An examination of the women's vaginal tissue also showed no differences between the two groups. Based on their study results, the researchers concluded that laser therapy was not an effective method of improving vaginal symptoms. Additional study and research will help to guide practice in the future.

Pusic. "Breast implant surgery has never been safer, because the implant technology has improved and leak rates are lower than ever. In addition, surgical complications are lower as well, thanks to new techniques and strategies. Now, women get some added assurance that the FDA is also actively engaged in making sure that breast implants are safe and that every woman is well informed," she says.

A meeting reveals problems

The FDA changes were prompted by a panel of surgeons, scientists, women, and advocacy groups convened in the spring of 2019. Immediately following

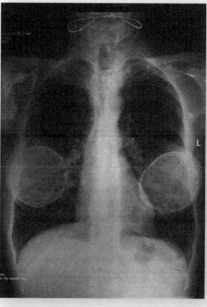

You may not think of breast implants the same way you do a cardiac pacemaker, but they are also medical devices and can bring risks.

the meeting, the FDA moved to ban the sale of textured breast implants, which were linked to an elevated risk of a rare cancer called anaplastic large-cell lymphoma. Women with the implants were not advised to remove them, but were told to watch for breast changes.

Another lesson learned from the meeting was that some women who have opted to get implants may have done so without clearly understanding all the potential drawbacks associated with the procedure. One of the risks the panel focused on is breast implant illness, a collection of symptoms including fatigue, anxiety and depression, chest pain, and hair loss that some women believe are linked to their implants.

"There is no question that a

ASK THE DOCTORS

by **HOPE RICCIOTTI, M.D., AND TONI GOLEN, M.D.**

Can you recommend strategies to help me manage my posterior vaginal prolapse?

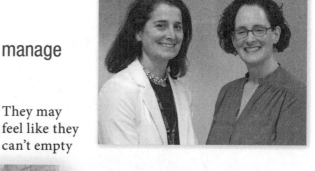

Q *I was recently diagnosed with rectocele. My doctor says I don't need surgery. How can I manage some of the discomfort that I experience during bowel movements?*

A Rectocele (formally known as posterior vaginal prolapse) occurs when the wall of tissue separating the vagina and rectum weakens over time, sometimes because of the strain of childbirth. This allows the rectal tissue to bulge into the back wall of the vagina. Some women with this condition find it more difficult to have a bowel movement, in addition to having other symptoms.

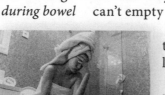

Bowel problems caused by pelvic organ prolapse are manageable.

They may feel like they can't empty their bowels completely, or they may leak stool unexpectedly.

Rectocele can often be successfully managed by making lifestyle changes to soften stool and avoid constipation, such as eating a high-fiber diet and drinking enough water. You might also want to discuss other options with your doctor, including pelvic floor physical therapy, to strengthen the pelvic muscles, or a support device called a pessary.

minority of women with breast implants are reporting symptoms. It's not yet clear whether these symptoms are caused by breast implants or if they are caused by something else completely," says Dr. Pusic. But researchers are trying to find out. In the meantime, the FDA wants women considering implant surgery to be aware that some women are experiencing these symptoms after the procedure.

The new checklist helps to inform women about this and other potential risks, such as surgical complications and breast implant rupture.

"The biggest takeaway is that we can do better in terms of informing patients about the risks and benefits of breast implants," says Dr. Pusic.

Monitoring for problems

In addition to requiring the checklist, the FDA changed its recommendations for screening women with silicone implants for leaks in an effort to encourage more women to get checked. "Silicone implants were reintroduced in the United States in 2006," says Dr. Pusic. They had been taken off the market after issues arose around breast implants leaking and

allowing the silicone to seep into the body.

To quickly identify and treat this problem before it becomes a health risk, the FDA recommends that women with silicone implants be screened for leaks every two years. Officials initially recommended that this be done using MRI. While this strategy was certainly effective in identifying breast implant rupture, many women didn't adhere to the recommendation. Not only was it costly—up to $2,000 out of pocket for each MRI scan—but for some women, MRI scans were also a source of anxiety, says Dr. Pusic. The FDA now recommends an easier, cheaper alternative—ultrasound examinations. Ultrasound can be used for routine surveillance, and potential problems, confirmed using MRI.

These new measures should ensure that women are informed and inspire confidence in those considering implants. Breast implants can bring benefits to the right patient—one who is well informed about the pros and cons of the procedure. But women should be clear that the procedure is still surgery and that breast implants are medical devices, and they need to be considered as such, she says.

Can a daily scoop of collagen powder really improve your skin?

There is evidence that collagen supplements help improve your skin, but individual studies have been small, and supplement quality varies.

Can a scoop of powder stirred into your drink really make you look younger? That's the claim made by manufacturers of collagen supplements, which are being widely promoted as a way to improve skin health and to banish wrinkles and other signs of aging.

Collagen is a crucial protein that serves as a building block not only for your skin, but also your tendons, ligaments, bones, and cartilage. It acts as scaffolding, giving your skin structure, which is why your skin starts to sag and wrinkle as collagen levels decline with age.

Collagen supplements, which also take the form

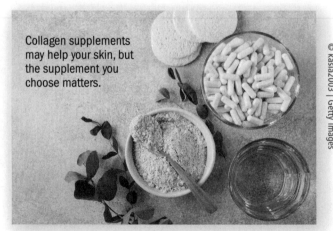

Collagen supplements may help your skin, but the supplement you choose matters.

© kasia2003 | Getty Images

of capsules, liquids, and gummy chews (among others), were a $3.71 billion market in the United States as of 2016, according to a 2019 review in the *Journal of Drugs in Dermatology*. But some of the claims surrounding these supplements sound too good to be true.

So, we wanted to know, is there any evidence that collagen supplements can really improve skin health and reverse signs of aging? More importantly, are they safe? We reached out to Dr. Peter Chien, an instructor in the Department of Dermatology at Harvard Medical School, to find out. Below is a summary of his responses.

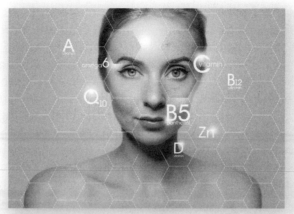

Collagen supplements are thought to be safe, but there are no long-term studies in this area.

Is there a scientific basis for these claims that collagen supplements can improve the skin?

Dr. Chien: It's biologically plausible that collagen supplements could produce an effect inside the body. When a collagen supplement is ingested, the protein is broken down into smaller parts, called dipeptides and tripeptides, which are absorbed by the intestines. Researchers know that the body absorbs them because these substances can be detected in the blood after someone takes a supplement. In mouse studies, researchers have found that dipeptides, in particular, quickly make their way into the skin, where they can be found for up to two weeks at a time. In people, collagen supplements do appear to have some effect in stimulating collagen production.

What is the evidence that collagen supplements work?

Dr. Chien: In the 2019 *Journal of Drugs in Dermatology* review, authors searched for randomized controlled trials that tested the effects of collagen supplements on the skin. They included 11 different trials that lasted an average of almost 70 days each. Overall, the combined number of trial participants was small—805 people total, 699 of them women.

The authors concluded that there was evidence that short- and long-term use of collagen supplements reduced wrinkles and other signs of skin aging, sped wound healing, boosted collagen density, and improved skin elasticity and hydration.

What types of collagen supplements were tested?

Dr. Chien: There were three types of collagen supplements studied in the various trials. Eight trials used a supplement called collagen hydrolysate. People in those studies took anywhere from 2.5 grams per day to 10 grams per day for eight to 24 weeks. Researchers in those studies were looking to see whether the supplement could help improve pressure ulcers, dry skin, signs of skin aging, or cellulite.

In two studies, participants took 3 grams per day of collagen tripeptide for 12 weeks to see if it would improve skin hydration and elasticity. A final study looked to see if collagen dipeptide could help improve age-related changes to the skin. Eighty-five women were divided into three groups and given either 5 grams of fish collagen hydrolysate with high dipeptide content (10 milligrams) daily for eight weeks, fish collagen hydrolysate with 0.5 milligrams of dipeptide for the same period of time, or a placebo pill. They determined that women who took the high-dipeptide supplement showed more improvement on measures such as skin moisture, elasticity, wrinkles, and roughness than women who took the low-level dipeptide supplement or the placebo.

What are some other specific examples from the studies that show improvement?

Dr. Chien: One study tested the effects of 10 grams of daily collagen hydrolysate in a group of 106 women between the ages of 40 and 65. Researchers found that collagen density increased by nearly 9% in women who took the supplement for 12 weeks. Density did not change in women who took a placebo.

In an eight-week study involving 114 women ages 45 to 65, researchers said those who took 2.5 grams a day of collagen hydrolysate saw a "significant" reduction in eye wrinkles compared with women who took the placebo pill. The women who took the supplements also saw an increase in skin collagen and elastin.

Another study testing collagen hydrolysate documented faster healing in pressure ulcers among long-term care residents who took the supplements, compared with those who did not.

How did researchers determine that supplements reversed signs of aging?

Dr. Chien: The studies included in the review used different methods to gauge improvements in skin aging. Some used devices to mark out wrinkles on the surface of the skin, charting how they changed over time. Others asked investigators (who weren't told who took the supplement and who didn't) to compare before-and-after photos of the study participants and to rate their skin quality.

Can someone achieve the same benefits from eating collagen-rich foods and skipping the supplement?

Dr. Chien: Collagen can be found in many foods, such as chicken and fish. Unfortunately, you probably can't eat enough collagen-rich foods to reach the amounts of collagen you would get in a supplement or to see an effect on the skin.

Do you have any overall recommendations regarding the use of collagen supplements?

Dr. Chien: Keep in mind that not all supplements are created equal. The business of making these products is very much the Wild West, with little regulation or quality control. For example, manufacturers may derive collagen from different sources, ranging from pigs and cows to marine animals. Collagen only occurs naturally in animals, but some brands claim to use plant-based collagen. It's not clear whether this type of product is effective.

Because of these variations, some supplements may help your skin, while others may do nothing. The lack of oversight also raises the risk that some formulations might not contain what's listed on the label, or they may include contaminants or other harmful ingredients. Choosing a product that uses an independent organization to verify quality, such U.S. Pharmacopeia, NSF International, or Consumer-Lab.com, can help provide some assurances. Even so, there is still room for caution.

Independent testing has found that even verified products may still have inconsistent quality. These are all things to keep in mind when considering a supplement. In addition, while there is some evidence that collagen supplements can help improve skin quality, the studies conducted so far are all small. More research is needed to confirm the results and also to determine the optimal dose as well as what skin conditions they are most effective in treating.

Are collagen supplements safe?

Dr. Chien: As of now, collagen is thought to be safe. The 2019 review published by the *Journal of Drugs in Dermatology* noted that nobody in any of the studies that they examined reported any ill effects after taking the supplements. But there aren't any studies that have examined long-term safety.

Are there other options that can provide anti-aging benefits for the skin, similar to the ones claimed by collagen supplement manufacturers?

Dr. Chien: Some cosmetic procedures that might be more effective in improving signs of aging are fractional laser resurfacing (which causes microinjuries to the skin to stimulate a healing response that boosts collagen), or skin microneedling (which uses a device to poke pinprick holes in the skin to stimulate collagen production). But these procedures also tend to cost more than supplements, so they aren't an option for everyone.

The bottom line

Ultimately, if you want to try a collagen supplement, it is likely safe and could help your skin. But the chance of seeing an improvement may depend on the product that you choose. The lack of regulation means that quality is highly variable.

Can we prevent urinary tract infections?

These are the steps to take when you're trying to ward off UTIs.

If you haven't experienced a urinary tract infection (UTI) before, take note: while the infections are uncommon in older men, they can be common in older women, occurring in 10% of women ages 65 or older, and in 30% of women ages 85 or older. For up to a third of women who have a UTI, the infection comes back within six months.

"*E. coli* bacteria [which live in the intestines] cause approximately 80% of all recurrent UTIs and continue generating microbe strains that are resistant to antibiotics. The ability of the bacteria to stick to the urinary tract can sometimes make them very difficult to eliminate," says Edward Doherty, who spent 10 years working on potential vaccines for recurrent UTI and other conditions at Harvard's Wyss Institute and is now CEO and co-founder of vaccine maker Attivare Therapeutics.

UTI causes

UTIs can arise anywhere in the urinary tract—the kidneys, bladder, ureters (the tubes that take urine from the kidneys to the bladder), or urethra (the tube that carries urine out of the body).

Female anatomy—specifically the short urethra, which opens to the outside world just above

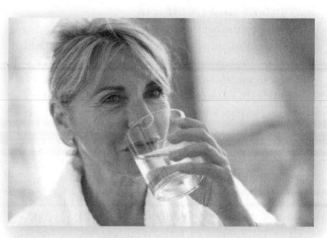
Drinking lots of water throughout the day will help flush bacteria out of the urinary tract.

the vagina—affects women's susceptibility. That's because bacteria from the rectum, especially *E. coli* (formally called *Escherichia coli*), can be pushed to the opening of the urethra through wiping or sexual intercourse. Then, they can travel up the urethra to the bladder.

"Men rarely get UTIs because of their longer urethra," explains Dr. Michael O'Leary, a urologist at Harvard-affiliated Brigham and Women's Hospital. "But sometimes a man's enlarged prostate gland impedes

IN THE JOURNALS

Migraines linked to high blood pressure after menopause

Is there a link between migraine headaches and high blood pressure (hypertension)? A study published online April 21, 2021, by *Neurology* found a connection. Researchers set out to determine if women who have had migraines were more likely to develop hypertension after menopause. They looked at 56,202 postmenopausal French women who were part of the French E3N cohort, a tracking project that began in 1990 to provide data for studies of lifestyle and disease. None of the women had high blood pressure or cardiovascular disease at the start of the study. The researchers asked women in a series of surveys if they had migraine headaches or hypertension. After controlling for migraine medications and lifestyle factors that could affect cardiovascular risk, the researchers found that high blood pressure was more common in women who had migraines than in those who did not.

the flow of urine from the bladder, causing urine to pool and creating a breeding ground for bacteria.

Symptoms and treatment

UTI symptoms usually include a burning feeling with urination, an urgent need to urinate, frequent urination, bloody or cloudy urine, or fever.

Sometimes doctors treat UTIs based only on symptoms. But the most accurate diagnosis requires a urine test to check for white blood cells and bacteria, and then a urine culture to grow bacteria in a lab and see which types are present. A course of antibiotics should clear up the infection.

One complication: older women can carry bacteria in their bladders without an infection or symptoms, a condition called asymptomatic bacteriuria. "Women with asymptomatic bacteriuria should not be treated," Dr. O'Leary says. "It's not necessary, and this causes antibiotic resistance."

Vaccines in the works

Doherty and his team started their company to license the vaccine technology developed at Harvard and then test it in humans. This vaccine and others being tested generally aim to prevent recurrent UTIs by targeting the mechanism bacteria use to stick to the lining of the urinary tract.

Some doctors, including Dr. O'Leary, are skeptical a vaccine could ever completely prevent UTIs. "There are many different bacterial causes, and one vaccine may not cover them all," he says. Still, given how commonly the responsible bacterium is *E. coli*, a vaccine targeting *E. coli* could go a long way toward preventing many, if not all, recurrent UTIs.

UTI prevention

Some women are prone to frequent or recurrent UTIs. Here are strategies that can help ward them off:

- Drink lots of water each day to flush out the urinary tract.
- Empty your bladder immediately after sexual intercourse.
- If you're a postmenopausal woman, consider using vaginal estrogen cream to help inhibit "bad" bacteria from living near the urethral opening.
- If you're a woman of any age, wipe front to

IN THE JOURNALS

Early menopause linked to higher risk of stroke

Women who go through menopause before they turn 40 may be more likely than women who undergo the transition between 50 and 54 to have a stroke, according to a study published in the August 2021 issue of the journal *Stroke*. Researchers identified this elevated risk after looking at data collected from 1993 to 1997 from 16,244 postmenopausal women, ages 26 to 70, who were part of a large database. Participants were asked about their age at menopause, as well as about their overall health, reproductive history, diet, and lifestyle.

Some 830 women went on to have a stroke within the next 15 years. After adjusting for risk factors, such as smoking, blood pressure, and body mass index, the researchers found that women who went through menopause before they turned 40 had a slightly higher stroke risk than those who were older at the time of menopause. For each year after age 50 that passed before a woman entered menopause, the risk of a later stroke dropped by 2%.

Higher risk was only seen for the most common type of stroke—ischemic stroke, which is caused by a clot or other obstruction that blocks blood flow to the brain. Risk was not higher for hemorrhagic stroke, which occurs when a weakened blood vessel in the brain bursts. The link between stroke and an earlier menopause was highest among women who entered menopause naturally, but risk was still elevated in women who entered menopause when they had their ovaries surgically removed. Researchers speculated that risk rises because of a decline in a female hormone called estradiol, which may either directly harm the blood vessels or elevate other risk factors for stroke.

back after going to the bathroom; wiping from back to front carries "bad" bacteria toward the urethral opening.

- Consider a daily long-term, low-dose antibiotic (although this has a risk of encouraging antibiotic resistance).
- If your UTIs often follow sexual intercourse, take a single dose of an antibiotic after sex.

What about supplements that claim to ward off UTIs? There's mixed evidence that cranberry products can help. Cranberries contain natural chemicals that may keep bacteria from adhering to the urinary tract lining. "But cranberry juice is very high in sugar. Stick with tablets instead," Dr. O'Leary says.

The American Urological Association notes it's okay to try cranberry to avoid UTIs. But the group has not found evidence that any other supplements—including D-mannose, herbs, hyaluronic acid, or chondroitin—will help prevent UTIs.

Bracing for incontinence

As a woman gets older, she's more likely to experience certain forms of unintended urination.

Incontinence often sneaks up on women, becoming gradually more common with age. And recent numbers suggest that certain types of incontinence are sneaking up more than usual.

A study published in the August 2021 issue of the *American Journal of Obstetrics and Gynecology* found that between 2005 and 2018, among U.S. women ages 60 or older, the prevalence of urge incontinence (a sudden, unprovoked need to urinate) jumped from about 41% to 50%, stress incontinence (leaking urine with physical activity or pressure on the bladder) went from about 51% to 53%, and mixed urinary incontinence (a combination of urge incontinence and stress incontinence) went from about 24% to 31%.

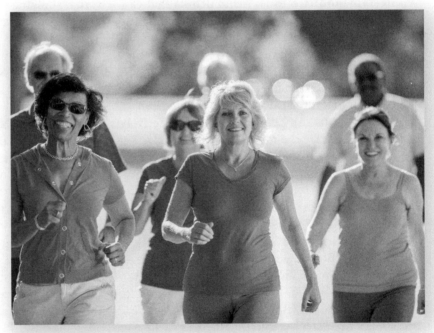

© FatCamera | Getty Images

Exercising, laughing, or coughing can cause women with stress incontinence to leak urine.

It's not clear what caused the increases. The authors noted that all types of incontinence were higher among women with obesity, other health conditions, and a history of vaginal delivery.

Since most women report some kind of incontinence by age 70, it may help to learn about symptoms so you can identify them and seek help if needed. "These conditions can worsen over time, especially if they go untreated," notes Dr. Mallika Anand, a urogynecologist and director of the Center for Intimate Health and Wellness at Harvard-affiliated Beth Israel Deaconess Medical Center.

Urge incontinence

With urge incontinence, the overwhelming feeling that you need to empty your bladder can be followed by leakage before you make it to the bathroom. The upper part of the bladder, called the detrusor muscle, initiates urination when your bladder is full. In urge incontinence, this muscle squeezes involuntarily even if your bladder is not full. "A small portion of women have a type of urge incontinence called 'neurogenic bladder,' when nerves have been damaged in some way—for example, from a stroke or diabetes," Dr. Anand says. "But most women with urge incontinence have 'non-neurogenic overactive bladder,' when the bladder is very sensitive to fluid."

Treatments for urge incontinence include the following:

Lifestyle modifications. Avoid drinks that can irritate the bladder (caffeinated drinks, sodas, and alcohol) and schedule regular bathroom breaks. If you wake up at night to urinate, try to reduce fluids for an hour or two before bed. Managing constipation can also reduce urge incontinence.

Pelvic floor exercises. A trained pelvic floor physical therapist can help you learn to effectively squeeze and release the muscles near your bladder so you can retain urine until you can reach the bathroom.

Medications. Anticholinergic medications, such as oxybutynin (Ditropan), inhibit the tightening of the bladder muscle; sympathomimetics, such as mirabegron (Myrbetriq), increase bladder capacity. "Both types of drugs can have side effects, so you'll need to monitor them carefully," Dr. Anand advises.

Botulinum toxin (Botox) injections. Injections relax the detrusor muscle for three to 12 months. "There are potential side effects, such as bladder infection or temporary urine retention. You'll have to learn to catheterize yourself three

times a day, until the Botox wears off slightly and your bladder empties more normally," Dr. Anand says.

Nerve stimulation. Your doctor can stimulate certain nerves with a needle or an implanted nerve stimulator to calm non-neurogenic overactive bladder.

Stress incontinence

If you leak urine when you cough, laugh, or exercise, it might be due to stress incontinence—leakage that occurs with pressure or physical force on the bladder. "This is a mechanical problem," Dr. Anand says.

"The tissues that support the urethra [the tube that carries urine out of the body] have weakened, and when pressure on the bladder pushes urine toward the urethra, the weakness in the tissues allows urine to leak out. Another type of stress incontinence occurs when the lining of the urethra thins, allowing urine to drip out like an open pipe."

Treatments are designed to stabilize the urethra. They can include pelvic floor exercises, weight loss, and the following:

A vaginal pessary. This is a silicone device, professionally fitted and worn inside the vagina, that pushes against the urethra to keep it in place. There are also disposable over-the-counter pessary-like devices you can try.

Urethral bulking agents. Your doctor can inject fillers into the lining of the urethra to tighten the opening. It works immediately and may be helpful for people who can't tolerate surgery, but it's not permanent.

Bladder sling surgery. Your surgeon can attach a polypropylene sling to your connective tissues to support and stabilize the urethra. "This is done through a two-centimeter vaginal incision under the urethra. A trained surgeon should place the sling, and the sling will need time to stabilize," Dr. Anand says. "In about six weeks, you should be able to laugh with your friends again, without worrying that you'll have to run to the bathroom."

Understanding menstrual changes

Here's a guide to perimenopausal bleeding to help you to decide when to call the doctor.

When it comes to menstruation, normal can be a little difficult to define. What's typical for one woman might not be for another. For example, while the typical interval from the start of one menstrual cycle to the next is 28 days, a healthy cycle can range anywhere from 21 to 35 days.

As you approach menopause—defined as one year since your last menstrual period—what's usual for you can also change. During the years just before menopause, which doctors refer to as perimenopause, women's cycles often change in length. Bleeding may become heavier or lighter. You may even miss a period from time to time. Add these changes on top of existing individual variation, and it can be hard to know what's a problem—and what's not.

We asked Dr. Karen Carlson, an internal medicine specialist and associate professor at Harvard Medical School, for some guidelines that women can use to determine how to tell which changes are normal variations and which should be brought to the attention of a doctor. Here are her answers.

Is it common for women to experience changes to menstruation during perimenopause?

Changes in menstruation are to be expected during perimenopause, which starts on average four years before the last menstrual period.

What kind of changes are typical in the years before menopause?

Cycles often get shorter as a woman enters the late reproductive years in her 40s. With the onset of perimenopause, the intervals between periods start to get longer. More dramatic changes in menstruation can also occur, including skipped periods and occasional episodes of heavier bleeding. After several years of irregularity, menstrual periods stop altogether. It's important to note that there is no typical pattern, so women should not hesitate to report a concern to their physician.

Are there certain types of bleeding that should be brought to the attention of your doctor?

In general, heavier or prolonged bleeding (more than seven days) is a greater concern than absence of bleeding. Continued irregular bleeding or spotting between periods is not typical and should be reported. Keep in mind that pregnancy is still a possibility if you miss a period, even though fertility declines with the approach of menopause.

How long should you wait before reaching out to your doctor? Is one abnormal cycle enough, or should you wait a few cycles?

It depends on how marked the change is. A single episode of very heavy premenopausal bleeding out of the blue should prompt a call to report the event. For a woman who is experiencing longer cycles or who skips a period (if there is no possibility of pregnancy), it's reasonable to keep a menstrual diary for a few cycles and then check in with the doctor.

What conditions may cause abnormal bleeding? Can any of these conditions be successfully treated?

Abnormal bleeding in perimenopause is often caused by the dramatic hormonal changes that take place during this phase of reproductive life. Other common causes of bleeding include problems in the uterus, such as fibroids (benign growths of muscle or fibrous tissue that can develop inside or on the uterus), polyps (noncancerous areas of endometrial tissue overgrowth inside the uterus), and adenomyosis (a condition where tissue that normally lines the uterus migrates into the uterine wall). In adenomyosis, the tissue continues to respond to hormones, leading to thickening and bleeding with menstrual periods, which can cause discomfort or irregular periods.

Bleeding may also arise from problems with blood clotting or be triggered by certain medications. Less commonly, bleeding may be caused by cancer of the cervix or by precancerous changes (hyperplasia) or cancer of the uterine lining. All of these conditions can be treated.

If you have abnormal bleeding, what type of tests should you anticipate?

Your doctor may want to order blood tests, such as a complete blood count, to check for anemia and to rule out pregnancy. She may also want you to undergo a pelvic ultrasound to look for a structural problem within the uterus (such as a fibroid or polyp), and to measure how thick the lining of the uterus is. Sometimes a biopsy of the uterine lining is necessary.

Routine blood tests to check hormonal levels are often not helpful.

Is bleeding a problem if you have already gone a year since your last menstrual period?

Any bleeding after menopause, even a tiny spot or brownish staining that looks like old blood, should never be ignored. Always report it to your doctor.

Although most cases of bleeding after menopause are not due to cancer, even a single episode can be a symptom of cancer of the endometrium (the uterine lining) and needs to be thoroughly evaluated.

Easing summer swelling

Tips to help you reduce puffiness in your feet and ankles and learn to recognize when it might be a sign of something more serious.

It's hot, you've been on your feet all day, and you know what's coming—uncomfortably swollen feet and ankles. This common problem is not unexpected if you spend a lot of time on your feet, particularly during the summer months.

"It becomes more common as you age because some of the conditions that cause it tend to occur as you get older," says Dr. Jennifer Cluett, a doctor of internal medicine at Harvard-affiliated Beth Israel Deaconess Hospital.

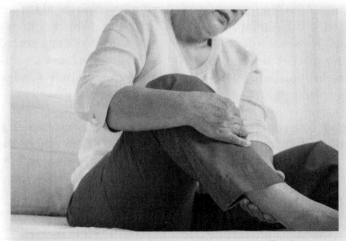

In the summer months, you might be more prone to swollen legs and ankles.

retention can be triggered by many things, including eating too much salt, heat, drinking alcohol, or standing for a long period of time.

You might be more prone to swelling if you are older, overweight, or have a condition that is increasingly common with age, called venous insufficiency, in which the veins in your leg have difficulty pushing blood against gravity back toward your heart.

Certain medications may also cause edema. The more common culprits are antidepressants, steroids, some types of blood pressure medications, and hormones, like those found in postmenopausal hormone therapy or birth control pills. Medications are a common cause, says Dr. Cluett, an assistant professor at Harvard Medical School.

Understanding edema

Lower leg and foot swelling is most often the result of an abnormal fluid buildup. Doctors call it edema. Because fluid flows downhill, it pools in the lowest parts of your body. Excess fluid

"Medication-associated swelling usually goes away when the medicine is stopped or the dose is lowered," she says.

But even if you suspect that a drug you are taking is at the root of your edema, always consult your doctor before you stop taking it. Swelling is sometimes triggered by a medical problem, such as a blood clot in your leg, an infection, an injury, or—less commonly—heart, kidney, or liver failure.

Signs of trouble

While in most instances, swelling has a harmless cause, signs that it should be brought to the

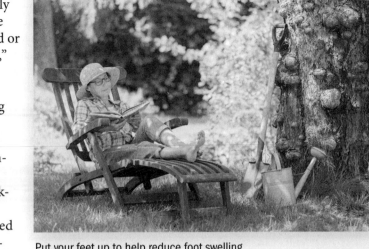
Put your feet up to help reduce foot swelling.

attention of your doctor include the following:

Swelling develops in only one leg. "In general, asymmetric swelling is often a red flag that there is something more going on," says Dr. Cluett. "Certainly, serious things can cause swelling in both legs, but when a single leg swells, it really suggests something local affecting only one leg, such as an infection, a blood clot, or an injury."

The change is sudden. Another thing to look out for is if the change in swelling is abrupt or different from what you typically experience.

Swelling is accompanied by other symptoms. You

IN THE JOURNALS

Pregnancy problems may foretell future heart disease

Women who develop health problems such as high blood pressure or diabetes while they're pregnant face an increased risk of heart disease later in life, according to a scientific statement from the American Heart Association published May 4, 2021, in the journal *Circulation*.

Up to 15% of women experience what doctors refer to as adverse pregnancy outcomes. In addition to high blood pressure and diabetes (known as gestational hypertension and gestational diabetes, respectively), four other pregnancy-related conditions also are associated with cardiovascular risk: preterm birth (giving birth before the 37th week of pregnancy), delivering

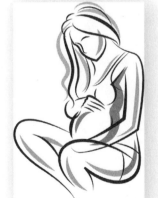

a small baby (one that weighs less than 5 pounds, 8 ounces), placental abruption (when the placenta separates from the uterus before birth), and stillbirth (death of a baby before delivery).

During pregnancy, a woman's heart pumps about 50% more blood than usual, and the demands on her body are akin to a cardiac stress test. Women who had pregnancy complications—even if they gave birth decades ago—should share that information with their physicians. The added cardiovascular risk may warrant more vigilant screening and treatment of factors related to heart health, such as blood pressure, blood sugar, and cholesterol.

should also call your doctor if in addition to swelling you have redness and pain, a fever, shortness of breath, chest pain, or pressure.

Treating edema

If your edema is not caused by a medical problem, there are some at-home strategies that you can use to get some relief.

Cut down on your salt intake. Sodium can cause your body to retain water, so focus on eating less of it. You can achieve this both by putting away the salt shaker and by carefully reading labels to avoid high-sodium foods.

Put your feet up. If you have a few minutes, elevate your feet above your heart when you are seated or lying down. This can help reduce swelling, as can putting a pillow under your feet at night while you sleep.

Wear support stockings. If you have venous insufficiency, wearing support stockings, which provide pressure to the veins in your legs to help move blood back up toward the heart, can help reduce swelling.

Get moving. Exercises such as walking, moving your ankles, and stretching can also reduce swelling by helping to push blood back toward your heart.

Prevent related problems. Chronic swelling leads to skin problems in some instances. "Taking good care of your skin will reduce your risk of infection. Use moisturizers to prevent dry, cracked skin that can be a portal for infection," says Dr. Cluett.

Chapter 10

—

Men's Health

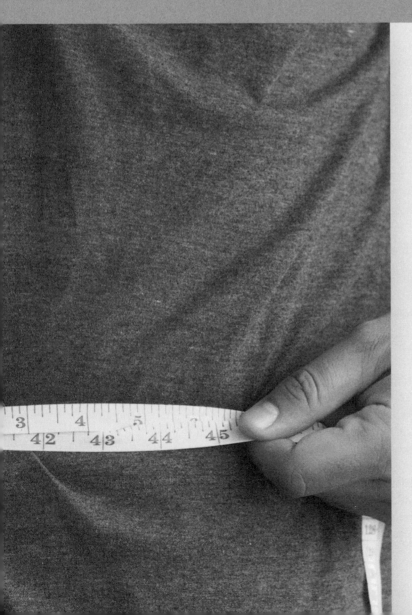

Take Action!
5 Things You Can Do Now

1 **Review your screening tests.** These are the ones you definitely should have. (page 245)

2 **Eat extra produce.** The foods could help combat erectile dysfunction. (page 255)

3 **Walk up two flights of stairs.** If you can do so without symptoms, your heart is healthy for sex. (page 258)

4 **Hire a trainer.** The investment goes a long way to reaching your weight training goals. (page 262)

5 **Cut some daily calories.** Eating a little less may lead to a longer life. (page 265)

A healthier way to look at body fat

You need some body fat for optimal health. However, where it's stored may affect your risk of health problems.

Americans have a big weight problem. According to the CDC, about 42% of men ages 60 and older are obese, storing excess body fat. "But body fat in itself is not the issue, as your body needs a certain amount of fat to stay healthy," says Dr. Caroline Apovian, co-director of the Center for Weight Management and Wellness at Harvard-affiliated Brigham and Women's Hospital. "Rather, excess stored fat and especially its location in the body have the greatest impact on health."

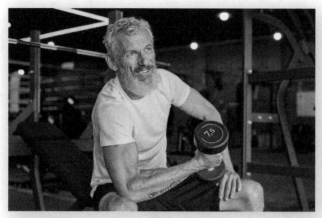

Resistance training has been shown to help older men lose excess fat by increasing muscle mass.

Body fat facts

Here is how your body stores fat. When you eat, the main components of food—protein, carbohydrates, and dietary fat—are broken down and mostly metabolized as energy to fuel the basic biological processes that keep you alive and kicking.

Any unused fuel gets stored as lipids (fatty molecules) in fat cells, called adipocytes, all around the body. The amount of that stored fuel—measured in calories—determines how much fat cells grow. In fact, fat cells can expand or shrink in size by up to a factor of 50.

You never lose fat cells, and once you reach adulthood, the number more or less stays the same. You also can't control where your body stores fat. "Factors like body type, age, hormones, and genetic predisposition all determine where excess fat ends up," says Dr. Apovian.

Stored fat in itself is not bad. The body needs fat reserves for emergency energy, and fat helps insulate the body and protect vital organs. Fat cells also release leptin, a hormone that acts on the brain to decrease appetite and help regulate body weight.

It's how much body fat you have, and where, that makes a difference to your health. In most people, about 90% of body fat is subcutaneous, meaning it lies in a layer just beneath the skin. The remaining 10% is visceral fat, which lies beneath the abdominal wall and in the spaces surrounding the liver, intestines, and other organs. Of the two, visceral fat is the most troublesome: having too much increases the risk for type 2 diabetes, heart disease, and a fatty liver. While fat is practically everywhere in the body—chest, back, stomach, glutes—the midsection is where most men see (and feel) excess amounts

Too many calories

Why does body fat build up? It's a myth that eating fat makes you fat, and in fact, it can be the opposite. "Many natural foods high in healthy mono- and polyunsaturated fats can make you feel fuller faster because fats are slow to digest," says Dr. Apovian. She points out that the highly touted Mediterranean diet, which was recently ranked the healthiest diet, contains 40% to 50% fat.

Weight gain is caused by eating too many calories, no matter the source. The biggest calorie culprits are ultra-processed foods, such as frozen pizza, soda, fast foods, and salty snacks. Americans eat more of them than ever, according to a study published online Oct. 14, 2021, by *The American Journal of Clinical Nutrition* that examined the daily eating habits of about 41,000 adults over a period of 18 years.

Other research has found that people whose diets contain high amounts of ultra-processed foods eat around 500 extra calories per day compared with people who eat few of these foods. "The research suggests that ultra-processed foods 'fool' your brain into eating more calories than if you are eating whole foods or unprocessed foods," says Dr. Apovian. "If your body doesn't use those extra calories, they get stored as fat, and that is why people gain weight."

Using the fuel

There are different ways to burn excess stored fat. The first is to reduce your calorie intake. When you consume fewer calories than your body needs, your body converts stored fat into usable energy for fuel. As a result, fat cells get smaller, and you lose weight.

Low-carb diets follow this approach since carbohydrates are the body's primary source of calories. Research has shown low-carb diets can help jumpstart weight loss, but the effect can wane after about six months to a year. "Part of the problem is that low-carb diets are tough to maintain for long periods," says Dr. Apovian.

This is why many nutritionists promote an all-around healthy diet that includes adequate amounts of protein, carbohydrate, and fat as well as essential vitamins and minerals. "A low-carb diet can help in the short term, but if you don't adjust your overall eating habits, you can gain it all back," says Dr. Apovian.

The other way to burn fat and shrink fat cells is with exercise. Moderate-intensity aerobic exercise like brisk walking, cycling, and swimming can force the body to tap into stored fat for energy. (Guidelines suggest you get at least 150 minutes per week of moderate-intensity exercise.) However, how quickly your body burns fat depends on your body size and exercise intensity.

Resistance (weight) training also can help older men lose excess stored fat by increasing muscle mass. "Men naturally lose muscle mass as they age, and increasing muscle can make their body burn more calories," says Dr. Apovian.

An analysis published online Sept. 21, 2021, by *Sports Medicine* found that people who engaged in 45 to 60 minutes of resistance training two to three times a week for five months reduced both their visceral fat and total body fat.

"But if you want to lose weight, you can't count on exercise alone. You will also need to reduce your calorie intake," says Dr. Apovian. "And to help keep it off, you need to do resistance training at least two to three times per week."

Do BMI numbers add up?

Body mass index has had a mixed reputation for estimating obesity and possible health risks. Are there alternatives to measuring body fat?

How much body fat do you have? The number on a bathroom scale usually offers a clue, but it doesn't always tell the complete story.

For decades, researchers have used body mass index (BMI) to determine whether a person's weight is optimal and as an estimate of a person's proportion of body fat. The BMI formula uses body weight in kilograms divided by the square of height in meters—or, in American measurements, body weight in pounds divided by the square of height in inches and then multiplied by 703. (If you want to avoid doing math, use an online BMI calculator like the one at

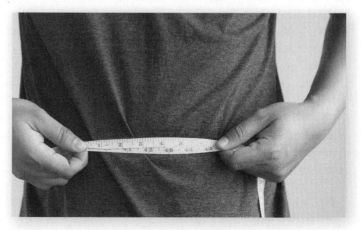

Measuring waist size is a simple way to identify changes in fat mass.

www.health.harvard.edu/bmi.)

There are four categories of BMI:

- underweight: less than 18.5
- normal weight: 18.5 to 24.9
- overweight: 25 to 29.9
- obesity: 30 or higher.

"BMI provides a good estimation of a person's amount of body fat, and the number can offer guidance on whether people should make lifestyle changes, like modifying their diet and adopting more cardio and strength training," says Dr. Frank Hu, a professor of nutrition and epidemiology at the Harvard T.H. Chan School of Public Health.

Still, BMI is far from an ideal measuring system, and for many older adults, it may not be the best way to gauge body fat.

Fat problems

It's essential to keep tabs on body fat as you age. Our bodies need some fat to perform everyday functions. But carrying too much can raise your risk of heart disease, diabetes, and certain cancers. In general, the higher the BMI number, the greater the risks.

While research has found BMI a strong predictor of health risks, it has its faults. First, while it has some correlation to overall fat mass, BMI can't distinguish between subcutaneous fat (the kind that lies just below the skin) and the more dangerous visceral fat, which lies deep in the body and surrounds organs.

Studies also have suggested the BMI scale may be less accurate for certain ethnic groups, like Asians, who tend to naturally carry more body fat than people of European descent, and Black men, who tend to have lower body fat percentages than white men.

BMI also can't be adjusted to account for normal physical changes. "As men age, they naturally lose muscle mass, which can get replaced with fat," says Dr. Hu. "So, even though their weight may be about the same, they may have added extra fat that BMI won't recognize."

Measure of success

Are there any alternatives to BMI? The most accurate way to measure fat mass is with computed

The line on waist size

Waist circumference is the distance in inches around the abdomen. Here's how to accurately measure it:

1. Stand and place a tape measure around your bare waist—at or just below your belly button.

2. Keep the tape snug but not so tight that it compresses the skin.

3. Relax and let your breath out before measuring.

4. Do it at least twice to get an accurate reading.

Ideally, your waist size should be no more than one-half of your height in inches. For example, a man who is 6 feet tall could feel good about a waist size of 36 inches or less. Even if you're above your ideal goal, track your measurement monthly to see if you're headed in the right direction.

tomography (CT) and magnetic resonance imaging (MRI) scans. These imaging techniques also can identify amounts of subcutaneous and visceral fat.

Another high-tech approach is dual energy x-ray absorptiometry (DEXA), which measures fat via x-ray beams that pass through body tissues at different rates. However, DEXA cannot distinguish between subcutaneous and visceral fat. "The major downside to these is that they require specialized machines, which makes the tests expensive," says Dr. Hu. "They also are not widely available to most people."

The solution? Grab a measuring tape.

"It's not highly technical, but measuring your waist circumference is an easy way to identify increased fat mass, since most men accumulate extra fat around their midsection," says Dr. Hu. (See "The line on waist size.")

This doesn't mean BMI is useless. In fact, Dr. Hu suggests older men use both BMI and waist circumference to measure and monitor their fat mass.

"Neither one is perfect, but taken together, they can help create a more accurate reading of your accumulated fat," he says. "Perhaps best of all, they help you stay mindful about your weight so you can note any increases before they escalate."

Answers to prostate cancer questions

Confused about the latest guidelines on testing and screening? Here's what you need to know.

Postate cancer is the second most common cancer among American men, behind skin cancer. Most men can live long and fruitful lives with the disease if it's properly managed and treated. Still, new studies and evolving guidelines have made the testing and screening process unclear.

So what are the current procedures for getting checked for possible prostate cancer? And what new options are now available? We asked Dr. Marc Garnick, editor in chief of the 2022 *Annual Report on Prostate Diseases* from Harvard Health Publishing, to address the questions men commonly ask.

The role of PSA

Is the prostate-specific antigen (PSA) test still the best screening option for men?

A PSA test is still controversial, since the vast majority of studies suggest it's not associated with better quality of life or lower risk of death from prostate cancer. And the results may not always tell the whole story about whether or not you have prostate cancer. Still, it can provide some helpful information.

The test measures the amount of PSA in your blood. PSA is a protein produced by both cancerous and noncancerous tissue in the prostate. While small amounts of PSA normally circulate in the blood, large amounts could suggest cancer. A PSA number less than 4 nanograms per milliliter [ng/mL] is considered to signify a very low risk for cancer. A score of 4 to 10 ng/mL is the gray area where the risk is higher but not

---

IN THE JOURNALS

Warning: Hidden ingredients in supplements for weight loss and male enhancement

Think twice before buying dietary supplements that claim to help you lose weight or rev up your sex life. The FDA is seeing an increase in sales of over-the-counter supplements that contain hidden and dangerous prescription drugs, controlled substances, or untested and unstudied components. Such ingredients may cause serious side effects and interact with medications you're taking. The tainted supplements are widely available and sold online from sellers on eBay or Amazon or through large retail stores such as Walmart. In December 2021, for example, the FDA identified nine sexual

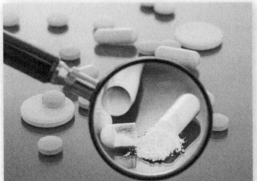

© unpict | Getty Images

enhancement products with dangerous ingredients sold on Walmart's website.

Remember: unlike pharmaceuticals, over-the-counter supplements are not tested by the FDA, and companies can sell anything they like until the FDA proves they're unsafe. Also, know that many types of supplements contain dangerous ingredients—including some products claiming to promote better sleep or relieve pain. Talk to your doctor before taking any supplement, and do your homework: check out the FDA's tainted products database (www.health.harvard.edu/tainted) to see if supplements in your medicine cabinet (or some you're eyeing) are listed.

conclusive. A PSA score higher than 10 ng/mL is the most concerning.

In men with a high PSA score, the test is usually repeated for accuracy. For example, PSA levels can temporarily spike if you had sex in the previous 24 to 48 hours. An enlarged prostate, which affects most men over time, can also influence PSA. Depending on your PSA score, your doctor may suggest retesting anywhere from four weeks to six months later to check for rising levels.

A digital rectal examination [DRE] is often given if your score is higher than 4 ng/mL. Here, your doctor feels your prostate for any hardness or irregularities in the tissue, which may indicate cancer. It's best to discuss the pros and cons of PSA testing with your doctor.

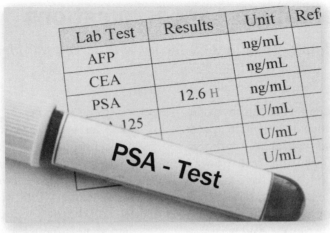

© jarun011 | Getty Images

Lab Test	Results	Unit	Ref
AFP		ng/mL	
CEA		ng/mL	
PSA	12.6 H	ng/mL	
A 125		U/mL	
		U/mL	
		U/mL	

PSA tests can provide valuable information, although their overall role is still debated.

Biopsy guidelines

If my PSA continues to rise, or gets higher than 10 ng/mL, what will my doctor order next? Is it time for a biopsy?

For rising or high numbers, there are a few additional tests that could be offered. One is a test that looks for prostate cancer biomarkers in the urine. The kind of biomarker and the amount can indicate the likelihood that cancer exists and may spread.

Another is a blood test for what is known as free PSA. PSA circulates in the blood in two forms—either bound to other proteins, or unbound, also called free. A regular PSA test measures both bound and unbound PSA. The free PSA blood test gets reported as a percent of the total PSA.

A lower percentage suggests a higher risk of cancer. For example, cancer is more likely if a free PSA level is 15% or lower and less likely if it's higher than 25%. Depending on the results of these tests, your current PSA score, and the findings of a DRE, your doctor may suggest a biopsy to analyze prostate tissue

samples for cancer.

However, before a biopsy, you may get a prostate MRI scan. This helps determine the size and location of tumors for a more targeted biopsy with the possibility of having fewer samples taken. Still, during the first biopsy, many doctors will recommend taking biopsies from the entire prostate gland in addition to the abnormal areas suggested by the scan.

Also, keep in mind that even if an MRI scan doesn't suggest cancer, your doctor may suggest a biopsy depending on the results of the other tests.

New technologies

Are there new diagnostic tests available?

There are two new FDA-approved imaging technologies—the Axumin and gallium-68 PSMA-11 scans. Both are game changers, as they can help identify previously undetectable cancer that even MRI can't always pick up.

Axumin is the trade name for fluciclovine F 18, a radioactive agent that is injected into your body. You then undergo a scan with positron emission tomography [PET] and CT. Prostate cancer cells absorb amino acids at a more rapid pace than healthy cells. Axumin concentrates on these specific cells, which are highlighted under a PET and CT scan.

The gallium-68 PSMA-11 test also uses an injectable radioactive agent in conjunction with a PET scan. Once injected, the agent binds to prostate-specific membrane antigen [PSMA], high levels of which are found in prostate cancer cells. This makes any PSMA-positive lesions in the prostate easier for a PET scan to see.

Additional research will guide how doctors might use these new diagnostic tests in the evaluation of men with possible prostate cancer.

A look at health screenings

Which screening tests do you really need?

Men are less likely than women to get regular diagnostic screenings and tests, especially when they are younger. But as men age, these screenings become even more essential. "Screenings and tests are still one of the best ways to find potential problems before they become serious," says Dr. Paul Heinzelmann, a primary care physician at Harvard-affiliated Massachusetts General Hospital.

There are all kinds of screening tests available for an array of potential health problems. So which ones do you need? Most of them fall into two categories: tests that almost all men should get and ones men should consider.

Get these

Most doctors follow screening guidelines from the U.S. Preventive Services Task Force (USPSTF), an independent panel of experts that reviews the value of tests based on the latest scientific evidence. "There are certain ones that men should definitely have at some point," says Dr. Heinzelmann. Essentially everyone should be screened for the following conditions.

Colon cancer. The USPSTF recommends people ages 45 to 75 get screened for colon cancer. For people ages 76 to 85, the decision should be based on life expectancy, overall health, and results of past screenings. After age 85, routine screening is more likely to cause harm rather than benefit. There are several ways to screen for colon cancer:

- Colonoscopy is the gold standard for screening. A doctor eases a thin, flexible tube mounted with a tiny video camera into the rectum. He or she examines the entire colon looking for, and possibly removing, growths called polyps. If no polyps are found, you repeat the exam in 10 years. If precancerous polyps are removed, your doctor may suggest another colonoscopy in three to five years.
- Flexible sigmoidoscopy is similar to a colonoscopy, but the doctor examines only the bottom third of the colon, where most polyps develop. This option is repeated every

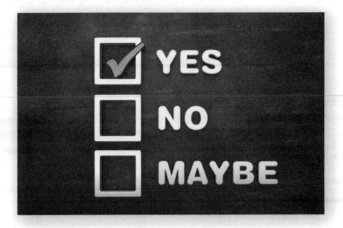

All men should get specific health screenings at certain points in their lives.

five years. If precancerous polyps are found, you will need a colonoscopy.
- CT colonography uses a CT scan to view the entire colon. While this test can spot polyps, it takes a colonoscopy to remove them. This test is repeated every five years.
- Stool-based tests are a less-invasive option; if the result is positive, you'll need a colonoscopy. There are several kinds. A guaiac-based fecal occult blood test (gFOBT) and fecal immunochemical test (FIT) work similarly. You place stool samples on test cards, put them in a supplied container, and send to your doctor for analysis. These should be done yearly. A multitargeted stool DNA test—also known by its brand name, Cologuard—combines the FIT with a test that looks for altered DNA in a stool sample you send to a lab. It is given every one to three years.

Diabetes. While it's a good idea for all adults to have at least one blood sugar test, almost 75% of men in America are considered overweight or obese (a body mass index of 25 or higher). This puts them at higher risk for diabetes, and they should get screened for type 2 diabetes starting at age 35.

Other candidates are those with a blood pressure reading of 135/80 millimeters of mercury (mm Hg) or higher or who currently take blood pressure medication. To diagnose diabetes (and prediabetes), doctors most commonly order a blood glucose test after fasting, or a non-fasting hemoglobin A1c level that reflects the average blood glucose over the prior two to three months.

Hepatitis C. This virus causes an infection that can damage the liver. All adults up to age 79 should get a blood test for hepatitis C, especially those who use injected drugs or have done so in the past. "This is a one-time screening for people with normal liver function and no special risk factors," says Dr. Heinzelmann.

High blood pressure. Adults should have their blood pressure checked at least annually. Current guidelines define elevated blood pressure as having a systolic measurement (the first number in a reading) of 120 to 129 and a diastolic measurement (the second number) lower than 80. A reading of 130/80 mm Hg or higher is considered high blood pressure.

Dr. Heinzelmann says getting your blood pressure check at the doctor's office can offer an accurate baseline reading. "But you should also use a home blood pressure monitor to compare the numbers, as some people suffer from white-coat syndrome, a condition where a person gets high blood pressure when they are around doctors," he says.

If you have elevated or borderline high blood pressure, your doctor may suggest checking it again after four to six months.

HIV. The USPSTF recommends at least a one-time blood test for HIV infection for all men up to age 65

Give these tests a pass

The U.S. Preventive Services Task Force (USPSTF) recommends against routine screening for several conditions, including pancreatic, testicular, and thyroid cancers and chronic obstructive pulmonary disease (COPD). "These screenings don't have any evidence to support their effectiveness in people who don't show symptoms," says Dr. Paul Heinzelmann with Harvard-affiliated Massachusetts General Hospital.

The USPSTF recommends against prostate-specific antigen (PSA) testing to screen for prostate cancer in men ages 70 and older. However, PSA testing for men ages 55 to 69 remains an individual decision, so check with your doctor.

The USPSTF has also weighed in regarding some routine screening tests with insufficient evidence that they offer more benefit than potential harm. These tests include routine electrocardiograms (ECGs), mouth exams to look for cancer, and tests for vitamin D deficiency, hearing loss, sleep apnea, osteoporosis (men only), and celiac disease. Of course, these tests may be appropriate for men with special risks or symptoms.

---

and for men older than 65 who continue to have more than one sexual partner or who have entered a new relationship.

Consider these
Men should also consider the following screening tests if they are at increased risk for a specific condition. "Talk with your doctor about whether these apply to you," says Dr. Heinzelmann.

Abdominal aortic aneurysm (AAA). This is a swelling in the lower section of the body's main blood vessel. The condition can worsen over time and cause the aorta to burst. Men ages 65 to 75 who have ever smoked should get a one-time ultrasound. Most people won't have symptoms, but they can include a pulsating feeling near the navel and pain in the chest, lower back, or above the kidneys.

Hepatitis B. People who are more likely to have been infected with the hepatitis B virus should get screened with a blood test, since many who have the virus don't show symptoms until the liver becomes inflamed or they develop cirrhosis (liver scarring). High-risk people include those who are HIV-positive, have used injected drugs, share a household with someone with the virus, and men in same-sex relationships.

Lung cancer. Adults ages 50 to 80 who have smoked the equivalent of a pack of cigarettes a day for 20 years and who currently smoke or have quit within the past 15 years should consider an annual lung low-dose CT scan.

Steps to treating an enlarged prostate

Drugs can often help, but sometimes surgery is needed.

As men age, they often experience a new kind of growth spurt, known as benign prostatic hyperplasia (BPH) or an enlarged prostate gland.

Your prostate is located just below the bladder. Over time, it can grow from about the size of a walnut to as large as a lemon. It weighs about 30 to 35 grams in your 50s, but can balloon to as much as 100 grams. A growing prostate can place pressure on the urethra, the tube that carries urine from the bladder through the penis and out of the body (see image).

This can lead to all kinds of urination problems. The most common are trouble beginning to urinate, dribbling, and the feeling that you have not fully emptied your bladder. Urine that doesn't get expelled and collects in the bladder may be prone to becoming infected. You also may make extra bathroom trips, especially at night, and even potentially lose bladder control.

"While BPH won't raise your prostate cancer risk or necessarily lead to serious sexual problems, it can cause bothersome urination problems," says Dr. Martin Kathrins, a urologist with Harvard-affiliated Brigham and Women's Hospital.

Drugs of choice

The first line of treatment for BPH is lifestyle

Benign Prostatic Hyperplasia

Bladder

Urine

Enlarged prostate

Compressed urethra

For more information on BPH and other prostate problems, read the *2022 Annual Report on Prostate Diseases* from *Harvard Health Publishing*, available at www.health.harvard.edu/prostate.

© Sakurra | Getty Images

Tips for relieving BPH symptoms

These simple steps can help alleviate some of the symptoms of BPH:

▶ Reduce stress by exercising regularly and practicing relaxation techniques such as meditation. Some men who are nervous and tense urinate more frequently.

▶ When you go to the bathroom, take the time to empty as much of your bladder as you can. This will reduce the need for subsequent trips to the toilet and minimize the chances that urine will collect and become stagnant in the bladder, leading to possible infections and bladder stones.

▶ Talk with your doctor about all your prescription and over-the-counter medications; some, such as antihistamines and decongestants, may affect urination. Your doctor may be able to adjust dosages, change your schedule for taking these drugs, or prescribe different medications that cause fewer urinary problems.

▶ Avoid drinking fluids in the evening, particularly caffeinated and alcoholic beverages. Both can affect the muscle tone of the bladder and stimulate the kidneys to produce urine, leading to nighttime urination.

▶ On long airplane flights, avoid drinking alcohol, and try to urinate every 60 to 90 minutes.

changes to help manage symptoms. These include maintaining a healthy weight, avoiding medications like antihistamines and decongestants, adopting a healthy diet, and limiting caffeine, which can irritate the bladder and increase urination frequency.

If these are not helpful, medication may be needed. Drugs help manage symptoms or shrink the prostate. There are two main classes: alpha blockers and 5-alpha-reductase inhibitors (5ARIs). Your doctor may prescribe one or both types, depending on your symptoms.

Alpha blockers. These relax the muscles around the prostate and bladder neck so urine flows more easily. Symptoms often improve within a few days. They are most effective for men with mild to moderate prostate enlargement. The common drugs include tamsulosin (Flomax), alfuzosin (Uroxatral), and silodosin (Rapaflo).

5ARIs. These shrink the prostate, so it puts less pressure on the urethra. They can reduce the prostate's size by one-fifth or more after six months, which is usually sufficient shrinkage to improve symptoms. The two drugs often prescribed are finasteride (Proscar) and dutasteride (Avodart).

"Low daily doses of the erectile dysfunction drug tadalafil [Cialis] also have shown to help with BPH symptoms," says Dr. Kathrins.

It may take time for men to notice improvement with these drugs, so doctors recommend sticking with them for about three months. But sometimes medication is not enough.

"For some men, drugs simply don't work, or they have trouble taking them as required," says Dr. Kathrins. "In these cases, minimally invasive surgery may be helpful."

For details on BPH drug side effects, please see "Medications for BPH" on page 250.

Know your options

Surgical procedures can treat BPH in three ways: remove excess prostate tissue that disrupts the flow of urine, adjust the position of the prostate so it's no longer obstructive, or shrink the prostate. Procedures last about one to two hours. Some can be performed in the office or a surgical center, while others require a short hospital stay. "Depending on the procedure, most men can see improvements in their symptoms in a few weeks, on average," says Dr. Kathrins.

There are possible side effects to BPH surgery. Some men experience short-term erectile dysfunction, although this could become an ongoing problem. Another potential issue is retrograde ejaculation, where semen discharges into the bladder instead of out through the penis. "This may bother some men, even though it doesn't affect sexual performance and is often the cost of surgically treating an enlarged prostate," says Dr. Kathrins.

The type of surgery you need depends on several factors, such as your prostate's size and shape and your comfort level. (Your doctor can use a digital rectal exam, ultrasound, or MRI of the pelvis to find out the size and shape.) Here's a look at the most common choices, as well as some new options. Talk with your urologist about which one is best for you.

Transurethral resection of the prostate (TURP). TURP is the go-to surgery for BPH and treats a broad range of prostate sizes—from 30 grams to 100 grams. Here, an instrument called a resectoscope, which contains a light and an electrical loop for both cutting tissue and sealing blood vessels, is inserted into the urethra via the penis. The surgeon then uses the wire loop to hollow out the enlarged tissue blocking the urethra and impeding urine flow. Most men need a catheter for a few days to urinate.

Vaporization. These approaches, which are also suitable for medium-range prostate sizes, include photo-selective vaporization of the prostate (PVP) and bipolar plasma vaporization (BPV). PVP uses a high-powered laser to vaporize prostate tissue. BPV uses energy to heat a button-shaped electrode that destroys the excess tissue. Both options are less invasive than TURP and have a quicker recovery time. "Some men experience more irritative symptoms after this surgery compared with TURP," says Dr. Kathrins.

Holmium laser enucleation of the prostate (HoLEP). HoLEP helps with larger prostates (60 grams or more). It involves using a tiny laser threaded through the urethra to destroy excess prostate tissue. The procedure usually causes minor bleeding and has a relatively fast recovery time. However, it's not available everywhere.

5-alpha-reductase inhibitors, alpha blockers, and cancer

In addition to treating BPH, 5-alpha-reductase inhibitors have also been tested as a means of preventing prostate cancer. In two separate trials, finasteride and dutasteride were shown to lower the overall risk of prostate cancer by about 25% to 30%. Here's the catch (and it is an important one): both medications were also associated with a small, but statistically significant, increase in risks for high-grade prostate cancer. As a result, the FDA put a cancer warning on the drugs. In 2019, scientists followed up with findings showing that alpha blockers similarly reduce the likelihood of developing prostate cancer—in this case, by 11%. But increased risks of high-grade prostate cancer among diagnosed men were also observed.

If you are taking a 5-alpha-reductase inhibitor, an alpha blocker, or the combination pill Jalyn (which contains dutasteride along with the alpha blocker tamsulosin) for BPH, talk with your doctor about the cancer risk and what you should do.

Sources: Thompson IM Jr, Goodman PJ, Tangen CM, et al. Long-Term Survival of Participants in the Prostate Cancer Prevention Trial. *New England Journal of Medicine* 2013;369(7):603–10. PMID: 23944298.

Van Rompay MI, Nickel JC, Ranganathan G, et al. Impact of 5a-Reductase Inhibitor and a-Blocker Therapy for Benign Prostatic Hyperplasia on Prostate Cancer Incidence and Mortality. *BJU International* 2019;123(3):511–18. PMID: 30216624.

Walsh PC. Survival in the Prostate Cancer Prevention Trial. *New England Journal of Medicine* 2013;369(20):1967–68. PMID: 24224633.

Prostatic urethral lift. This procedure, known by the trade name UroLift, is often used on prostates 30 grams to 80 grams in size. The doctor passes small implants through the urethra and places them in the prostate so that they pull back on the obstructive tissue and hold it out of the way. UroLift's advantage is that it tends to reduce the risk of erectile dysfunction and retrograde ejaculation.

Water vapor thermal therapy. For this procedure, known by the trade name Rezum, the doctor inserts a tool with an attached camera through the urethra into the prostate, where it delivers small amounts of steam. The steam damages the obstructing tissue cells and shrinks the prostate. "This procedure is used for similar size ranges as UroLift and limits the risk of sexual side effects after surgery," says Dr. Kathrins.

Aquablation. This procedure, which uses a robotically controlled water jet to remove excess tissue, is often a choice for prostates larger than 80 grams. Aquablation has been found to limit the risk of sexual side effects compared with TURP, but it is not widely available.

Prostate artery embolization (PAE). The FDA approved PAE for use in the United States in 2018, although Europeans have used it for years. A small catheter is inserted into the upper thigh or wrist and threaded into the arteries that supply blood to the prostate. Using the catheter, the doctor deposits small particles into the arteries, where they partially block blood flow. This will eventually cause the prostate to shrink.

The advantage of PAE is that it's an outpatient procedure and has a lower risk of causing erectile dysfunction. However, the American Urological Association, citing a lack of supporting studies, has not yet endorsed it.

"Depending on the initial procedure a man chooses, he may need another surgery later," says Dr. Kathrins. "Some men will continue to take a 5ARI indefinitely to reduce the risk that the prostate will regrow."

Also, keep in mind that surgery won't completely improve all urinary problems, and you need to have some realistic expectations. "Your doctor can explain what to expect so you can prepare for the outcome," says Dr. Kathrins.

Medications for BPH

MEDICATION	SIDE EFFECTS	COMMENTS
Alpha blockers (nonselective)		
doxazosin (Cardura) terazosin (Hytrin)	Dizziness, headache, and fatigue are most common. Nasal congestion, dry mouth, and swelling in the ankles can also occur. Low blood pressure (hypotension), although rare, may pose a danger for some people.	Should be used carefully by those with high blood pressure (hypertension) or heart disease. May increase risk of aggressive prostate cancer; important to monitor PSA (see "5-alpha-reductase inhibitors, alpha blockers, and cancer" on the previous page).
Alpha blockers (selective)		
alfuzosin (Uroxatral) prazosin (Minipress) silodosin (Rapaflo) tamsulosin (Flomax)	Dizziness, headache, and fatigue are most common. Nasal congestion, dry mouth, and swelling in the ankles can also occur. Can cause rash.	Do not lower blood pressure, but men taking silodosin may notice a drop in blood pressure upon standing.
5-alpha-reductase inhibitors		
dutasteride (Avodart) finasteride (Proscar)	Although uncommon, decreased libido, decreased ejaculate volume, and impotence may occur. (Problems with libido may continue after you stop taking finasteride.) Cardiovascular effects and depression may occur in some men. Minor reports of rash. New data suggest a heightened risk of osteoporosis.	Help shrink larger prostate glands. Reduce need for surgery. Not beneficial for small prostates. Slow to act; can take up to two years to see full benefits. Can lower PSA levels by 50%. May increase risk of aggressive prostate cancer; important to monitor PSA (see "5-alpha-reductase inhibitors, alpha blockers, and cancer"). In some men, finasteride can lead to problems in sexual function, depression, and other changes in mood.
Combination therapy		
dutasteride and tamsulosin (Jalyn)	Dizziness, headache, and fatigue are most common. Low blood pressure, although rare, may pose a danger for some.	Can lower PSA levels considerably. May increase risk of aggressive prostate cancer; important to monitor PSA.
PDE5 inhibitor		
tadalafil (Cialis)	Headache, flushing, upset stomach, and nasal congestion can occur. Temporary disturbances in color vision are possible. In rare cases, may cause priapism, an erection that lasts too long.	Do not take more than one pill in 24 hours. Do not take if you are also taking alpha blockers or nitrate medications, to avoid risk of low blood pressure that can cause fainting.
Antimuscarinics		
fesoterodine (Toviaz) oxybutynin (Ditropan) tolderodine (Detrol)	Dry mouth, dilation of pupils and sensitivity to light, increased fluid pressure in the eye, and dry skin may occur.	May accelerate existing cognitive decline in the elderly.
Antidiuretic hormone		
desmopressin acetate (Noctiva)	Dizziness is the most problematic, potentially leading to falls. Others include nasal discomfort, cold symptoms, increased blood pressure, and back pain.	Nasal spray to limit nighttime urination. Can depress sodium levels in blood. Should not be taken by men with low sodium levels, as excessively low values can lead to dizziness, fainting, and coma in rare instances. Should not be taken by men with heart failure or uncontrolled hypertension.

Your urinary symptom score

To evaluate the severity of your benign prostatic hyperplasia (BPH), your doctor may ask you to complete a questionnaire like the International Prostate Symptom Score (IPSS). Choose one number to respond to questions 1 to 7, and then calculate your total urinary symptom score. Question 8 is separate and indicates how bothered you are by the condition.

Urinary symptom scores of 1–7 indicate mild symptoms. Scores of 8–18 are considered moderate. And scores of 19 or greater are severe. If you have moderate to severe symptoms, and if your answer to question 8 is a 3, 4, or 5, you may want to discuss treatment (either medication or surgery) with your physician.

1. Over the past month, how often have you had a sensation of not having emptied your bladder completely after you finished urinating?

0	Not at all
1	Less than 1 in 5 times
2	Less than half the time
3	About half the time
4	More than half the time
5	Almost always

2. Over the past month, how often have you had to urinate again less than two hours after you last finished urinating?

0	Not at all
1	Less than 1 in 5 times
2	Less than half the time
3	About half the time
4	More than half the time
5	Almost always

3. Over the past month, how often have you stopped and started again several times while urinating?

0	Not at all
1	Less than 1 in 5 times
2	Less than half the time
3	About half the time
4	More than half the time
5	Almost always

4. Over the past month, how often have you found it difficult to postpone urination?

0	Not at all
1	Less than 1 in 5 times
2	Less than half the time
3	About half the time
4	More than half the time
5	Almost always

5. Over the past month, how often have you had a weak urinary stream?

0	Not at all
1	Less than 1 in 5 times
2	Less than half the time
3	About half the time
4	More than half the time
5	Almost always

6. Over the past month, how often have you had to push or strain to begin urination?

0	Not at all
1	Less than 1 in 5 times
2	Less than half the time
3	About half the time
4	More than half the time
5	Almost always

7. Over the past month, how many times, typically, did you get up to urinate between the time you went to bed and the time you got up in the morning?

0	None
1	Once
2	Twice
3	Three times
4	Four times
5	Five times or more

Urinary symptom score: _____

8. How would you feel if you had to live with your urinary condition the way it is now, no better, no worse, for the rest of your life?

0	Delighted
1	Pleased
2	Mostly satisfied
3	Mixed
4	Mostly not satisfied
5	Unhappy

Quality of life score: _____

Help for erectile dysfunction

Pills help many men maintain an active sex life. But if you need more assistance, there are other options.

Taking erectile dysfunction pills is still the easiest way for most older men to manage their ED. The drugs work quickly to increase blood flow to the penis to help produce and maintain an erection, and the effect can last several hours, usually with minimal side effects. With more generic versions available, ED drugs are now more affordable.

But ED pills don't work for everyone, or the results are inconsistent. Men also could be bothered by the side effects, such as headaches, flushing, upset stomach, or dizziness. This doesn't mean you have no other options.

"There are other methods that may be just as just as effective as taking traditional ED drugs," says Dr. Michael O'Leary, a urologist and director of men's health at Harvard-affiliated Brigham and Women's Hospital's Division of Urology, and the editor in chief of the Harvard Special Health Report *Erectile Dysfunction* (www.health.harvard.edu/mens-health/erectile-dysfunction).

Here is a look at some alternative therapies that may be more effective and tolerable, and some devices that can offer much-needed support.

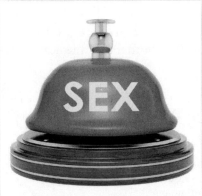

It's normal for older men to sometimes require a little extra help with their erections.

Injection therapy

The thought of injecting drugs into your penis with a needle may make you squeamish, but this approach can get medication quickly to where it needs to go. The needle is about a half-inch long, like the ones used to inject insulin. Your doctor can show you how to perform the injections yourself. "They are surprisingly painless," says Dr. O'Leary.

The injection usually contains alprostadil combined with one or two other medications, all of which work to relax the smooth muscle tissue of the penis and allow blood to flow more freely. An erection usually occurs within five to 20 minutes after injection and lasts for approximately 30 to 60 minutes.

The effectiveness varies according to the drug used and the dosage. Doctors usually prescribe a combination of drugs, which often works better than a single drug.

Side effects are rare but can include mild bruising or scarring. A rare complication is priapism—an erection that lasts too long. You should go to the emergency room to get a counteracting drug if an erection lasts for more than three hours after injection.

MUSE therapy

If you're not keen on injections, you could try a therapy called MUSE (medicated urethral system for erection).

Here, a drug called alprostadil (the same medication used with injections) comes in a tiny pellet that is inserted about an inch into the urethra with a disposable plastic applicator. You usually do this about five to 10 minutes before intercourse. The drug is quickly absorbed by the surrounding tissue and dilates blood vessels, increasing blood flow to the penis. As with injection therapy, your doctor will prescribe the best dose. A potential downside is that some men find the application process uncomfortable.

Penile band

For a man whose main problem is sustaining an erection once he has one, a penile band, also known as an ED ring, may be helpful. The band works by compressing the penile veins. These ring-like devices fasten around the base of the erect penis to keep blood from escaping.

They are usually made of rubber, plastic, or silicone. You don't need a prescription to get one, and they can be bought online. "Bands also can be used in conjunction with traditional ED drugs," says Dr. O'Leary.

Vacuum pump

With this therapy, you lubricate your penis and place it into an airtight plastic cylinder that's attached to a handheld pump. Air is pumped out of the cylinder to create a vacuum, which increases blood flow to the penis. Some pumps are manual, while others operate on a battery. You can find them at many pharmacies and online.

It takes about five minutes to get an erection. You then remove your penis from the cylinder and fit a penile band around its base to prevent blood from draining.

The erection lasts until the ring is removed. Men who take blood thinners or who are being treated for a blood disorder should check with their doctor before using a vacuum device.

The main advantages of penile bands and vacuum pumps over medication is that they are noninvasive and can be used as often you want.

Still, men may feel that their erections aren't as natural and firm as they would like, or they encounter problems ejaculating.

To help assess your erectile function, see the table below.

The Abridged International Index of Erectile Function (IIEF) questionnaire

The full-length IIEF questionnaire includes 15 questions to assess erectile function, orgasm ability, sexual desire, satisfaction with sexual intercourse, and overall satisfaction. An abridged version of the questionnaire with five questions, called the IIEF-5, focuses specifically on erectile function and satisfaction. A higher point total means better erectile function, and therefore less ED. Because the answers to some questions are subjective, clinicians also rely upon your medical history, a physical exam, and lab tests to diagnose and treat ED.

RATE YOUR SYMPTOMS IN THE PAST SIX MONTHS:	1 POINT	2 POINTS	3 POINTS	4 POINTS	5 POINTS
How do you rate your confidence that you could get and keep an erection?	Very low	Low	Moderate	High	Very high
When you had erections with sexual stimulation, how often were your erections hard enough for penetration (entering your partner)?	Almost never or never	A few times (much less than half the time)	Sometimes (about half the time)	Most times (much more than half the time)	Almost always or always
During sexual intercourse, how often were you able to maintain your erection after you had penetrated (entered) your partner?	Almost never or never	A few times (much less than half the time)	Sometimes (about half the time)	Most times (much more than half the time)	Almost always or always
During sexual intercourse, how difficult was it to maintain your erection to completion of intercourse?	Extremely difficult	Very difficult	Difficult	Slightly difficult	Not difficult
When you attempted sexual intercourse, how often was it satisfactory for you?	Almost never or never	A few times (much less than half the time)	Sometimes (about half the time)	Most times (much more than half the time)	Almost always or always

Your score
Add up your points from each question

_____ + _____ + _____ + _____ + _____ = _____

What do the numbers mean?
5–7: severe ED
8–11: moderate ED
12–16: mild to moderate ED
17–21: mild ED
22–25: no ED

Sources: Rosen RC, Cappelleri JC, Smith MD, et al. Development and Evaluation of an Abridged, 5-Item Version of the International Index of Erectile Function (IIEF-5) as a Diagnostic Tool for Erectile Dysfunction. *International Journal of Impotence Research* 1999;11(6):319–26. PMID: 10637462.
Rosen RC, Riley A, Wagner G, et al. The International Index of Erectile Function (IIEF): A Multidimensional Scale for Assessment of Erectile Dysfunction. *Urology* 1997;49(6):822–30. PMID: 9187685.

How cardiology experts fight heart disease

Three Harvard doctors share what they do to lower their risk.

Doctors advise that the best ways to lower risk for heart disease are to exercise, eat right, and adopt healthy lifestyle habits, like stress management, social engagement, and adequate sleep.

But do you ever wonder what heart specialists do to practice what they preach? We asked three Harvard doctors to share their heart-healthy habits and how they work to overcome the same challenges patients face.

Our three experts are Dr. Jona Ludmir, critical care cardiologist at Harvard's Massachusetts General Hospital; Dr. Kyle Pond, chief of cardiology at Harvard's Mount Auburn Hospital; and Dr. Stephen Juraschek, a clinical researcher of cardiovascular disease epidemiology for Harvard-affiliated Beth Israel Deaconess Medical Center.

Here's what they had to say.

Exercise

Dr. Ludmir: No matter how crazy the day gets, I squeeze in at least 15 to 20 minutes of exercise.

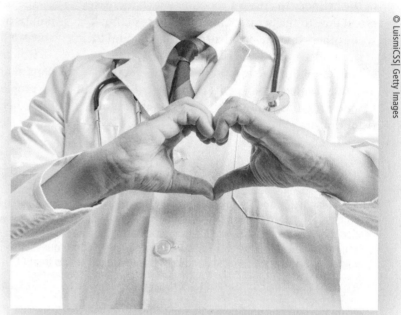

Regular exercise, a plant-based diet, and stress management are the foundations for heart health.

I enjoy high-intensity interval training (HIIT)—one favorite fitness website is Fitness Blender (www.FitnessBlender.com). I can elevate my heart rate and sweat and feel like I had a great workout

---

IN THE JOURNALS

Less may be more when treating urinary tract infections

A shorter duration of antibiotics may be better when treating urinary tract infections (UTIs), according to a study published online July 27, 2021, by *JAMA*. The randomized study involved two groups of men with UTI symptoms (average age 69). Half of the men took antibiotics for 14 days, while the other half took them for seven days.

Both durations had similar outcomes. The seven-day treatment had an average 92.5% success rate, while the 14-day treatment had an average 90.3% rate. Both groups also had a similar percentage of UTI recurrence (9.9% for the seven-day treatment and 12.9% for the 14-day treatment). Participants taking the shorter course reported fewer medication side effects, such as diarrhea and nausea.

According to the researchers, a shorter duration of antibiotics may have other advantages that the study did not explore. For instance, it can make medication easier to manage, reduce out-of-pocket costs, and possibly help lower antibiotic resistance.

in only 10 minutes. Plus, the HIIT workouts focus on the four principles of fitness: aerobics, strength training, stretching, and balance. Peloton is another favorite exercise app.

Dr. Pond: People often have trouble fitting in daily exercise. What has worked for me—and I encourage my patients to follow—is having an exercise "hour" in your day. This doesn't mean that you have to exercise for the full 60 minutes. Instead, commit to whatever amount of time you realistically can do, even if it is only 30 minutes or less. Pick a time that works for you (my exercise hour is 5 a.m. to 6 a.m.).

Consistency is vital for fitness, and that begins with committing time every day. And while you want variety in your fitness, doing one thing is always better than doing nothing. Also, don't hesitate to transition away from activities because of age or health issues. I used to run marathons, but now it's easier to ride a stationary bike, lift weights, and do more stretching.

Dr. Juraschek: Like many people, I, too, find it sometimes challenging to get in the recommended 150 minutes of weekly exercise. So I've focused on being consistent with short bouts of about 15 minutes on a stationary bike, five days a week, and supplement with walking.

For instance, I try to use public transportation, which encourages me to walk more. I also like the bike as I can always watch TV or read, which helps the time pass faster and overcomes the motivational barrier to exercise.

Diet

Dr. Ludmir: My interest in nutrition was sparked by my brother-in-law, Avner. He had already adopted a plant-based diet and was an avid endurance athlete who did marathons and ultramarathons. He urged me to read *The China Study*, a best seller that explored the health benefits of a whole-food, plant-based diet.

After that, I jumped into similar readings and research. It became clear that a diet based on unprocessed, natural food with vegetables, fruits, whole grains, legumes, and nuts is a crucial backbone to healthy living. Two of my favorite plant-based cookbooks are *The Oh She Glows Cookbook* and *The Forks Over Knives Cookbook*. My go-to dishes include homemade lentil burgers, power bowls (rice, beans, sweet potatoes, and veggies),

---

IN THE JOURNALS

A plant-based diet may protect against prostate cancer and ED

Science has shown the power a plant-based diet has on heart health. Now, three new studies suggest the diet also may help protect men from prostate cancer and erectile dysfunction (ED). The results were presented at the American Urological Association meeting in September 2021.

In the first study, researchers looked at about 1,400 men, average age 54, who were part of the National Health and Nutrition Examination Survey (NHANES). Those who ate more fruits and vegetables were less likely to have elevated prostate-specific antigen (PSA) scores—an indicator of possible prostate cancer—than those who did not follow a plant-based diet. In a second study, researchers randomly selected 2,549 men from the NHANES and found that those who had a higher intake of fruits and vegetables also had a lower risk for ED.

For the third study, about 27,000 study participants filled out diet questionnaires every four years for 28 years. The results showed that those who followed a plant-based diet were less likely to get prostate cancer. And those who did get cancer were less likely to develop advanced cases.

These studies only showed associations and cannot verify causes, but men who follow plant-based diets have a potential win-win. The diet is also linked to other health benefits, including better blood pressure, a reduced risk of heart disease, and a healthier weight.

and breakfast smoothies (almond milk, frozen banana, spinach, chia seeds, almond butter, and oats).

Dr. Pond: I have the same cholesterol issues as my patients. While I don't follow a particular diet, I have made significant changes to my eating habits. Eating my greens is essential, and I try to have a daily salad layered with nutrients like vegetables, chickpeas, and lean meat like chicken or salmon.

Also, I used to skip breakfast, but now I begin each day with a healthy meal, such as plain yogurt with blueberries and a little granola. These small changes have improved my cholesterol numbers.

Dr. Juraschek: I follow the DASH (Dietary Approaches to Stop Hypertension) diet that is a bit modified to be higher in healthy unsaturated fat like salmon and avocado.

The DASH diet has been shown to help lower cholesterol and high blood pressure. I specifically try to make one or two vegetables a principal part of every meal and further avoid excess sodium by eating out less and staying away from canned and processed foods.

Lifestyle

Dr. Ludmir: Mental health is very much related to heart health, so anything I can do to manage stress is welcomed. One part of my stress management routine is daily prayer or meditation. It's a small action, but I can improve my mindset and be more present during the day.

Dr. Pond: I keep my mind active along with my body. For me, I read for personal interest and to manage stress. I choose topics with broad appeal that I find mentally engaging, like biographies and nonfiction. (A recent selection is a biography of famed Duke University basketball coach Mike Krzyzewski.) Reading also helps me wind down and prepare for sleep and avoid stimulating screen time in the evening, which makes falling asleep harder.

Social engagement is also essential for my well-being. I volunteer with several organizations. It allows me to not just help a cause I support, but meet other like-minded individuals, many of whom have become good friends.

Dr. Juraschek: I strive to make healthy sleep a priority as it's essential for heart health, but sleep needs differ substantially. If you are overweight or obese and snore, having a sleep study to screen for sleep apnea may be worthwhile.

I also try to avoid too much stimulation or stimulating substances, like caffeine, right before sleep and practice mindfulness or another type of de-stressing routine to eliminate negative thoughts and emotions that might disrupt my sleep.

IN THE JOURNALS

Erectile dysfunction drug may lower Alzheimer's risk

If you take sildenafil (Viagra, Revatio) to treat erectile dysfunction or pulmonary arterial hypertension, here's good news: the little blue or white pill may also be protecting you from Alzheimer's disease. Researchers analyzed insurance claims data of 7.23 million people and found sildenafil users were 69% less likely to develop Alzheimer's over a six-year period than non-users. The possible link? As part of the study, the researchers also examined brain cells from Alzheimer's patients and found sildenafil users had more brain cell growth and slower formation of neurofibrillary tangles in the brain, an early biomarker of Alzheimer's.

It's important to note that the results showed only an association between sildenafil use and lower Alzheimer's risk. Randomized controlled studies are needed to confirm the findings. But so far, it looks like sildenafil could have far-reaching health benefits. The results were published online Dec. 6, 2021, by *Nature Aging*.

by **HOWARD LEWINE, M.D.**

Managing premature ejaculation

Q *I am in a new sexual relationship and surprised that at age 63 I have premature ejaculation. My partner is understanding, but it bothers me. What might help?*

A Premature ejaculation is common in older men, especially when beginning a new relationship. Even men with erectile dysfunction (ED), who have difficulty getting and holding an erection, can experience premature ejaculation. It's great that your partner is so understanding, and it benefits you both to be open about the issue and discuss your options together.

The official definition of premature ejaculation is uncontrolled and unwanted ejaculation within a minute or less of penetration. Personally, I think this definition is too limiting. Of course, men need to be realistic about their expectations for staying power. But if a man is consistently ejaculating before he wants to, and it causes him distress, then he should speak with his doctor.

However, there are two techniques you and your partner can try right away that may help. They are the "stop-start" and "stop-squeeze" methods.

With stop-start, you begin sexual intercourse and keep going until you are close to the point of orgasm. You stop all sexual stimulation until the feeling passes and then resume intercourse.

Stop-squeeze is somewhat similar. When you approach orgasm, you pause, and you (or your partner) use the thumb and two fingers to gently apply pressure just below the head of the penis for about 20 seconds. Then release the squeeze, and resume sexual activity. Both techniques can be repeated as often as needed.

Another option is to apply a topical numbing agent to the head of the penis. The most convenient types are sprays that contain lidocaine or a similar anesthetic product. You will need to test this out to see if your partner finds it causes irritation. (Using condoms also might help by reducing sensation.)

Antidepressant medications, such as selective serotonin reuptake inhibitors (SSRIs), can counter premature ejaculation because delayed orgasm is a common side effect. Some studies suggest that paroxetine (Paxil) may be the most helpful, but any of the other SSRIs also should work, such as fluoxetine (Prozac), sertraline (Zoloft), citalopram (Celexa), and escitalopram (Lexapro). However, they need to be taken daily, since they don't work on an as-needed basis.

Men who have both ED and premature ejaculation should first address their ED. That usually entails taking medication like sildenafil (Viagra), tadalafil (Cialis), vardenafil (Levitra), or avanafil (Stendra). After this, they can add an SSRI.

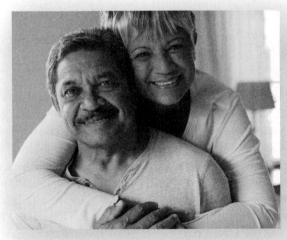

Practicing certain techniques with your partner during sex can help avoid premature ejaculation.

© Wavebreakmedia | Getty Images

Working around health issues and sex

You don't have to let age-related conditions stop you from enjoying an active sex life.

Studies show that regular sex is a significant health booster for men. But as men age, health issues can become a barrier.

While specific problems can affect men's sexual performance and stamina, it's how they respond to these obstacles that can pose the greatest challenge.

"The most important sex organ rests on your shoulders," says Dr. Michael O'Leary, professor of surgery at Harvard Medical School and director of Men's Health at Harvard-affiliated Brigham and Women's Faulkner Hospital. "Worrying about how conditions may cause physical limitations or possible health risks during intimacy can make sex stressful and less enjoyable."

What can you do? Here's a look at three common

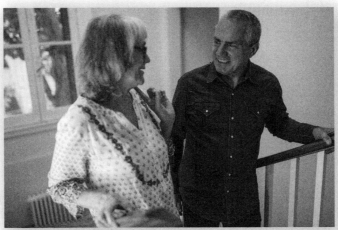

Your ability to safely climb stairs is a good indicator you are healthy enough for sex.

sex-related worries and how to counter them.

Heart disease

Men with heart disease often have one concern in the bedroom: will sex cause a heart attack?

The good news: it's highly unlikely. For men with heart disease, the odds of suffering a heart attack during sex is estimated at 1 in 50,000, according to some estimates.

"The risk is so low because the actual physical exertion from sex is quite small and lasts only a brief time," says Dr. O'Leary.

For instance, walking up two flights of stairs requires about 5.5 metabolic equivalents, or METs. (METs are one way to measure your body's energy expenditure.) Sexual activity averages

---

IN THE JOURNALS

Worry and anxiety linked to higher heart risk in men

Middle-aged men who often feel worried or anxious may be more prone to problems that raise heart disease risk as they age compared with their less-worried peers, a new study finds.

Begun in 1975, the study included 1,561 men without heart disease whose average age was 53. All the men completed tests to assess their levels of worry and neuroticism, a personality trait associated with feelings of fear, sadness, and anger. Every three to five years, researchers collected data to assess the men's risk of cardiometabolic disease (which includes

heart disease, stroke, and type 2 diabetes) until the men died or dropped out. The measurements included blood pressure, cholesterol, triglycerides, blood sugar, body mass index, and a blood marker of inflammation.

Over an average follow-up of nearly 23 years, researchers found that having higher levels of worry or neuroticism was linked to a 10% to 13% higher risk of having six or more risk factors for heart disease, stroke, or type 2 diabetes. The study was published in the February 2022 issue of the *Journal of the American Heart Association*.

between 2 and 4 METs, which is equal to brisk walking or doing housework like cleaning and sweeping.

This is why the "flights of stairs" test is used to gauge whether it's safe to have sex, especially after a heart attack. "If you can walk up two flights with no chest pain, labored breathing, lightheadedness, or extreme fatigue, you are good to have sex," says Dr. O'Leary.

Keep in mind that if you take a heart medication containing nitrates, like nitroglycerin or isosorbide dinitrate, check with your doctor before taking any erectile dysfunction drug. Combining them can make blood pressure drop dangerously low.

Arthritis

The pain and stiffness of arthritis sometimes interferes with intimacy. Trying different positions can help you work around any limitations. For example, people with arthritis in the hips, knees, or spine often find sex more comfortable when both parties lie on their sides.

Taking a pain reliever or a long, warm shower an hour before sex can ease muscle and joint stiffness. You can also place support under your joints to alleviate pain. Pillows work well, or you can get special angled wedges and cushions at medical supply stores and online.

Also, consider scheduling sexual activity when flare-ups are less likely—for instance, if pain is worse in the morning, plan on a romantic afternoon instead.

Chronic back pain

Back pain can make sex uncomfortable, and flare-ups sometimes strike at the wrong time. Here are a few ways to navigate around this problem:

- During sex, avoid bending your spine backward. Instead, try to keep it straight or bent slightly forward.
- During sex, avoid lying on your stomach or your back with your legs flat on the bed and extended straight out. If you can, try to keep your hips flexed, which can take some pressure off your lower back. Placing pillows under your thighs or knees also might help.
- Try sexual positions that are easier on your back, such as lying on your side with your hips and your knees slightly bent.
- Be reasonable and gentle. Don't aim for prolonged, vigorous lovemaking if your back is bothering you.
- Be patient and don't try to resume sex too soon after a backache. If you find that your back hurts when you continue sexual activity, wait a few days before trying again.

Battle of the bulges

Take these steps to avoid ailments that afflict your colon.

As you age, there's a good chance you'll develop diverticulosis, a condition that affects the walls of your colon. In fact, about 58% of people over 60 have diverticulosis, according to the National Institute of Diabetes and Digestive and Kidney Diseases.

Diverticulosis occurs when tiny bulges (called diverticula) form in weak areas of your colon's inner wall. These bulges occur naturally over time, but certain conditions and lifestyle habits can accelerate the process. For instance, people with frequent constipation or irritable bowel syndrome are more likely to develop diverticulosis, especially at an earlier age.

The bulges themselves usually don't cause symptoms or problems. Most people never know they have diverticulosis, as it's usually discovered after a colonoscopy or a CT scan for an unrelated issue.

However, diverticulosis can lead to a more serious condition called diverticulitis. This occurs when one or more of the bulges becomes inflamed or infected. It typically causes pain in the lower abdomen, most often on the left side, often with fever and fatigue. Diverticulitis requires immediate medical attention and sometimes hospitalization. In some cases, even surgery is needed.

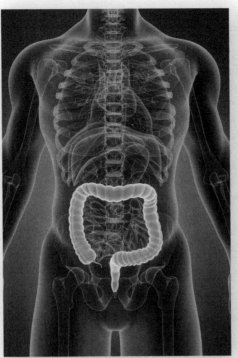

Diverticulosis and the more serious diverticulitis are disorders of the colon.

The other possible complication of diverticulosis is lower intestinal bleeding. As diverticula become enlarged, the wall of the colon weakens, which may lead to a break in one of the small blood vessels that feed the inner lining.

"The best way to protect yourself against diverticulitis and bleeding is to take steps to keep diverticulosis from occurring," says Dr. Matthew Hamilton, a gastroenterologist with Harvard-affiliated Brigham and Women's Hospital, and medical editor of the Harvard Medical School Guide *Diverticulosis and Diverticulitis*.

Lowering your risk

First, address the factors linked with a higher risk of developing diverticulosis. They include the following:

Being overweight. Research has found that men with a body mass index (BMI) of more than 30, classified as obese, have a 78% higher risk of diverticulosis than men who have a low normal BMI of less than 21.

Smoking. A recent analysis published in the *Journal of Postgraduate Medicine* found a 46% higher risk

of diverticulosis in smokers than in nonsmokers.

Taking certain medications. There are several drugs linked with an increased risk of diverticulosis and lower intestinal bleeding, such as corticosteroids, opiates, and nonsteroidal anti-inflammatory drugs (NSAIDs), like aspirin, ibuprofen (Advil, Motrin IB), and naproxen (Aleve). "This does not mean you should avoid these medications, especially if you use them to treat other conditions, but check with your doctor if you take them regularly," says Dr. Hamilton.

Keep your system smooth

You can further lower your risk of diverticulosis, and thus bleeding and diverticulitis, by improving your digestive system's overall health. Here are some strategies.

Get enough fiber. Fiber helps to bulk up stools and move waste through your intestines, so you can maintain regular and healthy bowel movements. Not eating enough fiber also raises your risk of constipation, which causes you to strain when using the bathroom. Over time, this excess pressure can weaken the colon walls and increase the chance diverticula will form.

How much fiber do you need? A recent review in the *European Journal of Nutrition* found that people who consumed 30 grams of fiber per day had a 41% lower risk of developing diverticulosis and diverticulitis than those who ate 7.5 grams daily.

However, on average, adults eat only about half this amount daily. One way to gauge your fiber intake is to base it on your daily calorie intake.

The National Academy of Medicine suggests people eat 14 grams of fiber for every 1,000 calories consumed. This comes to 34 grams based on 2,400 daily calories, 28 grams for 2,000 calories, and 22 grams for 1,600 calories.

There is a wide selection of high-fiber foods from which to choose. (Go to www.health.harvard.edu/fiber for a list of common fiber-rich foods from the Dietary Guidelines for Americans.) But here are some tips for adding more fiber to your diet:

- Include fruits, vegetables, or both with each meal.
- Eat beans, lentils, or peas at least three times a week.
- Choose pieces of fruit or a palm-sized serving of nuts or seeds as snacks. Also, add them to other foods like yogurt, oatmeal, and salads.
- Switch out traditional pasta for versions made from whole wheat, quinoa, chickpeas, or lentils.
- Eat more whole grains like brown rice or bulgur instead of white rice.

Make regular bathroom trips. Holding a bowel movement also can increase straining. Track your bathroom trips so you can better predict when they are most likely to occur. If you battle chronic constipation, talk with your doctor about taking laxatives or stool softeners.

Take a walk. Any kind of exercise and activity supports a healthy digestive system. Also, try walking for 15 minutes after eating. This can speed up how fast food travels from the stomach to the small intestine, which can encourage more regular bowel movements.

Getting through grief

Prolonged grief disorder can emerge after someone close has passed away. Here's how to recognize the signs.

For many people, the pandemic has caused long and often incapacitating feelings of grief and mourning. This has led, in part, to the American Psychiatric Association (APA) recently adding prolonged grief disorder to its official list of mental disorders.

Prolonged grief disorder can develop when someone close to you has died within the past 12 months. You may experience intense longing for the deceased or preoccupation with thoughts about him or her. These feelings often occur most of the day, nearly every day, for at least a month.

The disorder doesn't have to involve the death of a loved one, either, according to the APA. It also can occur after traumatic events like natural disasters and mass shootings.

"Grief and mourning are an expected part of life, but professional help may be required when it lingers for weeks and months," says David H. Rosmarin, director of the spirituality and mental health program at Harvard-affiliated McLean Hospital.

See the signs

Prolonged grief disorder can affect people in different ways. Which symptoms people experience and the severity of each can vary. The following are the most common:

- identity disruption (feeling as though part of oneself has died)

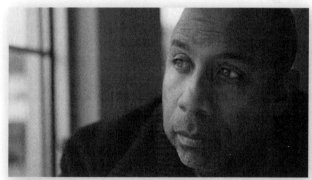

Many men have trouble acknowledging their grief, but it's the first step toward healing.

- a marked sense of disbelief about the death
- avoidance of reminders that the person is dead
- intense emotional pain (anger, bitterness, sorrow) related to the death
- difficulty moving on with life, such as problems engaging with friends, pursuing interests, and planning for the future
- emotional numbness
- feeling that life is meaningless
- intense loneliness and feeling alone or detached from others.

If not addressed, prolonged grief disorder can, over time, flood the body with high amounts of cortisol (the stress hormone). Too much cortisol can raise blood pressure and increase blood sugar and

Do men and women grieve differently?

Another way the sexes are different? How they grieve. Research suggests that men are more likely than women to suffer in isolation when grieving. They often seek out distractions like work and are more susceptible to addictive and risk-taking behavior. Men also are more likely than women to commit suicide following the death of a spouse.

This behavior may be related to the idea that admitting or showing grief is a form of weakness, says David H. Rosmarin, director of the spirituality and mental health program at Harvard-affiliated McLean Hospital. "Yet getting past this mindset and realizing you need assistance can help men deal with their grief before it worsens."

cholesterol levels. Indirectly, prolonged grief disorder also can change your usual healthy habits.

"You may be less likely to exercise and get routine screenings," says Rosmarin. People with the disorder also are more likely to abuse alcohol and drugs. "If left untreated, your condition eventually can turn into more serious concerns, such as chronic depression," he says.

Talk it out

Men may be less likely than women to recognize the signs of prolonged grief disorder or act on them. This may be due to how the two sexes naturally approach grieving (see "Do men and women grieve differently?").

"It can be difficult for men to be honest with themselves and accept they may have trouble dealing with a loss," says Rosmarin. "But they need to understand that it's okay to give themselves permission to not be okay."

Talking about one's feelings can be challenging for men. Yet it's often the best way for men to confront their grief. "Getting it off your chest can be a great relief," says Rosmarin. "When people have prolonged grief disorder, they can't expect everything to get better without finding someone to talk with."

It can help to open up to a close friend or someone you trust, but not everyone feels comfortable doing so. In most cases, professional talk therapy is a better option. This involves sessions with a licensed psychologist, psychiatric nurse, counselor, social worker, or psychiatrist. "Therapy is a safe place where you can explore your feelings without worrying about being judged or feeling embarrassed," says Rosmarin.

Working with a professional can enable you to examine the depth of your grieving and how to begin healing. "And in many cases, you don't need long-term therapy," says Rosmarin. "A few sessions could be all that is necessary."

Going through this process also can prepare you for the next traumatic event. "Chances are you will be exposed again to something that may trigger prolonged grief disorder, but now you will be better able to cope," says Rosmarin.

Building better muscle

These strategies can help maintain more muscle as you age.

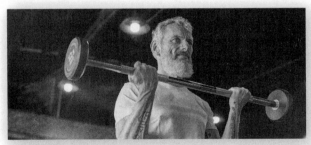

Regular weight training is the best way to increase and maintain muscle mass.

First, the bad news. Men tend to lose as much as 3% to 5% of their muscle mass per decade after age 30. The muscle-building hormone testosterone also drops gradually after age 40.

Now for the good news. You have the power to slow this natural decline and perhaps even reverse it. The solution is to lift weights—often enough, long enough, and heavy enough.

"Weight training is the best way to keep the muscle mass you have and even increase muscle mass you may have lost with aging," says Shawn Pedicini, a physical therapist at Harvard-affiliated Spaulding Rehabilitation Hospital.

So how should you approach weight training in your later years? Here are some strategies.

Invest in a trainer. A licensed and credentialed trainer can design a personalized program. A trainer can also teach you proper form and technique. Check with your local gyms for referrals. If you're not ready for in-person sessions, many trainers now offer virtual workouts. After you learn the basics, you can work out on your own.

Get free. Training with free weights, like dumbbells, kettlebells, and barbells, is often better for muscle building than machines, says Pedicini. "However, machines are ideal if you have balancing issues or other limitations that make it safer to sit during weight training," he says. You can also go back and forth between free weights and machines depending on the type of exercise and which muscles you are working on.

Leg up. While you need full-body workouts that address all your major muscles, older men should pay special attention to their leg muscles: quadriceps and hamstrings (in the thighs), the gluteals (in the buttocks), and the calf muscles. "These are involved in many daily functional movements like squatting and climbing stairs," says Pedicini. Compound exercises that work different muscles in one movement—like squats, deadlifts, and lunges—are great for building leg muscles.

Weight, reps, and sets. Pedicini says older men should do fewer repetitions (reps) with heavier weights to gain the most muscle. "An ideal routine would be eight repetitions for each exercise for three sets total." But you can adjust this as needed. "People with movement issues might need to use lighter weights and do more repetitions."

Find your tempo. Lifting should be done at a seven-second tempo. That means three seconds to lift the weight, a one-second pause, and three seconds to lower it. You also want to use enough weight, so the last few reps are a challenge. If you can't lift the weight at least eight times, use a lighter weight. When you can comfortably perform eight reps without completely tiring the muscle, increase the weight. "Muscles grow stronger only if you keep adding resistance," says Pedicini.

Two days is plenty. Ideally, you should do weight training at least twice a week. "Two days of full-body training can produce measurable changes in muscle strength," says Pedicini. You often can feel results after four to six weeks of consistent training.

Give it a rest. Always allow at least 48 hours between sessions for muscle recovery. Some people prefer to break their workouts into two parts: upper body and lower body. In that case, you can perform upper-body exercises one day and lower-body the next.

Always raise the bar. "Don't forget to consistently challenge yourself as you progress," says Pedicini. "It's necessary to gain the muscle and strength changes you want and need."

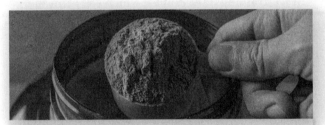

The power of protein

Does consuming more protein help you make more muscle? The answer is yes for younger people, and some evidence suggests that the combination of higher protein intake plus resistance training also can build muscle mass in older men.

How much extra protein is enough? A sedentary adult needs only 0.8 grams per kilogram of body weight per day. However, if you want to build muscle, the goal of daily protein intake should be 50% higher, or 1.2 grams. So, a 175-pound man doing weight training should aim for about 95 grams a day.

If possible, divide your protein intake equally among your daily meals to maximize the body's ability to create muscle. Also, consume about 20 to 40 of those daily grams within an hour after a workout to help with muscle repair. An easy way to meet your daily protein quota is to mix 1 to 2 scoops of whey- or plant-based protein powder to into oatmeal, a smoothie, yogurt, or a glass of water. (Check the label for specific protein amounts.) Other good protein sources: 3 ounces lean chicken (24 grams), 8 ounces plain Greek yogurt (23 grams), 1 cup cooked lentils (18 grams), 3 ounces salmon (17 grams), 2 eggs (13 grams), and 1 ounce (28) peanuts (7 grams).

by **HOWARD LEWINE, M.D.**

Why am I so tired after exercising?

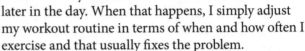

Q *I used to get invigorated after exercising. Now, if I exercise three days in a row, I actually feel more fatigued the rest of the day. What might have changed?*

A With so much emphasis placed on increasing physical activity, we hear little about the downside of doing too much.

Overtraining is the point at which you train so hard and for so many hours that recovery does not occur after regular periods of rest. It's a problem that competitive and recreational athletes sometimes face, but it can affect regular people too.

For serious athletes, optimal performance demands a balance of extreme effort and recovery. Therefore, they must expend a tremendous amount of energy on some days, along with adequate, but not excessive, rest days or at least time spent exercising with less intensity.

But what about the average man who just wants to increase his fitness?

I am not an athlete and don't compete in events. However, I exercise almost daily, mostly because I feel good while doing it. I really miss it if I go more than one day without working out. But if I overdo it, or don't occasionally skip a day, I sometimes feel fatigued either after my workout or later in the day. When that happens, I simply adjust my workout routine in terms of when and how often I exercise and that usually fixes the problem.

While fatigue is often the main symptom of over-exercising, people might experience injuries, aches and pains, anxiety, irritability, and restless sleep. Too much exercise also can lessen sexual desire.

Because many health issues can cause these problems, you should examine what else could cause your post-exercise fatigue, such as anxiety, depression, an unhealthy diet, or poor sleep. Some heart and blood pressure drugs, like beta blockers, also can make you feel sluggish and less energetic after exercise.

I suggest taking some time off. Spread out your usual exercise days and see if that improves your condition. If not, make an appointment with your doctor.

Besides reviewing your medication, your doctor might suggest blood tests to look for other common causes of fatigue, including anemia, an underactive thyroid, liver or kidney disease, or an imbalance of blood electrolytes.

Achieving a higher level of fitness requires pushing yourself physically. However, too much exertion breaks down muscles, uses lots of energy and makes you weak. It is the rest and recovery periods that allow you to get stronger. In general, it's best to limit intense aerobic exercise to no more than three days in a row, and for resistance training the intervals of muscle rest be no more frequent than every other day.

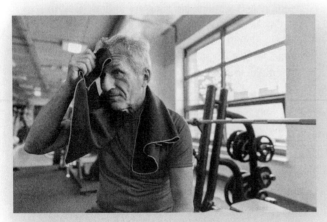

Proper rest and recovery time can help with post-exercise fatigue.

Live long and prosper

Can you predict how long you will live? And what can you do to make sure you reach that number?

As the saying goes, there are two certainties in life: death and taxes. A good accountant can estimate your taxes due, but what about your life span? Is it possible to predict how long you have left?

Health calculators are available that can estimate a person's 10-year risk of having a major cardiovascular event, such as a heart attack or stroke. But that's not the case for almost all other diseases. And when it comes to predicting your own longevity, there are too many individual variables.

"Calculating longevity is complex because there are multiple factors at play," says Dr. David Sinclair, professor in the Department of Genetics and co-director of the Paul F. Glenn Center for Biology of Aging Research at Harvard Medical School. "A person's age, past health issues, current health status, geography, and lifestyle all have a significant role."

All in the family

It turns out that the most significant predictor of longevity is something people have zero control over—their DNA. "Longevity tends to run in the family, and your genetic makeup can often provide the best chance to live a long time," says Dr. Sinclair.

How do your genes help you live longer? Science believes their primary role is to help protect the body against age-related diseases.

A study in the Dec. 3, 2020, issue of *Nature*, led by Dr. Sinclair, explored this concept. The researchers created a virus that carried three "longevity genes" into mice—a technique known as gene therapy. They found that these longevity genes protected the mice from becoming obese (even when fed a high-fat diet), developing type 2 diabetes and heart failure, and suffering kidney failure. This was an animal study and may or may not apply to humans. Still, it suggests how people born with good genes can avoid serious health problems.

What can you do now?

This type of gene therapy resides only in the lab. So, what can you do even if you haven't inherited good

DNA? No surprise: the habits that keep you healthy right now also can help you live longer.

A recent study in *Circulation* led by researchers at the Harvard T.H. Chan School of Public Health found that maintaining five healthy habits can increase life expectancy. They include not smoking, having a healthy body mass index (18.5 to 24.9), doing at least 30 minutes of daily moderate-to-vigorous activity, consuming no more than moderate amounts of alcohol (up to two 5-ounce glasses of wine per day for men), and following a heart-healthy diet. The researchers looked at how these factors affected people starting at age 50. They found that men who didn't adopt any low-risk lifestyle factors had an average

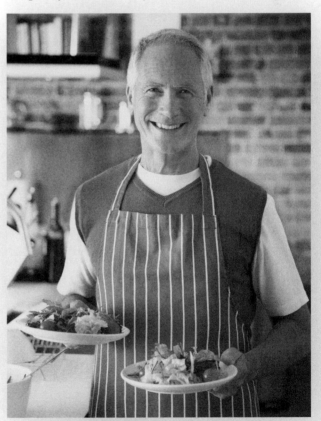

Watching your caloric intake is one of the best ways to live healthier and longer.

estimated life expectancy of 25.5 more years. Yet, those who adopted all five factors had a life expectancy of 37.6 more years.

Eat less, live longer

This study, and similar ones, point to weight management as perhaps the biggest controllable influence on longevity. Excess weight is linked to various health problems that can shorten one's life. Keeping your weight down with a proper diet and exercise goes a long way.

Of course, that's always easier said than done. Dr. Sinclair says one way people can address this issue is to focus on calorie reduction. One study showed that lowering average daily calories by only 12% helped overweight people reduce their high blood pressure and cholesterol levels. They also had significant drops in levels of C-reactive protein, an inflammatory factor linked to cardiovascular disease.

If tracking daily calories is difficult, you could try a system called intermittent fasting, which helps with overeating and late-night snacking.

A popular pattern is the 16/8 method, where you eat during an eight-hour period—for example, from noon to 8 p.m.—followed by 16 hours of fasting, in this case from 8 p.m. until noon the next day, when the pattern repeats. Researchers have found that people who followed 16/8 intermittent fasting lowered their blood pressure, cholesterol, and inflammation levels.

The end result of all these lifestyle changes—proper diet, adequate exercise, watching weight and alcohol, and not smoking—is that they help keep the body healthy. In essence, this is the basic formula for longer life. "Longevity is simply a side effect of not getting sick," says Dr. Sinclair. "Doing everything you can to be healthier now can pay off down the road."

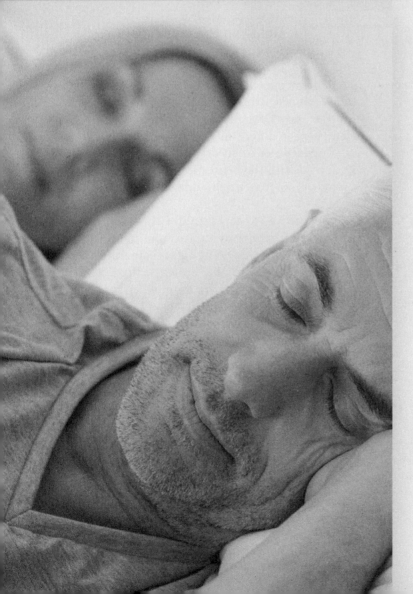

Chapter 11

—

Healthy Habits

Take Action!
5 Things You Can Do Now

1 **Jazz up your drinking water.** Adding flavorful slices of fruit helps you drink more. (page 268)

2 **Take a 10-minute brisk walk.** A little more daily movement could help you live longer. (page 269)

3 **Share a chuckle.** Laughing with buddies is associated with reduced disability. (page 272)

4 **Become a volunteer.** Volunteering is associated with longevity, happiness, and more purpose in life. (page 273)

5 **Try a yoga class.** This mind-body practice can be a gateway to healthier habits. (page 280)

How to hydrate

Proper hydration is vital all year round. Here's how to keep your daily water intake flowing.

Humans can live for about three weeks without food, but they can last only three or four days without water. Even though the liquid is essential for life, an estimated 40% of seniors are chronically underhydrated, and adults ages 65 and older have the highest hospital admission rates for dehydration.

Part of the problem is that the sense of thirst diminishes with age. "Older people don't sense thirst as fast as when they were younger, and by the time they do feel thirsty, they are probably already quite dehydrated," says Dr. Howard LeWine, assistant professor of medicine at Harvard Medical School and Editor-in-Chief of *Harvard Men's Health Watch*.

Watering your health

Drinking enough water is crucial for many reasons. It helps deliver nutrients to cells, regulates body temperature and blood pressure, lubricates joints, prevents infections, and keeps organs functioning correctly. Water also keeps food moving through your digestive tract and supports kidney health.

On the other side, prolonged dehydration raises the risk of certain conditions like urinary tract infections, kidney stones, and constipation.

Dehydration also affects brain health. A study recently published online by the *European Journal of Nutrition* found dehydration weakens cognitive skills like sustained attention and working memory.

The National Academy of Medicine suggests healthy

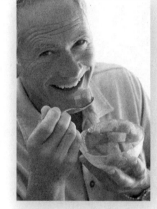

Eating water-rich foods like melon counts toward your daily requirement of fluids.

men consume 13 cups of fluid per day and women nine cups, not all of which needs to be water or even liquids; many foods contain a significant amount of water. Drinking a bit more or less day to day is not a problem because your kidneys do a great job of keeping your body's water balance where it should be. There are times when you need extra fluids, like when you sweat from exercise or in hot weather, or when you lose bodily fluids from vomiting or diarrhea.

Going to the well

Besides lack of thirst, adults are prone to dehydration because they simply forget to drink enough water. "One way to overcome this is to make drinking water part of your daily routine," says Dr. LeWine. "Start your day with a glass of water and drink with every meal."

If plain water turns off your taste buds, boost its appeal with flavorful slices of lemon, lime, orange, or cucumber, or add some mint, berries, or ginger.

Another way to stay mindful about hydration is to drink from a water bottle, aiming to empty it once or twice a day. The right temperature also may help increase intake. Research suggests that people tend to drink more water when it's served at room temperature.

Water is not the only way to stay hydrated. "All beverages containing water contribute toward your daily needs," says Dr. LeWine. This includes coffee, tea, and juice. (For regular coffee or tea drinkers, caffeine does not make your kidneys lose water, but you may want to watch your intake if too much makes you jittery.)

Unsweetened carbonated water is fine; however, avoid sweetened beverages, energy drinks, sports drinks, and so-called vitamin waters as your primary fluid sources, as they can be high

The color of hydration

Urine color is a simple way to monitor water intake. When you're hydrated, your urine should be between clear and the color of light straw. A darker yellow or amber color is a sign you need to drink more water.

Hydrated
Ideal
Good
Fair
Lightly dehydrated
Dehydrated
Very dehydrated
Severely dehydrated

in sugar. Beer and wine don't count because they can have a diuretic effect, so you can lose as much or more fluid as you take in.

Food also counts toward your daily quota. In fact, about 20% of people's total daily water intake comes from water-rich foods. Try to add more of them to your diet, like cucumber, iceberg and romaine lettuce, tomatoes, zucchini, spinach, strawberries, and melons.

Take a breather

Breathing exercises can help you counter stressful situations.

Every day, the average person takes about 22,000 breaths. Each inhalation fills the lungs with oxygen-rich air that fuels every bodily function, from your pumping heart to your flexing muscles and everything in between.

Most often breathing follows a smooth, steady rhythm. When you are active, your breathing rate increases to meet the demand for extra energy. But sometimes, normal breathing turns erratic. For example, when you are stressed or panicked, breathing becomes shallow, making it feel as if it is hard to take in air. When your fight-or-flight response kicks in to confront perceived danger (real or imagined), your breathing pace quickens to prepare the heart and muscles for a quick getaway. If you overexert yourself, your breathing becomes labored as you attempt to "catch your breath."

"These are natural responses to stimuli, and usually breathing returns to normal after the stress recedes," says Dr. Darshan Mehta, medical director at the Harvard-affiliated Benson-Henry Institute for Mind Body Medicine at Massachusetts General Hospital. "But sometimes you are too quick to react to these moments and need help resetting your breathing rhythm."

IN THE JOURNALS

Adding 10 extra minutes of daily activity linked to a longer life

Moving for an extra 10 minutes a day may add years to your life, suggests a *JAMA Internal Medicine* study published online Jan. 24, 2022. Researchers pulled information on 4,840 participants in the ongoing National Health and Nutrition Examination Survey. The people ranged in age from 40 to 85 and wore an activity monitor for a week. The researchers divided the people into groups based on how many minutes they moved each day on average, and then checked how many died over the next 10 years.

Using the results as a sample, the researchers created what-if scenarios by calculating how

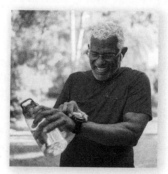

A quick scheduled walk or run is an easy way to squeeze in extra daily exercise.

increasing a person's average daily movement might affect death rates. They estimated that adding 10 more minutes of moderate-intensity exercise per day, like brisk walking or any similar activity, could mean 7% fewer deaths per year. Increasing daily activity by 20 or 30 minutes could lower the rate by 13% or 17%, respectively.

The results of this study add to the growing body of evidence supporting the health benefits of moderate-intensity exercise. However, it's an observational study, meaning it can only show an association between more exercise and longer life, but not prove cause and effect.

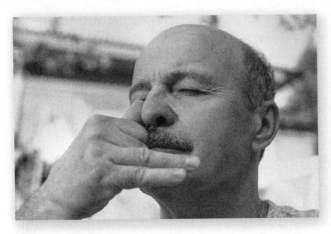
Alternate nostril breathing helps you take deep breaths when you are anxious or stressed.

Change your ways

Stressful breathing, whether triggered by physical or emotional tension, is often more challenging to control as you age. "The muscles in your chest walls can weaken over time, which makes inhales and exhales more difficult, especially when under stress," says Dr. Mehta. "You can't always breathe at your full capacity or easily control your breathing."

One way to overcome this problem and to manage stressful breathing when it arises is by practicing better breathing methods, which can bring in more oxygen and slow the rhythm of your breaths. Here are three breathing exercises that can help.

Belly breathing

Diaphragmatic (belly breathing) stimulates the vagus nerve, which runs from the head down the neck, through the chest, and into the abdomen. This nerve activates your relaxation response, reducing your heart rate and blood pressure and lowering stress levels. This kind of deep breathing can also help clear your mind. A study in *Frontiers in Psychology* found that diaphragmatic breathing helped people improve their performance on attention tests.

To start belly breathing, sit upright in your chair and place your palms on your belly just above your navel. Let the tips of your middle fingers touch. As you inhale, let your belly expand, so the middle fingers come apart. Exhale, letting your belly flatten slightly, so the tips of the middle fingers come back together. Continue for about five minutes or as long as necessary until you feel calm.

Alternate nostril breathing

Alternate nostril breathing, where you breathe through one nostril at a time, is believed to help reset an out-of-whack nervous system by slowing your breathing rhythm and forcing you to take deep, full breaths.

Using a finger or your thumb, close one nostril and then slowly breathe in and out through the open nostril (see picture). After about five to 10 breaths, switch and close the other nostril and repeat the breathing pattern. Another variation is to inhale through one nostril with the other one closed, and then change finger/thumb positions so you exhale through the previously closed nostril. Then inhale through that one, close it, and exhale through the other nostril. Go back and forth like this for several minutes.

Rhythmic breathing

This is a method designed to slow your breathing rate. Near the end of each inhalation, pause while you hold the air and mentally count to three before fully exhaling. Repeat about 10 times or as long as needed.

Breathing new life into heart health

A breathing exercise known as high-resistance inspiratory muscle strength training (IMST) could help protect older adults from cardiovascular disease, says a study in the July 6, 2021, issue of the *Journal of the American Heart Association.* IMST involves inhaling vigorously through a handheld device. Researchers recruited 36 healthy adults, ages 50 to 79, with systolic blood pressure (the top number in a reading) above normal levels, at 120 millimeters of mercury or higher. Half did IMST for 30 breaths, six days a week, for six weeks. The other half followed a placebo regimen where they did the same breathing exercise, but at a low resistance. Systolic blood pressure fell by an average of 9 points in the IMST group, a reduction similar to the effect produced by some blood pressure drugs. The placebo group had no change. The IMST group also showed a 45% improvement in artery function.

Health and happiness go hand in hand

Happy people are generally healthier. So how can you be more joyful?

People who describe themselves as happy tend to have fewer health problems, a lower risk of depression, and longer lives. Yet what if you're not a naturally cheerful person? Is it possible to make yourself happy, especially during trying times?

It turns out that most people can increase their happiness. Research suggests that, on average, 50% of people's general level of happiness is determined by genetics. However, 40% is under people's control, and the remaining 10% depends on the circumstances.

"This implies that even if you don't consider yourself happy, there is a good chance you have some power to change it," says Dr. Robert Waldinger, director of the longest-running study on happiness, the Harvard Study on Adult Development.

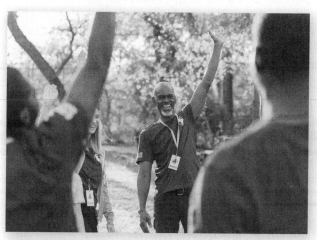

Volunteering is just one way for older adults to increase their levels of happiness.

Working on happiness

Of course, it's a challenge for even the most happy-go-lucky person to constantly remain upbeat. Happiness, like any aspect of wellness, is a constant work in progress. But no matter your current state of happiness, there are ways to boost your outlook and give your mental and physical health a lift. Here are some strategies to try.

Stay connected. The Harvard study led by Dr. Waldinger found a strong link between happiness and close relationships with family and friends. "Personal connection creates emotional stimulation, which is an automatic mood booster, while isolation is a mood buster," says Dr. Waldinger.

Raise your hand. Volunteering provides a sense of purpose and improves your mood. A BMJ Open study found that the effect was especially strong in adults older than age 70.

Perform regular acts of kindness. Pick a day and focus on performing acts of kindness toward others that you would not otherwise do. "It can take considerable planning in advance," says Tyler J. Vander-Weele, director of the Human Flourishing Program at Harvard's T.H. Chan School of Public Health. "But the planning itself and the deliberate intention to do good for others can also have important effects on one's own well-being."

Find your inner child. When you are older, you have a chance to revisit the activities that gave you joy as a child or young adult. What made you happy when you were younger? Pick up those hobbies, games, sports, or other interests from your youth.

Buy more time. A study in the *Proceedings of the National Academy of Sciences* suggested that people who spend money on time-saving purchases, such as paying to delegate household chores, rather than material goods have greater life satisfaction. The effect was similar no matter a person's income.

Invest in experiences. Another way money may buy happiness is through life experiences. It doesn't have to be a big-ticket adventure either. For instance, opt for dinner in an ethnic restaurant, a matinee at the theater, or an art exhibit. The investment can have a lasting impact, too. According to some studies, people who spend money on experiences have longer-term satisfaction, as they create happier memories. In comparison, buying material objects often provides only temporary happiness.

Hang out with happy people. Happiness can be contagious. One study found that happiness can spread through social networks. Your upbeat feeling can trigger a chain reaction, whereby your contacts become happier being around you, and they, in turn, help their contacts feel more joyful, and so on. The researchers also found that sadness does not spread as robustly as happiness.

© SDI Productions | Getty Images

See more green. A study published online May 30, 2021, by *EPJ Data Science* looked at urban green spaces and their effect on citizens in 90 cities worldwide. It found that people's happiness correlated with their area's amount of urban green space, such as parks, gardens, and riversides, regardless of the country's economic state. Creating your own green space can have a similar effect. Other research has shown that gardening at home improves emotional well-being in much the same way that activities like cycling and walking do.

Break up your routines. People feel happier when they have more variety in their daily routines, according to a recent study published by *Nature Neuroscience*. Even small changes can have a big impact. The results found that altering one's regular pattern—such as by trying a new exercise program every couple of weeks, listening to podcasts on some days and music other days, or just taking a different route to the grocery store or pharmacy—can add spice to your life.

Count your blessings. Set aside time to write down items for which you are grateful. It could be something you usually take for granted (a roof over your head and a supportive family) or something simple like receiving a heartfelt compliment, a book you enjoy, today's good weather, or a great-tasting meal you had yesterday.

Make fewer decisions. Research has found that people given more options have more opportunities for regret and worry. A simple strategy can help you ease your choice burden and protect your happiness. If a decision doesn't bring significant consequences, try limiting the amount of time you give yourself to pick, or choose between fewer options. Don't allow yourself to second-guess the decision once it's made. Save the serious deliberations for more significant issues. However, even when making those choices, try to avoid looking back.

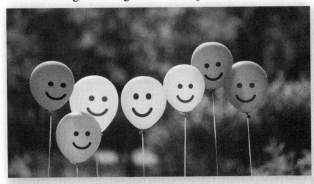

Put on a happy face

Researchers reporting in a recent issue of *Psychological Bulletin* combed data from 138 studies testing more than 11,000 people worldwide on how facial expressions affect emotions. They found that smiling makes people feel happier, just as scowling makes them feel angrier, and frowning makes them feel sadder. The impact was small, but smiling can have broad appeal.

Laughing with friends linked to lower risk of disability

Laughter is good for the soul, and it's great for health, too—including your heart, lungs, and stress control. Now, a study published in the February 2022 issue of *Preventive Medicine* suggests that laughing with friends is associated with a reduced risk of developing functional disability—that is, problems performing essential everyday activities (such as bathing or dressing).

Researchers evaluated the self-reported laughing habits of more than 12,000 people in Japan ages 65 or older. Scientists asked which types of situations made participants laugh, how often they laughed, and with whom they laughed. Compared with people who typically laughed alone, people who typically laughed in a conversation with friends had a 30% reduced risk of being functionally disabled.

The study was observational and doesn't prove that laughing was the cause of people's improved physical function. But we know that a sense of social connectedness is tied to many aspects of good health. And what better way to feel connected than sharing a laugh with friends?

The benefits of volunteering, without leaving home

By helping others as a virtual or remote volunteer, you'll still reap the rewards of this labor of love.

Dr. Martin Luther King, Jr., once said that "life's most persistent and urgent question is, 'What are you doing for others?'" Those words from 1957 are still relevant in our world full of inequities and people in need. And interestingly, helping others—particularly volunteering—also appears to boomerang back to us with significant health and wellness benefits.

But how can you volunteer if you're homebound due to disability or transportation issues? Take heart: there are lots of opportunities, and many reasons to consider them.

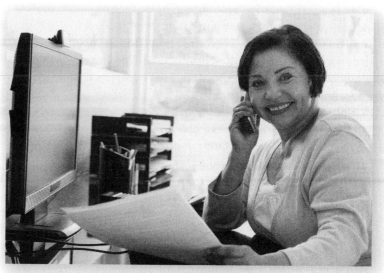

You can volunteer by phone, without leaving your home.

Volunteering benefits

Research suggests that volunteering is good for the mind and body. For example, a Harvard study of 13,000 older adults, published in the August 2020 issue of the *American Journal of Preventive Medicine*, found that people who volunteered at least two hours per week said they were not only happier, more active, and more optimistic than people who didn't volunteer, but also less depressed, hopeless, or lonely.

Volunteers reported more contact with friends and more purpose in life than the non-volunteers. Volunteers even had greater longevity by the end of the four-year study period: they were 40% less likely to die prematurely than non-volunteers. The findings echo other studies that associate volunteering with health, wellness, or longevity.

Why is volunteering so powerful?

A combination of the following factors may make volunteering good for us.

You gain a sense of purpose. "You feel like you're part of a broader cause, contributing to a process that helps a lot of people and making a difference in the world. That's enormously energizing. It enhances the motivation to get out of bed and be active," says sociologist Dr. Matthew Lee, an author

of the *American Journal of Preventive Medicine* study and a research director at Harvard University's Human Flourishing Program.

People who have a sense of purpose also have greater levels of physical activity, better sleep quality, healthier diets, and lower rates of cardiovascular disease.

You connect with others. "When you interact with other people, even if it's not in person, you're likely to build relationships and feel more engaged," Lee points out.

You get a break from your own problems. "You stop worrying about your own situation when you start helping others improve theirs," Lee says.

It develops your sense of virtue. "By design, human beings want to become better people," Lee notes. "When we nurture others, we flourish and grow."

It just feels good. "Feeling like you're making a contribution lights up reward centers in the brain and gives you the 'helper's high,' the warm feeling you get when you're helping others. It leads to a strong sense of personal well-being and positive emotions," Lee says.

Ways to pitch in

Even if you can't leave home, you can still volunteer your time for a good cause. Here are some ideas.

Volunteer online. Thanks to computers, it's common to be a "virtual" volunteer. For example, you can provide administrative, accounting, or marketing assistance via computer, or you can tutor or mentor someone via video chat. There are opportunities in the arts, business, education, health, medicine, and many other fields. Think about your life experience and who might benefit from it.

Volunteer by phone. Telephones are still important in volunteer work. For example, you can use a phone to help raise money for nonprofits, answer a hotline, or make check-in calls to homebound adults.

To find opportunities:

- Call an organization you like and ask if it has any "remote" or virtual volunteer opportunities.
- Search online for volunteering opportunities in your ZIP code on websites such as Volunteer Match (www.volunteermatch.org) or Idealist (www.idealist.org).

If you can leave your home but you're not ready to be part of a group, consider assisting neighbors. Someone you know may need help getting the daily mail or paper, walking a dog, preparing meals, helping in their garden, or taking garbage to the curb.

Or get creative and come up with other ways to contribute. For example: "If you were an art teacher, offer free Zoom classes. If you like writing, send cards or letters to soldiers, nursing home residents, or children in hospitals to brighten their day," Lee suggests.

Will helping from home confer the same benefits as volunteering in person? "In many ways, it should. You're still connecting deeply with people and being part of something larger than yourself that's meaningful to you. Distance doesn't diminish the story that you become part of," Lee says. And you get to answer the profound question Dr. King posed so long ago.

IN THE JOURNALS

The best bedtime for heart health?

People who fall asleep between 10 and 11 p.m. may be less likely to develop heart disease than those who start their slumber earlier or later, according to a recent study. For the study, more than 88,000 people ages 45 to 79 wore devices on their wrists that tracked when they fell asleep and woke up for one week. They also completed assessments and questionnaires about their health and lifestyle habits. Researchers then tracked heart attacks, strokes, and other cardiovascular problems in the participants for an average of 5.7 years.

Compared with a sleep start time of 10 to 10:59 p.m., cardiovascular disease rates were 25% higher when sleep began at midnight or later, 12% higher when sleep started in the 11 o'clock hour, and 24% higher when people fell asleep before 10 pm. The findings don't prove that early or later bedtimes promote heart disease. But nontraditional sleep times may disrupt the body's 24-hour internal

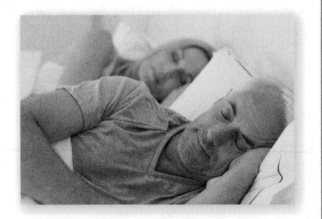

clock, or circadian rhythm, which plays a key role in regulating physical functioning. People who stay up past midnight may have the highest risk because they're less likely to see morning light, which resets the body clock, say the authors. Their study was published Nov. 9, 2021, in the *European Heart Journal–Digital Health*.

New ways to think about sex

An enjoyable sexual relationship can happen without traditional intercourse.

People's bodies change over time. Probably nowhere is this most telling than with their sex lives.

For men, sexual drive can slow as hormone production naturally drops, and it's common to experience erectile dysfunction or health issues that can interfere with sexual performance.

Women can have their own physical barriers to sex, such as vaginal dryness and lower libido after menopause. All of these issues can make conventional sex problematic and stressful for both parties.

"Even though older adults go through physical changes, they often expect their sex life to stay the way it was decades earlier, and that is just not always realistic," says Dr. Sharon Bober, director of the Sexual Health Program at Harvard-affiliated Dana-Farber Cancer Institute. "Still, there are many ways to continue a strong, healthy sexual relationship without always relying on regular intercourse. Couples should see this new phase of their sex lives as an opportunity to explore different and exciting ways to satisfy each other."

Redefining sex

The first step older couples should take is to re-examine their definition of "sex." "Don't give in to the idea of a so-called normal sex life being narrowly defined," says Dr. Bober. "Sex refers to a broad spectrum, and there are many places you can land."

Examine what sex now means to you and your partner. This could mean changing how you pleasure each other, routines you follow, and frequency—as well as making compromises about expectations. "Don't assume there is only one way to have a sexual relationship," says Dr. Bober. "It doesn't have to be all or nothing."

Your relationship status also can shape this new idea of sex. For instance, some couples may enjoy a connection based more on companionship, where the emphasis is on emotional bonding and spending quality time together and less on the physical side.

Language of love

As with most aspects of a strong relationship, communication is vital. "The more you avoid talking about your sex lives, the bigger the issues become," says Dr. Bober.

Of course, talking about sex isn't always easy, but most partners are open and willing to discuss and share if given a chance. "Often partners aren't sure how to begin the conversation, so it never happens," she says. There are many ways to initiate a sex dialogue. Here are some suggestions:

Seek permission. Begin the conversation positively. For instance, say something like "I want to find ways to reconnect that feel good for both of us" or "Our sex life has been on my mind and I have been wondering if I could share some of my thoughts. Is it okay to talk about it?"

By asking for permission, you can broach the topic without intimidating your partner. "This initial conversation is not about making demands, but about finding ways to explore mutual goals," says Dr. Bober.

Invite a response. Make it clear you want to hear your partner's feelings too. For example, say, "I've been wondering how you feel about our sex life. What has sex been like for you?" Inviting partners to participate can prevent them from feeling defensive and shows you care about their experience and input, says Dr. Bober.

Express what you both want. Talk about what you both hope to gain from this new sexual relationship,

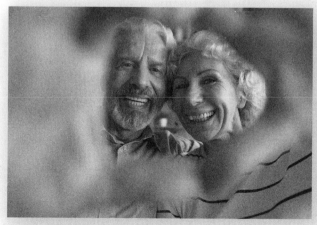

Sharing goals and desires about your sex life can open up new opportunities to explore.

such as more excitement, greater closeness, or even reconnection. "Sharing your needs and expectations helps your partner express theirs, so you both can come to some kind of mutual understanding," says Dr. Bober.

Different ways to satisfy

Once you've had these talks, then you both can look for different ways to approach your new sex life. Dr. Bober says a good place to begin is with "outercourse." Here, the attention and energy are directed toward foreplay and manual stimulation with your partner, like massages, hugging, petting, kissing, or just snuggling naked in bed.

"The emphasis is on intimacy and closeness without any big expectations of intercourse," says Dr. Bober. "This can take the pressure off both partners and eliminate some of the stress and anxiety of having regular sex. It also shows that you can interact with your partner in various satisfying ways."

Penetration is not always needed to achieve pleasure or orgasm for both people. Instead, try sexual aids like vibrators as well as manual stimulation, masturbation, and oral sex.

As you explore ways to stay intimate, be mindful that every couple is unique. "A sexual relationship is defined by the two people in it and nobody else," says Dr. Bober. "Focus on what matters to you and your partner. Your sex lives may have changed, but together you can discover what's best for each other and your relationship."

Learning to right a wrong

Forgiving yourself for past actions is a powerful healing tool.

You may still struggle at times when you think about how someone mistreated you. But what about when you were in the wrong? It's not unusual to revisit memories of when you bullied someone, wronged a person at work, or insensitively broke off a relationship with a friend or family member.

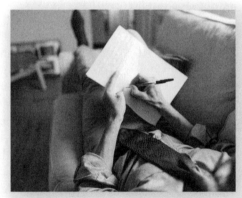

Penning a letter to someone you wronged is good therapy whether or not you send it.

is the misconception that it is a sign of weakness. But it actually takes courage. "Forgiving yourself can culminate in self-growth," says Cowden. "So, when things come back that we regret having done, we can approach it as an opportunity to learn about ourselves and grow in beneficial ways."

"This can occur more often as people age and suffer personal loss or setbacks," says Richard Cowden, a social-personality psychologist with the Human Flourishing Program at Harvard's Institute for Quantitative Social Science. "They begin to have regrets. But when these memories arise, it's usually a sign you need to work through those feelings and not push them down. They may affect you in ways you don't realize, and this is a chance to address your past mistakes and finally move on by forgiving yourself."

Practicing self-forgiveness can have a range of health benefits. Studies have shown that self-forgiveness is associated with reductions in guilt, shame, stress, depression, anxiety, and substance abuse, as well as greater self-esteem and life satisfaction.

"We are often harder on ourselves than on others," he says. "But once you can forgive yourself and break away from self-punishment, you can begin the process of healing and positive behavior change."

Change is good

The challenge many people face with self-forgiveness

The four R's of forgiveness

There are four parts to the self-forgiveness process: responsibility, remorse, reorientation, and renewal.

Here are some ways to approach each one.

Responsibility. Facing what you have done is often the most challenging part of self-forgiveness. "It's uncomfortable to admit you've done something wrong, and it's natural to protect one's self-esteem by dismissing what happened or making excuses for your behavior," says Cowden.

What you can do: Write a letter. Using pen and paper or a computer keyboard, outline your errors and acknowledge your misgivings. "You don't have to send it to the person," says Cowden. "Just the act of expressing yourself and writing it down can help you process your emotions about your past behavior."

Remorse. Once you take responsibility for your past, you may experience negative feelings, such as shame and guilt. "This is normal, so don't bottle them up," says Cowden.

What you can do: Talk it out. Always remember that you are not alone, and others struggle with similar issues. "Sharing these feelings with a trusted friend could help you work through them and gain valuable insight, and you often can return the favor," says Cowden.

Reorientation. One of the most crucial parts of self-forgiveness is to make amends (if that is possible) and to try your best not to transgress again in the same way.

What you can do: Apologize. Apologize if it's called for (or send that letter, if that's easier). Use expressions of regret like "I wish I could take it back," or "I wish I had been more thoughtful." Another approach is to ask the person what you can do to make amends. If you can't communicate with the person, have an imaginary conversation with him or her, or share your apology with someone you both know. "This exercise can help you commit not to engage in the same behavior in the future," says Cowden.

Renewal. This is the self-healing stage where you let go of what you did wrong and move forward with the lessons you've learned.

What you can do: Reconnect with your spiritual side. If you follow a religious or spiritual practice, have thought about it, or are looking to return to a lapsed practice, this is an opportunity to explore self-forgiveness through prayer or meditation. "This often facilitates internal reflection, which can help you realize that everyone makes mistakes and that you are not beyond repair," says Cowden.

Self-forgiveness is not easy and may take time and extra effort, but it's worth it, adds Cowden. "It can free you from your past mistakes and help you live more fully in the here and now. You might be surprised how much better you feel if you can work through the process of forgiving yourself."

The senior's guide to dental care

Avoiding problems like gingivitis and tooth loss may help protect against other serious health issues.

The eyes may be the gateway to your soul, but oral health is a window into overall health. "Good dental health not only protects against gum disease, gum inflammation, and tooth loss, but also can protect against many other age-related diseases," says Dr. Len Brennan of the Harvard School of Dental Medicine. "A healthy mouth really can lead to a healthier body."

A healthy smile

Poor oral health can have severe consequences.

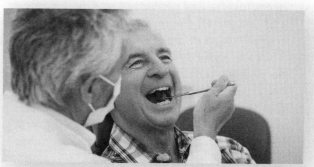

Routine dental check-ups can catch problems early and help you avoid costly treatments.

© alvarez | Getty Images

Research has shown that gum inflammation (gingivitis) raises the risk for lung disease, heart disease, blood vessel blockage, and strokes.

Tooth loss from gum disease (periodontitis) may raise your risk of dementia. In the October 2021 issue of the *JAMDA: The Journal of Post-Acute and Long-Term Care Medicine*, researchers looked at 14 studies and found that older adults who had lost more than one tooth had an almost 50% higher risk of developing cognitive impairment and a 28% higher risk of being diagnosed with dementia.

Poor dental health also can affect your social life. "Insecurities about your smile can make you feel less attractive and less likely to socialize, which can increase isolation," says Dr. Brennan.

Rinse, brush, floss

Like other aspects of health care, prevention is the best medicine when it comes to your teeth and gums. "Investing in proper dental care and upkeep is relatively inexpensive," says Dr. Brennan. "Dental treatments are where it can get costly."

He recommends seeing your dentist every six months for check-ups, x-rays as needed, and cleanings. In between, you should follow a daily dental hygiene routine to reduce plaque buildup, gingivitis, and cavities. There are three basic steps: rinsing, brushing, and flossing.

Rinsing. Before you brush, rinse with plain water to dislodge food particles. After brushing, you can rinse again with an over-the-counter alcohol-free mouthwash with fluoride, which can help protect against tooth decay. Some products can reduce tooth sensitivity. Ask your pharmacist for a suggestion. If you have trouble controlling plaque, gingivitis, bad breath, or dry mouth, speak with your dentist about a therapeutic mouthwash.

Brushing. Brush at least twice a day for no less than two minutes each time. Choose a toothpaste with the American Dental Association (ADA) Seal

IN THE JOURNALS

Eating more olive oil linked to longer life span

Consuming a small amount of olive oil every day may help you live longer, according to an observational study. Researchers looked at health data from about 90,000 people over a period of nearly 30 years. Participants were free of heart disease and cancer and completed dietary questionnaires every four years. They were asked how often, on average, they ate specific foods, including types of fats and oils. The results showed that those who consumed more than ½ tablespoon of olive oil per day (more than 7 grams) had a 19% lower risk of dying from any cause than those who rarely or never had olive oil. Looking at specific conditions, the researchers

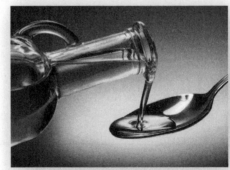

A little daily olive oil serves up big health benefits.

found the olive oil group also had a 19% lower risk of cardiovascular disease, a 17% lower risk of dying from cancer, and a 29% lower risk of dying from a neurodegenerative disease such as Alzheimer's disease. The researchers suggested that substituting olive oil for unhealthier fats could have a more significant effect. They estimated that replacing 10 grams per day of fats like margarine, butter, and mayonnaise with the same amount of olive oil could lower the risk of overall death and disease by as much as 34%. The study was published online Jan. 12, 2022, by the *Journal of the American College of Cardiology.*

of Acceptance, which verifies it contains decay- and plaque-fighting fluoride.

Toothpastes come in gel, paste, or powder forms. While the ingredients can differ slightly, all toothpastes contain the same general components: mild abrasives, humectants, flavoring agents, thickening agents, and detergents. Some brands also contain other ingredients that might reduce tooth sensitivity or tartar buildup, prevent enamel erosion, or whiten teeth. Ask your dentist for a recommendation for these specific issues.

"Natural" toothpastes also are popular, but again look for the ADA seal. Natural means certain ingredients are omitted, such as artificial flavors, colors, preservatives, and sweeteners. It also means that certain active ingredients that help with cleaning are derived from plant sources.

Select a brush with soft or extra-soft bristles. Replace toothbrushes every three to four months, or more often if the strands are visibly matted or frayed.

When brushing, tilt the brush at a 45° angle. Beginning with the upper teeth, take several up-and-down short strokes from the gum line to the bottom of the tooth. Do one tooth at a time before moving on to the next. To clean the inside surfaces of the front teeth, hold the brush vertically and make several up-and-down strokes. Repeat the process for the lower teeth.

If you have arthritis that makes it hard to brush or hold a toothbrush, or if it's difficult to reach the back teeth, invest in grip aids that slide over your brush's handle. Another option is an electric toothbrush. You can get more strokes from the brush's vibrations than from your hand motion. Some brands come with timers that tell you when you've brushed long enough.

Flossing. It doesn't matter if you floss before or after brushing, according to Dr. Brennan. "But also try to floss more than once daily, if possible,

Making sense of sensitive teeth and dry mouth

Two common dental problems many older adults face are sensitive teeth and dry mouth. Tooth sensitivity often occurs when you eat or drink hot or cold food. A typical cause is gum shrinkage, which exposes more of a tooth's root. Grinding your teeth when you sleep also can cause sensitivity, so you may need to use a mouth guard at night. A dry mouth means you produce less saliva, which makes tasting, chewing, swallowing, and even talking difficult. Dry mouth also is a common side effect of many medications and is linked with such health conditions as diabetes, stroke, Alzheimer's, and autoimmune diseases. Because both sensitive teeth and dry mouth have many different causes, check with your dentist to find the source of your problem.

preferably after a meal to reduce bacteria buildup in the mouth." You can use either waxed or unwaxed floss. People with particularly tight teeth may find waxed floss easier to use, but both kinds work the same.

Wrap the floss around your middle fingers, which helps you to reach the back teeth. Loop the floss around each tooth, so it makes a C shape. Beginning at the gum line, slide it up and down the tooth several times. Avoid just moving the floss back and forth in a sawing motion. Not only do you miss cleaning the entire tooth, but the friction can irritate the gums. "If gum bleeding occurs, that doesn't mean you should stop flossing," says Dr. Brennan. "Instead, just be more gentle around that area."

If traditional flossing is difficult, you can try over-the-counter tools, such as dental picks, floss picks, pre-threaded flossers, tiny brushes that reach between the teeth (which are especially helpful to get under crowns and bridges), and water flossers.

Yoga: A gateway to healthier habits?

This mind-body practice may improve heart-related risks by helping you manage stress and lifestyle changes more easily.

Popular culture often depicts yoga as an exercise for slender, flexible, younger women. But scores of older people have been practicing yoga for thousands of years. Today, yoga's popularity among the general population continues to rise, along with evidence supporting possible benefits for people with heart disease (see "Yoga and heart disease: The latest data").

"The beauty of yoga is that it addresses multiple factors that underlie heart disease," says yoga researcher and neuroscientist Dr. Sat Bir Singh Khalsa, assistant professor of medicine at Harvard Medical School. Whether you have chest pain from narrowed heart arteries (angina) or an irregular, fast heartbeat (atrial fibrillation), yoga can cultivate physical changes that may improve these and other cardiovascular conditions, he says.

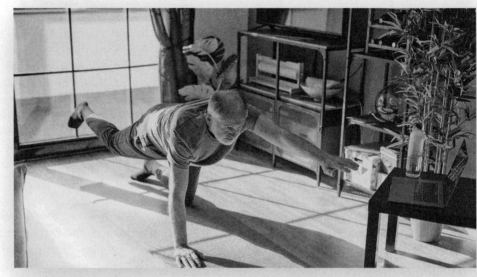

A regular yoga practice can enhance mind-body awareness as well as flexibility.

© Anchiy | Getty Images

Physical changes

All types of yoga (including gentle or beginner styles) can enhance your strength, flexibility, and balance—important but often overlooked aspects of overall physical fitness and well-being. Yoga fosters better sleep, which helps prevent or improve a host of health conditions linked to heart health, including depression and obesity. Yoga also encourages slow, deep breathing, which helps lower blood pressure and heart rate.

Yoga and heart disease: The latest data

Hundreds of studies have explored how yoga might improve heart health. But only a few have directly compared yoga to another treatment (usually standard medical care) in a randomized controlled trial—the gold standard of research studies. In 2021, researchers published a review of yoga's potential benefits in people with coronary artery disease in *Complementary Therapies in Medicine.* From more than 300 potentially relevant studies, they identified seven clinical trials that compared yoga—done anywhere from one to 14 times a week for at least a half-hour per session—to usual care or exercise.

Yoga was linked to improvements in blood pressure, cholesterol and triglyceride levels, body mass index, and quality of life. Yoga may also be an effective add-on therapy for people with heart rhythm disorders. For those with atrial fibrillation (a rapid, irregular heartbeat that usually occurs sporadically), some studies suggest that practicing yoga regularly may help reduce the number of episodes they experience. Another found that yoga may help reduce palpitations, a usually harmless condition that feels as though the heart is pounding or has skipped a beat.

And over time, a regular yoga practice trains your nervous system to be less reactive during periods of stress. Chronic stress is a major contributor to heart disease and many other health conditions.

Psychological benefits

But the added psychological benefits of yoga may be even more influential than the physical changes, says Dr. Khalsa. Doctors often warn heart patients about the dire consequences of eating a poor diet and avoiding exercise. Guilt and fear drive some people to make healthy lifestyle changes, but they usually don't stick with them, he says.

Yoga may help people make more lasting changes by cultivating greater mind-body awareness. In addition to leading you through a series of postures (called asanas), a good yoga teacher will also teach breathing exercises, relaxation, and meditation. Together, these practices can help you become more in tune with how your daily habits affect how you feel.

"Once you boost your mind-body awareness, you may start to realize that you don't feel so good after eating junk food," says Dr. Khalsa. Instead, try having some broccoli and really pay attention to the flavor.

Notice how your body feels healthier and lighter afterward compared with how you feel after eating highly processed, fat- and sugar-filled foods, he suggests. Yoga also may make it easier to quit other unhealthy habits, such smoking and excessive drinking, which people often use to cope with stress.

The underlying connection

Modern medicine often focuses on treating symptoms rather than the underlying condition, says Dr. Khalsa. "Most people would rather take a pill to treat their insomnia than commit to an eight-week yoga program," he says. Taking drugs to help you sleep isn't a good long-term solution, but doing yoga is.

What's more, a good night's rest may give you more energy and motivation to exercise and prepare healthy food. "In the end, everything's connected to everything else in our mind-body system," Dr. Khalsa says.

For more information on starting a yoga practice and its other health benefits, see the Harvard Special Health Report *An Introduction to Yoga* (www.health.harvard.edu/yoga).

Chapter 12

Health and Wellness Technology

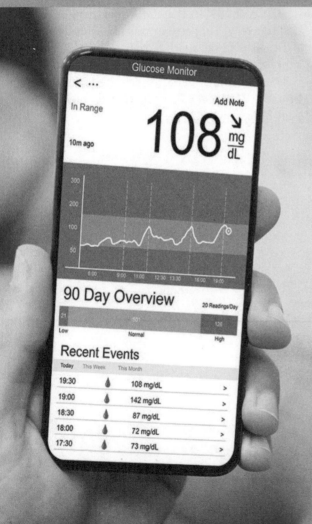

Take Action!
5 Things You Can Do Now

1 **Get a voice-recording pen.** This device is handy for making lists or capturing important points from a conversation. (page 284)

2 **Keep an eye on virtual reality to curb chronic pain.** Promising research shows this may be an effective way to get relief. (page 288)

3 **Use a fitness tracker.** The device has been shown to help people lose weight, even those with chronic disease. (page 289)

4 **Explore the heart rate alert settings on your smart watch.** Most devices will warn you if your heart rate is unusually low or high (page 291)

5 **Track your blood sugar.** People with diabetes are increasingly opting for the convenience of continuous glucose monitors. (page 293)

Gadgets to help you sleep better: Do they work?

These pill-free options may promote a better night's rest.

For many people, the nightly trip to dreamland is a difficult journey. Up to a third of all adults—including 30% to 48% of older people—have a hard time falling or staying asleep at some point, with about 10% developing chronic insomnia. So it's not surprising that a wide array of gadgets claim to help you get more Z's. Do they really help?

To find out, we turned to Dr. Lawrence Epstein, a sleep specialist with Harvard-affiliated Brigham and Women's Hospital and medical editor of the Harvard Special Health Report *Improving Sleep* (www.health. harvard.edu/is). Here are his takes on devices that promote sleep.

Sound or "white noise" machines

These small bedside machines play sounds from nature (like gentle waves or rain) or city sounds (such as traffic). "Sound machines can be very helpful if the person is in an environmentally challenging situation, where noise is disrupting sleep," Dr. Epstein says. "This can be anything from living near an airport to having the bedroom next to the garage or sleeping with someone who snores. The goal is to block out spikes in noise that can disturb someone's sleep."

Cost: Prices start at about $15.

Earbuds for sleep

These earbuds are designed for sleeping, not listening to music. They're comfortable enough for you to sleep on your side. They might mask noise with other sounds, or they might "cancel" noise by blocking it out with certain frequencies.

"As with sound machines, things that reduce noise will improve the sleep environment and can reduce unwanted awakenings," Dr. Epstein says.

Cost: Prices start at about $100.

A "sunrise" alarm

A sunrise alarm simulates the sun coming up by scheduling the timing of the first light you see. "It's very important to wake up and go to sleep at the same time every day, and a sunrise alarm can be very effective for people with circadian rhythm [sleep-wake]

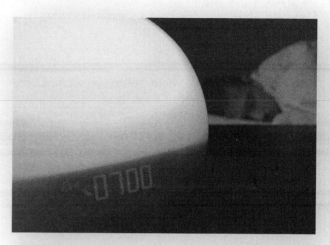

Setting a sunrise alarm too early in your sleep cycle can wind up worsening sleep quality.

disorders; light has the strongest effect in setting and shifting the circadian clock," Dr. Epstein says.

But be sure to set the alarm correctly: if it lights up too early, it will worsen the quality of your sleep.

Cost: Prices start at about $25.

A weighted blanket

Weighted blankets contain plastic or glass beads to make them heavier. Blankets range from 12 to 25 pounds and are intended to simulate a comforting hug or the swaddling we experienced as infants.

"There is little research on the effectiveness of the blankets, but some studies suggest they may be helpful in reducing anxiety. Less anxiety may help you fall or stay asleep, but we don't have enough evidence yet," Dr. Epstein says.

Cost: Prices start at about $50.

Smartphone apps

Applications ("apps") are programs you download to your smartphone. There are many apps that can help you sleep, including white noise makers, sleep activity trackers, relaxation and meditation guides, and even online programs for cognitive behavioral therapy for insomnia (CBTi).

"CBTi trains you to shift unproductive thinking patterns or habits that affect sleep," Dr. Epstein says. "Recently, Somryst became the first FDA-authorized prescription CBTi app for people with chronic insomnia."

Cost: For Somryst, costs are $700 for a nine-week program, which requires a doctor's prescription. Apps for white noise, sleep tracking, or meditation may be free or cost less than $10.

Cooling systems

Getting too hot at night can interrupt sleep. There are some elaborate ways to stay cool, such as using an expensive water-cooled system for your mattress or pillow. One newer, novel device that Dr. Epstein recommends is called the Ebb Cool Drift Versa Sleep System. It cools the forehead and is FDA-approved.

"The brain cools down during sleep, and the start of the temperature drop is one of the signals for impending sleep," Dr. Epstein says. Would a pillow or mattress topper with fabric that wicks away heat and moisture ease insomnia? Dr. Epstein says there's no evidence they'd help, but they wouldn't hurt if they keep you comfortable.

Cost: Prices for pillows with heat-wicking fabric start at about $25. The Ebb device is about $300.

What else helps

Proven methods to promote better sleep include seeking CBTi from a therapist and practicing good sleep hygiene: keep your room dark and cool; go to sleep and wake up at the same time each day; and avoid alcohol, meals, caffeine, exercising, and all electronic screens (bright phones, TVs, or computers) within two hours of bedtime.

Helpful gadgets for a fuzzy memory

Take advantage of tools to keep you organized.

Just because you experience a wee bit of forgetfulness from time to time, it doesn't mean your memory is failing; it's just prone to the effects of aging. "Memory starts to weaken once we hit our 30s. Add a few more decades and plenty of important information to keep track of—like busy schedules, medication regimens, and monthly bills—and you'll notice memory changes more keenly," says Dr. Andrew Budson, a neurologist and chief of Cognitive and Behavioral Neurology at VA Boston Healthcare System.

Fortunately, there are lots of gadgets that support memory. Get some for yourself or give a few tools to a friend. After all, who wouldn't want to unwrap a little memory boost?

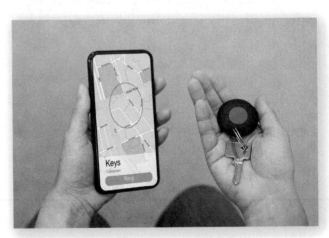

© AndreyPopov | Getty Images

Attach a tracker to an object, like a key, and you'll be able to see its location on a map.

Basic reminders

In the medical world, gadgets that provide reminders are known as external memory aids. Some examples:

A talking motion-activated sensor. (Cost: about $25.) This device allows you to record a reminder message that will play automatically when you walk by (and trigger) the sensor. For example, you could record, "Don't forget your wallet," and place the sensor by your front door; or "Drink more water," and keep the sensor by the refrigerator.

A voice recorder or a voice-recording pen or watch. (Cost: $30 to $50.) These devices record your voice, or someone else's, at the touch of a button.

That's handy for making lists or capturing important points from a conversation (perhaps with a doctor) that you can write down later. Make sure others in a conversation agree to being recorded.

Office supplies. (Cost: $5 to $50.) "There's no reason to memorize your to-do list or upcoming appointments. If an external memory aid can help you, take advantage of it," Dr. Budson advises. He suggests using wipe boards and dry-erase markers, pads and pens, colorful sticky notes, calendars, or daily planners. Get a nice selection of these tools to sprinkle throughout the house. When it comes to calendars, get one that's large, with easy-to-see numbers and extra room to write notes on each day of the week.

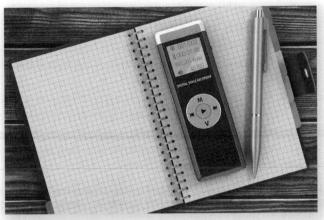

Simple tools like notebooks help support your memory, and so do digital voice recorders.

Homes for everyday objects

One of the best ways to remember where you've left objects like keys or glasses is to keep them in a predetermined spot. "If you put your wallet in the same place every day, it becomes a habit. Once it's a habit, you don't need to think about where it is, just like you don't need to think about how to ride a bike," Dr. Budson explains.

Here are two tools that support this habit:

Key hooks and mini shelves. (Cost: $10 to $20.) Install these by your door or another spot in your home, and use them regularly.

Doorknob organizers. (Cost: $10). These look like do-not-disturb signs with pockets on them. Hang one on your doorknob and store things you want to grab on the way out of the house, such as keys or driving glasses—remembering to return the items to the organizer when you get home.

Medication managers

Juggling a medication regimen is challenging, no matter how many pills you're taking. If a standard pillbox isn't working for you, consider using one of these:

Automatic pill dispenser. (Cost: $10 to $100.) Load pills into this organizer and it will dole them out at the right time and in the right amounts. Some dispensers sound alarms or use smartphone apps to alert you about pill-taking time.

Medication alarm. (Cost: $25 to $50.) If you prefer, skip automatic dispensing and just use a digital alarm to let you know when it's time to take various medications. Smartphones and watches also allow you to set regular alarms for different times throughout the day. Whichever style of alarm you choose, look for one with large numbers and backlighting, so you can see the numbers easily.

Trackers

If you often wind up hunting for your glasses, TV remote, or other objects, small tracking devices can help. You simply attach a tracker to an object, and then the tracker sends signals to your smartphone, showing the

---

Even more memory help

In addition to getting gadgets that help support memory, such as electronic reminders or automatic pill dispensers, consider taking a class to learn memory strategies.

Seek out memory training programs in group or individual sessions with a clinician. The best places to look for such training are medical centers. They'll have programs run by health professionals with expertise in cognitive rehabilitation.

Or consider taking the Harvard Health Publishing online class Cognitive Fitness (www.health.harvard.edu/cogfitcourse). The class explores decades of research on cognitive health and shares the pillars of brain health that help sustain good brain function and cognitive fitness (the ability to learn, reason, remember, and adapt your thinking processes) into old age.

object's location on a map.

If you're not tech-savvy, there are trackers that send signals to a remote control device; if you lose the object, you click the remote and it makes the tracker emit a loud sound, leading you to the lost item.

Trackers come in several forms:

Eyeglasses trackers. (Cost: $35 and up.) These are small strips you attach to the long part of the frame worn over your ear.

Keychain-style trackers. (Cost: $20 and up.) These are small, flat devices (an inch or two wide) with a large hole so you can add them to key rings or tie them to objects (like household tools, sports equipment, or a bicycle). You can also just slip a tracker into your luggage, purse, or backpack.

Wallet trackers. (Cost: $30.) These trackers are about the size and shape of a credit card and work well in a wallet, purse, or any bag.

Tracker stickers. (Cost: $25 and up.) These are small, flat round trackers (an inch or two wide) with adhesive backing. They're handy to stick on TV remotes as well as laptops, earbud cases, pillboxes, and more.

Note: Trackers have limited ranges, such as 150 to 400 feet. They also use batteries, which last a year or two.

Smartphones

If you're tech-savvy, smartphones already come loaded with many of the devices we've mentioned, such as calendars, notepads, voice recorders, and alarms.

You can also download apps designed to hold important information (such as passwords) or manage your medications. Popular medication reminder apps include Medisafe (www.medisafeapp.com) and My Therapy Pill Reminder (www.mytherapyapp.com). Both are available in the Android or Apple app stores.

Final advice

"Choose a memory aid that can make a difference in your life. Don't be seduced by a fancy appearance or features you don't need. Look for good, basic functionality," Dr. Budson advises.

"And if you're using these tools and you still can't find anything or track appointments, it may be time to talk to your doctor about your memory," Dr. Budson suggests. "It could be that an underlying condition, medication side effect, or vitamin deficiency is causing your cognitive challenges."

Do fitness trackers really help people move more?

These gadgets are popular with avid exercisers, but they may also encourage sedentary people to become more active.

About one in five people has a smart watch or fitness tracker, according to a recent survey. These wrist-worn monitors are a handy way to track your daily steps, and they're probably more accurate than the tally from your smartphone, which you might not carry with you every waking moment. Most wearable gadgets also offer an array of other data, such as your heart rate, walking pace, and more.

But does using one affect how active people are? According to the largest study to date on the topic, the answer is yes (see "Fitness trackers and activity levels: What's the evidence?" on the next page). Regular physical activity is vital for a healthy heart, and the improvements seen in this study could potentially

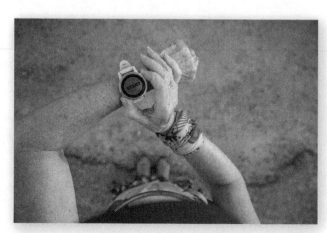

© Belinda Howell | Getty Images

Fitness trackers offer feedback that may help novice exercisers step up their game.

Fitness trackers and activity levels: What's the evidence?

To see how feedback from wearable fitness trackers affects exercise and activity levels, a team of Danish researchers reviewed and analyzed the evidence to date.

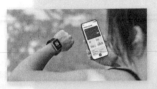

They identified 121 separate studies involving a total of nearly 17,000 mostly healthy adults ages 18 to 65. The median age of the participants was 47, and most were women. The median duration of the study intervention periods was 12 weeks.

Researchers found that on average, using physical activity monitors led people to take an extra 1,235 steps per day and do 49 additional minutes of moderate-to-vigorous physical activity per week. They also stood for an extra 10 minutes per day, although that amount wasn't significant. The study was published Jan. 26, 2022, in *The BMJ*.

make a difference, says Dr. Megan Wasfy, a cardiologist at the Cardiovascular Performance Laboratory at Harvard-affiliated Massachusetts General Hospital.

"The increase in moderate-to-vigorous physical activity was close to 50 extra minutes per week, which is one-third of the 150 minutes recommended by the federal activity guidelines," says Dr. Wasfy. The extra 1,200 daily steps taken when people were wearing trackers is about the same number that's been linked to a longer life in several studies. While 10,000 steps has long been touted as a daily goal, research suggests that 8,000 steps a day is nearly as effective longevity-wise, particularly in older populations.

No long-term data yet

The key, however, is to keep being physically active throughout your life, Dr. Wasfy says. Because many of the studies in the review lasted just a few months, it's impossible to know whether wearing a fitness tracker will promote lasting change in a person's behavior, she adds. And using a fitness tracker to change behavior requires a few more steps than simply being active—you also have to remember to keep the tracker charged, wear it consistently, and check your data.

Many people who might be motivated to use these devices are already regular exercisers, Dr. Wasfy points out. Such people tend to use them to step up their program or train for a race, rather than to transition from being mostly sedentary to more active. But if you're in that latter camp, a fitness tracker can be a useful tool, says Dr. Wasfy. "For people who are motivated to start exercising more, sometimes the day-to-day feedback on their progress helps keep them engaged," she says.

Tracker info

Activity monitors contain various sensors to track your movement and other health parameters. One basic feature is a sensor that shines a light through the skin to detect blood flow, revealing your heart rate. Another is the accelerometer, which tracks movement and velocity and enables the device to count steps. For people who want extra detail to help boost their performance, a global positioning satellite (GPS) sensor provides a more accurate assessment of your speed, distance, and pace during a walk, run, or ride.

For the average person, being able correlate how intensely you're exercising with your heart rate can be interesting, although it's certainly not mandatory, Dr. Wasfy says. If you're not interested in using a fitness tracker, the old-school "talk test" is an easy way to gauge exercise intensity. During moderate-intensity exercise, you should still be able to speak in full sentences but unable to sing.

However, if you've recently recovered from a heart attack or heart surgery or if you have other heart issues, you may need to monitor your exercise intensity more closely, and the heart rate function on a fitness tracker offers an easy way to do that. "High-intensity exercise may come with some added risk, so ask your doctor about a heart rate goal that makes sense for you," she advises.

Virtual reality for chronic pain relief

Virtual reality may have the potential to become a regular part of your treatment plan.

The latest tool to help reduce chronic pain sounds like it belongs in your grandkids' video game collection. It's called virtual reality (VR)—a computer-generated three-dimensional environment you can see with special goggles—and it's gaining traction as a promising therapy.

In November 2021, the FDA approved a prescription home-use VR device to help reduce chronic low back pain. And Harvard-affiliated Spaulding Rehabilitation Hospital has been studying VR for a few years now to see if the approach has the potential to manage any type of chronic pain.

"In the past, a lot of providers were using opioids as a way to treat chronic pain. As has become clear in recent years, opioids have many downsides, and providers are thirsty for alternative treatments. That's why there's increasing interest in this technology, and that's why we're studying it," says Dr. David Binder, a physiatrist and director of innovation at Spaulding Rehabilitation Hospital.

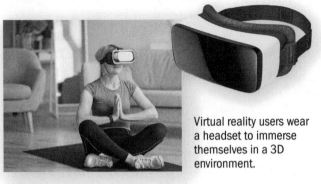

Virtual reality users wear a headset to immerse themselves in a 3D environment.

What is VR?

VR is an immersive technology that makes you feel as if you're in another world. While sitting comfortably, you put on a VR headset—goggles that give you a 360° view of a virtual environment. You can look anywhere in the virtual space—up, down, left, right, or behind—and you can hear sounds from speakers in the headset or headphones.

In a video game, you might put on a VR headset

IN THE JOURNALS

Mobile health and fitness apps pose privacy risks

Mobile health apps for your smartphone can help you recognize and manage health problems, provide nutrition advice, and count the number of steps you walk. But most aren't doing enough to protect your private information, according to a study published online June 16, 2021, by *The BMJ*.

Among millions of available apps (of any kind), researchers estimated that about 99,000 focus on health and fitness. Researchers downloaded almost 16,000 free mobile health apps and picked through their programming to see how the apps managed personal data (such as names, contact information, type of phone, and geographic location).

Most of the apps (88%) had the potential ability to share personal data (with Google and Facebook, for example). In brief tests, at least 4% of the apps collected and transmitted personal data, though researchers suspect this percentage could be much higher in real-world use. About a third of the apps didn't provide access to their privacy policies, and a quarter violated their own policies.

What that means for you: take the time to find out how an app might handle—or mishandle—your personal information before you start using it. Look for those details in an app's description, listed under "about this app" or "app permissions."

to ride on a virtual roller coaster. You'll see the track ahead of you, the amusement park to the sides, and the sky above. You'll experience the thrill of seeing your car bolt forward, twist, or turn—all while hearing the rattling of the car on the track and the shouts of other riders.

VR for chronic pain

For chronic pain reduction, VR isn't intended to excite you, but to calm you. The virtual environments are serene nature settings, such as a grassy field with a brilliant blue sky and a rolling stream nearby. You might hear sounds such as birds chirping and water gently bubbling along rocks. And the environments aren't always computer-generated. The system Spaulding Rehab experts are studying uses video of real places.

VR devices for chronic pain reduction incorporate other features as well, such as a narrator's voice guiding the wearer to take in the virtual surroundings, do breathing exercises, redirect negative thoughts about pain, or learn about pain responses.

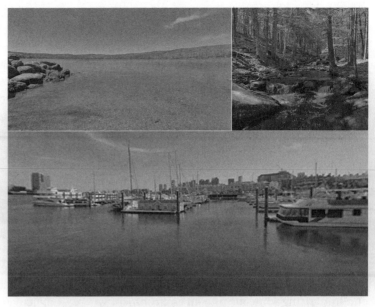

At Spaulding Rehabilitation Hospital, people using virtual reality for pain relief experience one of these 3D environments.

The device Dr. Binder's team is developing is accompanied by additional education. "Patients view the content in four sessions and use a workbook. And if they hear things in the educational content about pain that they don't understand, they have a trusted

Photo courtesy Spaulding Rehabilitation Hospital

IN THE JOURNALS

Wearable fitness trackers may aid weight-loss efforts

If you're starting a weight-loss plan, consider wearing a fitness tracker—like a smartwatch or bracelet that tracks steps, speed, and calories burned, and allows you to set goals, program reminders, and monitor your progress. A review published online March 17, 2021, by the *British Journal of Sports Medicine* found the devices helped overweight or obese people with chronic conditions (such as heart disease or diabetes) reduce body weight and lower their body mass index (BMI).

Researchers pooled data from 31 studies, involving more than 2,200 people. Studies required participants to wear a fitness tracker (many types were included) and set and meet weekly goals based on daily steps or minutes walked. Exercise programs that lasted at least 12 weeks were most effective.

People who wore research-grade fitness trackers (not available to the general public) lost the most weight (10 pounds), compared with people who did not use fitness trackers. People who wore commercially available fitness trackers (like Fitbit or Jawbone) lost an average of 6 pounds and two BMI points. Researchers say wearing a fitness tracker is a constant reminder to pursue health-related goals and be active.

© lucadp | Getty Images

clinician right there to talk about it and reinforce the concepts," says Lorna Brown, a physical therapist and lead clinical researcher for Spaulding's innovation team.

How it might help

The strategies used in VR for chronic pain reduction can include mindfulness (focusing on the present moment), meditation, guided imagery, or cognitive behavioral therapy (redirecting negative thoughts to positive ones). They're all used to control stress and mood. "Stress, anxiety, depression, and fear all contribute to pain," Dr. Binder says. "A lot of evidence suggests that if you're able to treat those, you can help reduce pain."

"Where VR might take these other therapies to a new level," Brown says, "is by putting them together and immersing someone into an environment where it's easier to focus."

It could also be that VR and its many stimuli simply distract your brain from receiving pain signals. "We already take advantage of this wiring all the time. For example, if you hit your elbow by accident, and it hurts, you rub the elbow and it feels better. You're tricking the brain by producing the sensory reaction of touching the elbow, which cancels some pain signals," Dr. Binder says.

Does it work?

The bulk of the evidence about VR for pain deals with treating sudden, severe pain—for example, using VR to distract people undergoing treatment for burns. VR is already used in many hospitals to ease pain after surgery, or during labor or cancer treatment.

While we don't have a lot of evidence yet that being in a VR environment reduces chronic pain, some studies are encouraging. For example, the evidence that swayed the FDA to approve the VR device for chronic low back pain (EaseVRx) was a randomized trial involving 179 people. Half used the three-dimensional VR device, and half used a sham device (with only a two-dimensional environment). After eight weeks of treatment, pain levels were reduced by more than half in 46% of

participants using the VR device compared with 26% of the other group.

The device Dr. Binder and his team are developing hasn't yet been tested in a randomized trial. So far, researchers have been trying it out in three Spaulding clinics to see if it's promising enough to do a large study. "We're learning how patients with persistent pain respond to the content. Based on that, we'll modify and improve it, and find out if there are any barriers to using the VR headset," Brown says.

Can you try it?

Spaulding's VR device isn't yet available, and the back pain VR device requires a doctor's order. It's not covered by insurance, and Dr. Binder doesn't anticipate that any VR device for chronic pain will be covered until VR becomes mainstream.

However, there are a number of VR devices with pain relief programs (not FDA-approved) available for purchase either online or through private physical therapy practices. Some hospitals and rehab centers also use VR for chronic pain.

And if you just want to try the technology, you can buy a VR device (starting at about $300) and download a meditation program for it. It won't have the same education and guidance found in a program designed for chronic pain reduction, supervised by a physical therapist. But it probably won't hurt—as long as you don't have any conditions that would make VR use dangerous, such as dizziness or balance problems.

What's the future for VR for pain reduction?

It's too soon to know if VR will become a standard part of chronic pain management. The answer depends on what happens with research, and how much value VR adds to treatment for chronic pain. "If VR content shows clear improvement, lower pain scores, and faster recovery, and if there's evidence from respected academic centers, the big technology companies would likely be interested. They're already investing heavily in VR," Dr. Binder says. "You might see VR being adopted at a level never imagined."

Listen to your heart

Knowing your heart rate at any time is easier than ever. What are the best ways to use this instant information?

There are many ways to track your heart rate nowadays, from fitness watches such as Garmin and Apple to activity trackers.

These devices use photoplethysmography sensors to measure your pulse. A light on the watch or tracker's underside shines onto the skin of your wrist and refracts off the blood flowing beneath. A sensor then translates that information into a pulse reading.

It's simple, fast, and reasonably accurate. But is this information valuable?

"Measuring your heart rate is an easy way to gauge your health in real time, as it provides a snapshot of your heart function," says Dr. James Sawalla Guseh, director of the Cardiovascular Performance Fellowship Program at Harvard-affiliated Massachusetts General Hospital. "Whether you are healthy and active or have a heart condition, these numbers can guide your workouts and at times highlight irregularities that you should have checked out."

Feel the beat

Traditionally, a normal resting heart rate—the number of heart beats per minute while at rest—ranges from 60 to 100 beats. But many healthy people have a resting heart rate in the 50s.

Knowing your heart rate at any given time, especially during workouts or any type of aerobic activity, is essential for people who need to be careful about overexertion and high exercise intensity, such as those diagnosed with coronary artery disease or other forms of heart disease.

"If you fall into this category, consider asking your doctor for a so-called 'exercise prescription' that specifies a good heart rate goal during exercise and an upper limit you should not exceed," says Dr. Guseh. For healthy older adults, monitoring heart rate can help maximize workout efforts. National guidelines recommend at least 150 minutes of moderate-intensity exercise per week.

Moderate intensity is 50% to 70% of your maximum heart rate, according to the American Heart Association, but the range can vary among individuals. In general, the greater your fitness level, the higher your moderate-intensity percentage range.

The most commonly used formula to calculate your maximum heart rate per minute is 220 minus your age. "For most people, increases in exercise intensity should be gradual," says Dr. Guseh. "As you exercise, you can use your heart rate monitor to see if your effort is adequate to stay within your desired target range, or if you need to increase the intensity or slow it down." (Some monitors let you program desired levels and sound an alarm if your heart rate suddenly goes too high or too low.)

You can also use this information to track your progress. "If your average heart rate begins to go

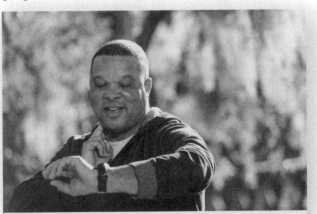

Pointing a finger at your heart rate

Don't have a heart rate monitor? Use your fingers. Lightly press the index and middle fingers of one hand on the opposite wrist, just below the base of the thumb. Or lightly press the side of the neck, just below your jawbone.

To calculate your heart rate, count the number of beats in 15 seconds and multiply by four. Repeat three times and average the number for a more accurate reading. Keep in mind that some situations can cause your resting heart rate to temporarily rise or fall. The best time to check it is right after you wake up before getting out of bed.

down, that's a sign of improved cardiovascular fitness," says Dr. Guseh.

Fast and slow

Another way to use heart rate monitoring is to look for values that are too high or too low, particularly at rest. Consistently unusual resting heart rates above 100 beats per minute or below 50 beats per minute, particularly if you feel unwell, require a conversation with your doctor.

A fast rate could be triggered by exertion, dehydration, stimulants, anxiety, or medication. It may also be a sign of infection, an overactive thyroid gland, or anemia. In addition, a fast heart rate may result from atrial fibrillation, a common heart rhythm abnormality that can emerge with age and is a frequent cause of stroke.

A slow heart rate is an expected side effect of certain heart and blood pressure medications, such as beta blockers and certain calcium-channel blockers.

Less commonly, an underlying heart condition, an underactive thyroid, or Lyme disease can be the reason. You also might experience nonspecific symptoms like lightheadedness, sudden fatigue, or brain fog.

"If you notice a slow heart rate along with new symptoms, it's worth discussing this with your doctor," says Dr. Guseh.

Screening for atrial fibrillation: An update

Wearable devices can detect this often-silent heart disorder. But as screening tools, they're not ready for prime time yet.

Nearly one in 11 people ages 65 and older have atrial fibrillation (afib), a heart rhythm disorder that causes bouts of rapid, irregular heartbeats. These unpredictable episodes—which may be fleeting or last for weeks or longer—may trigger symptoms such as dizziness and breathlessness, but not always.

However, the greatest threat from afib comes from the heightened risk of stroke that accompanies the condition. Because the heart's upper chambers (atria) don't contract regularly, blood may stagnate in the left atrium and form clots. If a clot escapes, it can travel to the brain and cause a stroke.

That potentially devastating outcome explains the ongoing effort to find an accurate, cost-effective method to detect afib—especially "silent" afib, which causes no symptoms and often remains unrecognized. "The idea is to catch afib soon enough so a person can start taking anti-clotting drugs to help prevent a stroke," says Harvard Medical School professor Dr. Peter Zimetbaum, director of clinical cardiology at Beth Israel Deaconess Medical Center.

Intermittent testing

Currently, doctors screen for afib during routine

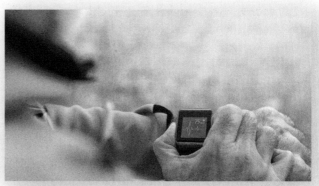

Electrocardiograms captured on smartwatches are not yet reliably accurate.

check-ups by asking people whether they have any afib symptoms and sometimes also with an electrocardiogram (ECG), a short recording of the heart's electrical activity. But because afib is usually transient, this strategy misses many cases. That's also true for other so-called intermittent screening strategies, which include simply monitoring a person's pulse at the wrist or neck for one full minute to check for a fast or irregular heartbeat. Home blood pressure monitors sometimes detect afib, as they also measure the user's heart rate.

Some smart watches and wrist-worn activity monitors feature programs that record ECGs. You open the app and touch sensors on the device, and it records your heart's rhythm for 30 seconds. If afib is detected, you receive an alert and a report you can share with your physician.

Current limitations

Sounds simple, right? It's more complicated than you might assume. For one thing, the algorithms to detect afib aren't completely accurate, and some reports can't be interpreted. Various things can throw off the recording, including movement (of either the person or the device), skin color, or environmental conditions such as lighting and temperature.

Another big issue: the reports can present an overwhelming amount of work for physicians, especially if they must sort through unusable data. "We don't have a system in place to manage all that information," says Dr. Zimetbaum.

Even if the device correctly identifies an episode of afib, that doesn't necessarily mean you need treatment. For now, experts don't know what burden of afib (that is, how frequently it occurs and for how long) warrants putting someone on anti-clotting medication, which points to another key message. "There is no point in screening people who don't have symptoms of afib unless they are prepared to consider taking blood thinners for the rest of their life," says Dr. Zimetbaum.

For people at high risk for afib (especially older people with underlying heart disease), doctors may use-longer-term ECG monitoring devices. An implanted loop recorder—a key-sized device placed under the skin of your chest—monitors your heart rhythm for up to three years. But this somewhat invasive and costly procedure is usually reserved for people with unexplained strokes or fainting spells. Another option is a Band-Aid-sized patch you wear on your chest for two weeks. If the patch doesn't detect any afib during that time period, however, that's no guarantee that you don't have afib.

Future promise?

"Within the next five to 10 years, wearable devices like the Apple Watch or Fitbit probably will be able to correctly identify afib without reporting false alarms. But we aren't there quite yet," says Dr. Zimetbaum.

Even your smartphone may one day be able to detect afib by recording your pulse when you press your finger on the camera, he says. But until these easy-to-use devices and accompanying programs or apps are available and affordable, widespread screening isn't feasible.

Meanwhile, to reduce your risk of afib, maintain a healthy weight, avoid alcohol (or drink only low to moderate amounts), and make sure your blood pressure is well controlled. If you snore loudly, get checked for sleep apnea, as this common sleep disorder is linked to a higher risk of afib.

Better blood sugar tracking: A benefit for heart health?

Continuous glucose monitors may help people better manage diabetes, a leading contributor to heart disease.

The high blood sugar levels that characterize diabetes—which affects about one in 10 American adults—are bad news for blood vessels. Elevated blood sugar can damage artery walls, making them more likely to narrow and stiffen; it also makes the blood stickier and more likely to clot. Having diabetes more than doubles your risk of heart disease.

Checking blood sugar has long required people to prick their finger and squeeze out a drop of blood. But growing numbers of people with diabetes are now using continuous glucose monitors (CGMs), which are small devices placed on your arm or belly with sensors inserted just under the skin. The devices measure a proxy for blood sugar every few minutes and transmit the readings to your smartphone or a portable monitor.

Awareness and availability

CGMs are already widely used by people with type 1 diabetes, the less common but more severe form of diabetes.

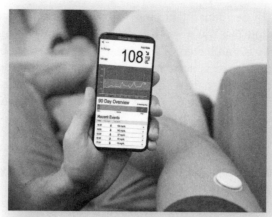

Continuous glucose monitors provide rapid feedback on how food affects blood sugar.

Recent research suggests that people with type 2 diabetes—who account for more than 90% of diabetes

cases—may also benefit from the technology. Meanwhile, television ads have boosted awareness of the devices among the general public.

"Many of my patients with type 2 diabetes are asking me about CGM devices," says Dr. Anna Goldman, an endocrinologist who specializes in diabetes at Harvard-affiliated Brigham and Women's Hospital. Currently, Medicare covers CGMs for people who inject insulin at least three times a day or use an insulin pump to control their blood sugar. Previously, people had to show they were

---

ASK THE DOCTORS

by HOPE RICCIOTTI, M.D., AND TONI GOLEN, M.D.

Can my phone and other devices interfere with my pacemaker?

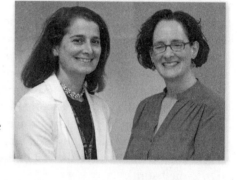

Q *I recently got a pacemaker, and I heard that some electronic devices might interfere with its operation. Are there certain things I should avoid?*

A While many electronic devices are safe to use if you have a pacemaker or an implantable cardioverter-defibrillator (ICD), there are some you should be leery of—primarily those that use magnetic chargers.

The magnets, if they are strong enough and held close to your device, can interfere with its operation, according to a 2021 report published in the journal *Heart Rhythm.*

Cardiac devices are equipped with something called "magnet mode," according to the FDA. This allows them to be temporarily disabled for safety reasons if someone is undergoing a test such as an MRI scan. In these situations, a doctor uses a strong magnet to temporarily deactivate the device. Once the magnet is removed, the device resumes its normal operation, says the FDA.

Magnets in devices, such as the iPhone 12 and

some wearable trackers like the Fitbit and Apple Watch, are sometimes strong enough to achieve this disabling effect if they are held close to the pacemaker. (Apple Support offers a comprehensive list of its products that contain magnets at https://support.apple.com/en-us/HT211900.)

The FDA recommends that pacemaker and ICD owners keep these electronic products at least six inches away from their cardiac device. For example, if you're talking on a smartphone, you might want to hold it against the ear that is farthest from your pacemaker and ensure that you don't hold or carry it close to your chest.

If you are uncertain about whether a device is safe for you to use, your best course of action is to discuss the issue with your doctor. She or he can help you determine if the product you are using presents any safety issues.

ASK THE DOCTOR

by **DEEPAK L. BHATT, M.D., M.P.H.**

Low heart rate warnings via smart watch

Q *Every once in a while, my smart watch informs me that my heart rate has dropped below 40 beats per minute. Is this any cause for concern?*

A The short answer is probably not—but there are a lot of caveats to consider. Are you experiencing any symptoms, such as feeling tired, dizzy, or weak, when these notifications appear? If the answer is no, that's reassuring. If yes, see a physician, as you might have a condition that warrants attention.

While you're awake, a normal resting heart rate is between 60 and 100 beats per minute (bpm), although it may drop well below 60 bpm when you're sleeping. Highly trained athletes and other people who exercise a great deal have very efficient hearts that beat more slowly when they're awake, sometimes even below 40 bpm.

But if you're not an elite athlete, there's another benign reason for an abnormally low heart rate reading. Remember that a smart watch is not a medical device, and the heart rate readings are not 100% reliable. Smart watches rely on optical sensors that detect light bouncing back from blood flow beneath the skin to measure your pulse. If the sensors aren't in close contact with your skin, the reading might be off. Of note: skin color does not appear to affect the accuracy of these measurements, according to one study.

Most smart watches include features that allow you to receive alerts when your heart rate dips below a certain level. For the Apple Watch, the default minimum heart rate setting is 40 bpm. However, doctors consider a slow heart rate to be less than 60 bpm when you're awake and active. Known as bradycardia, this condition usually results from a problem in the heart's natural pacemaker, the sinus node. The condition is fairly common in adults ages 70 and older and results from the normal wear and tear of aging. Other parts of the heart's electrical conduction system can also falter, causing a slow heart rate. Heart valve infections, a history of heart surgery, and certain blood pressure drugs may cause bradycardia. Other possible causes include obstructive sleep apnea and low thyroid function (hypothyroidism).

Episodes of bradycardia may come and go, so they're difficult to detect on an in-office electrocardiogram (ECG), a brief recording of the heart's electrical activity. People usually need to wear a portable heart monitor that records an ECG for 24 to 72 hours. Borderline or occasional bradycardia may not need to be treated. Other cases may resolve with medication adjustments. But severe or long-lasting cases—especially if the heart rate falls to 50 or less and causes symptoms or fails to increase with physical activity—often require an implanted pacemaker to regulate the heart's rhythm.

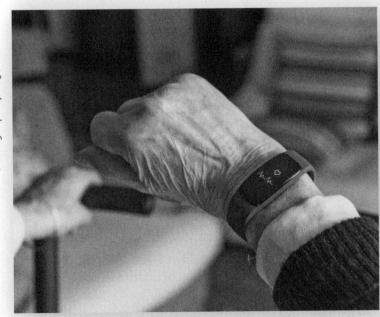

© deimagine | Getty Images

Smart watch pulse measurements may not always be accurate.

checking their blood sugar at least four times daily, but that requirement was eliminated in July 2021, removing one of the barriers to getting a CGM, says Dr. Goldman.

In 2021, two studies in *JAMA* found that for people with type 2 diabetes who take insulin, using a CGM led to better blood sugar control than traditional monitoring. One of the studies, which used real-world patient data, also documented fewer episodes of dangerously low or high blood sugar values among CGM users.

Feedback from food choices

Using a CGM can be very helpful by providing immediate feedback about how diet and exercise affects blood sugar. For example, people can see how bigger portions or poor food choices cause their blood sugar to rise—and how exercise helps lower blood sugar. "I've had patients tell me, 'Thank you for asking me to use this device; it really helped me change my habits,'" says Dr. Osama Hamdy, an associate professor of medicine at Harvard Medical School and director of the obesity clinical program at the Joslin Diabetes Center. Research suggests that

the more frequently people test their blood sugar, the more weight they lose, he adds.

One widely used test to assess diabetes control, hemoglobin A1c (referred to as A1c) reveals a person's average blood sugar levels over about three months. But A1c values can be misleading, says Dr. Hamdy. "You can have frequent episodes of very high and very low blood sugar and your average will still be fine. But that doesn't mean your blood sugar is well controlled," he explains. CGM readouts also show your blood sugar trends and tell you the percentage of time that your blood sugar is in a "good control" range (70 to 180 milligrams per deciliter for non-fasting levels). The higher your "time in range," the better.

Growing evidence suggests that frequent blood sugar fluctuations—known as glycemic variability—challenge your cardiovascular system. Sugar (glucose) is the fuel that provides energy for all the cells in your body. "Imagine you're driving a car and it's not getting a constant supply of fuel. Sometimes there's a lot, but sometimes there's not enough. That's hard on the motor," says Dr. Hamdy.

Another advantage of CGMs: they can be

© adamkaz | Getty Images

IN THE JOURNALS

Wearable devices may encourage enough exercise to prevent afib

Getting the recommended amount of physical activity appears to lower the risk of atrial fibrillation (afib), a heart rhythm disorder that raises the risk of stroke. The report relied on data from the UK Biobank, a long-term study that enrolled more than 500,000 people from 2006 to 2010.

From 2013 to 2015, nearly 94,000 of the participants wore wearable devices that tracked their movement for a week. Researchers then compared that data with afib diagnoses reported to the Biobank from 2013 to 2020. People who followed advice to get at least 150 minutes of moderate to

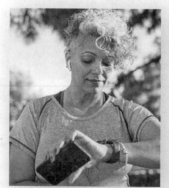

vigorous activity per week—as measured by the devices—had substantially lower risks of both afib and stroke.

By contrast, self-reported accounts of physical activity were not linked to a lower risk of afib or stroke. And the correlation between the amount of physical activity reported by the participants and what the devices measured was weak. According to the researchers, wearable devices such as smart watches and fitness bands may help people achieve the right amount of exercise to lower their afib risk. The study appeared May 25, 2021, in the *European Heart Journal*.

Breakthrough: AI and better medicines

Q *Do you think artificial intelligence will ever make a scientific breakthrough that leads to better medicines?*

A In fact, it's already happened. A remarkable recent example is called the protein structure breakthrough. The word "breakthrough" is often overused, but not in this case.

Proteins are the workhorses of every cell. How each protein does its work depends on its shape. Many diseases occur because of defects in particular proteins. To develop a drug that targets a defective protein, the scientist benefits from knowing that protein's shape.

The techniques traditionally used to determine a protein's shape are slow and difficult. For 60 years, however, scientists knew that there was a much faster solution: if you knew the structure of the specific gene that makes a specific protein, you should, in theory, be able to predict the shape of that protein. Unfortunately, the structure of very few genes was known.

However, beginning in the 1970s, scientists developed techniques for determining the structure of genes. By the early 21st century, the structure of every human gene, and many animal genes, had been determined. But scientists still struggled with translating theory into practice, with predicting the shape of a protein from the structure of its gene. In the 1990s, scientists began a competition to use mathematical models and computers to achieve that goal. Over time, predictions improved somewhat, but they still were pretty bad. In 2018, an artificial intelligence company owned by Google called DeepMind joined the competition. It did surprisingly well, but still not well enough to be useful. By the end of 2020, though, DeepMind's predictions had become accurate. The next question was whether its software was fast enough to determine the structure of very many proteins.

Indeed, very few protein structures were known. As of July 1, 2021, thousands of scientists working for nearly a century had determined the shape of only about 30% of the 20,000 human proteins, and the shape of only 0.01% of the 280 million nonhuman proteins. Could DeepMind really improve those dismal numbers?

On July 22, 2021, DeepMind published its answer. It reported a predicted structure for 98% of the human proteins, up from 30% on July 1. Now, that's a breakthrough.

Experts differ as to how rapidly this remarkable advance will lead to new treatments. Time will tell. For now, though, one thing is clear: the marriage of information technology and modern biology led to this breakthrough. These two fields may be the most important intellectual achievements of the past century. And they happened, and could only have happened, because societies invested in science.

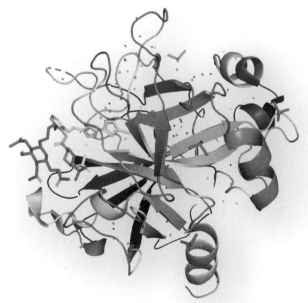

Proteins develop very complex shapes.

© sergunt | Getty Images

programmed to send an alert when your blood sugar is too high or too low, and they can send that data in real time to family or friends.

The future of CGMs

External CGM sensors (which are about the size of a quarter but thicker) need to be replaced every 10 to 14 days. An implantable CGM that lasts 90 days is also available, and one company is developing a version that lasts up to six months. As the technology improves and the costs decrease, use of these devices will continue to expand, says Dr. Hamdy. "Within 10 years, everyone with diabetes will have a continuous glucose monitor," he predicts.

Over-the-counter hearing aids are finally available

If you have difficulty hearing and you've been putting off doing anything about it, this is a good time to take action. In August 2022, the FDA finally approved a new category of safe, regulated hearing aids sold over the counter. You can get them without a prescription for thousands of dollars less than traditional prescription hearing aids (which can cost $5,000 or more per pair).

The move is meant to make hearing aids more widely available to people who otherwise couldn't afford them or who can't get to a doctor or an audiologist for a hearing evaluation and fittings. Instead, you can simply order over-the-counter hearing aids online or buy them at a store or pharmacy. They are "self-fitting," which means you'll adjust them yourself.

But note: the devices are meant only for people with perceived mild-to-moderate hearing loss who need to amplify the volume of sounds around them. If you're not sure what kind of hearing loss you have, it's a good idea to get an evaluation from an audiologist. And since getting the right fit and effectiveness takes trial and error, you might also want to consult an audiologist for advice on the right over-the-counter hearing aids for you.

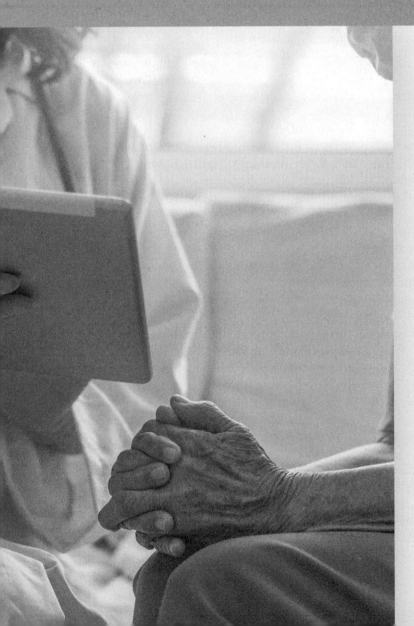

Chapter 13
—
Savvy Patient

Take Action!
5 Things You Can Do Now

1 **Make a cheat sheet.** Create and carry a list of questions for new medications. (page 304)

2 **Stop eating at night.** This may help you avoid heartburn. (page 306)

3 **Play background music.** It helps mask ringing in the ears. (page 309)

4 **Practice standing with one foot in front of the other.** It helps improve balance. (page 310)

5 **Dim your dashboard lights when driving at night.** This reduces some glare so you can see better. (page 316)

5 important blood tests beyond the basics

Bring this article to your next doctor appointment to ask if these tests are right for you.

Your next general check-up will probably include basic blood tests for levels of red blood cells, various types of white blood cells, fats (like cholesterol), and chemicals that indicate how your liver and kidneys are functioning. Some tests beyond the basics can also reveal important aspects of health, but your doctor might not offer them routinely. The following five tests may be worth pursuing in certain situations.

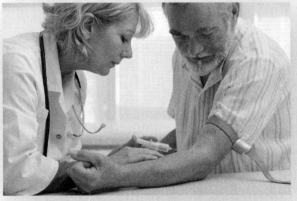

Ask your doctor if it makes sense to check your vitamin B_{12} level.

tested every few years. Low B_{12} levels can lead to anemia, memory problems, and walking difficulty," says Dr. Suzanne Salamon, associate chief of gerontology at Harvard-affiliated Beth Israel Deaconess Medical Center.

Normal B_{12} test results range from 160 to 950 picograms per milliliter (pg/mL). A low-normal test result in the range of 200 to 300 pg/mL may warrant a vitamin B_{12} supplement.

Vitamin B_{12}

B_{12} (cobalamin) is an essential vitamin we need for keeping our brain and nerves healthy, for producing DNA and red blood cells, and for lowering levels of homocysteine (an amino acid linked to chronic diseases such as dementia and heart disease).

Our B_{12} comes from food, including beef, eggs, poultry, and dairy foods (milk, yogurt). To absorb the vitamin, we need stomach acid to shake it loose from food. Then a protein called intrinsic factor (made in the stomach lining) binds to B_{12} so it can be absorbed by the small intestine and passed into the blood.

Some people have low B_{12} levels. There are several common reasons for this:

- They are vegetarians and don't eat B_{12}-rich foods.
- They produce less stomach acid than they used to.
- They use medications that reduce stomach acid, such as antacids for heartburn.
- They have a rare autoimmune disease (pernicious anemia) that leads to severe B_{12} deficiency.

Should you get the test? "I think everybody should get at least one B_{12} test after age 65, and then get

Vitamin D

We get a little vitamin D in our diet (from foods like fish, fortified milk, or yogurt), but most of it is manufactured by our bodies when the sun's ultraviolet B rays shine on our skin. That's why D is known as the "sunshine vitamin."

Still, many older adults are deficient in vitamin D, no matter how sunny their environment. "It doesn't matter if you live in Florida or California because, as you get older, your skin doesn't absorb sunlight as well," Dr. Salamon says.

You don't want to let vitamin D levels drop. Vitamin D is important for healthy bones, calcium absorption, inflammation reduction, immune function, and other body processes, and it may play a role in keeping cancer in check. Recent Harvard evidence suggests that taking a daily vitamin D supplement is associated with a reduced risk for advanced cancer in healthy-weight midlife or older-age people.

Should you get the test? Dr. Salamon recommends a baseline test at least once in your life, especially if you have brittle bones or a stomach condition that affects your ability to absorb vitamin D. But she points out that screening is hotly debated.

What if you have a high risk for cancer? "While

you may feel better knowing what your vitamin D levels are, an alternative is to skip the test and just start taking a supplement of 1,000 to 2,000 international units per day. If adding another pill to your regimen would overwhelm you, talk to your doctor about it first," says Dr. JoAnn Manson, Harvard's leading vitamin D researcher and chief of the Division of Preventive Medicine at Harvard-affiliated Brigham and Women's Hospital.

A normal result for a vitamin D test measuring a form of the vitamin (25-hydroxyvitamin D) is debated, but should be at least 20 nanograms per milliliter (ng/mL).

Hepatitis C

Hepatitis C is a viral infection that can lead to cirrhosis, liver damage, liver cancer, or liver failure. It's spread when a person comes in contact with the blood of an infected person, which can happen with intravenous drug use; having sex with an infected partner; getting a tattoo or body piercing with unsterile equipment; sharing razors, nail clippers, or toothbrushes; or having had a blood transfusion before 1992 (when the blood test for hepatitis C first became available).

Baby boomers (born between 1945 and 1964), who are five times more likely to have the virus than other adults, may have become infected in the 1960s through the 1980s. Yet only about 13% of baby boomers had been tested by 2015. "It could be due to the stigma, but I wouldn't be surprised if a lot of doctors don't offer the test. They may think their patients aren't at risk for hepatitis C," Dr. Salamon says.

Should you get the test? All U.S. adults should be tested at least once, and more often if they take part in risky behavior. The good news: "There's a cure for hepatitis C if you catch the infection early," Dr. Salamon says.

HIV

Since HIV (human immunodeficiency virus) and AIDS (the late-stage phase of HIV infection) first appeared decades ago, we've developed powerful antiviral medications to keep the infection from progressing.

But like hepatitis C testing, HIV testing also has a stigma. HIV is transmitted when someone is exposed to certain body fluids of an infected person. That can happen during vaginal or anal sex or the sharing of drug equipment such as needles.

Should you get the test? The CDC advises everyone ages 13 to 64 to get tested at least once, and warns that older adults are less likely to be screened because they (or their doctors) don't think they're at risk for HIV. Yet one in six people diagnosed with HIV in 2018 was age 50 or older. "Get this test if you've never had it before or if you're sexually active," Dr. Salamon advises.

Blood sugar

People with diabetes or prediabetes have elevated levels of glucose (sugar) in the blood. A blood sugar measurement taken after fasting may be ordered during a check-up and is covered by Medicare. But Dr. Salamon says primary care physicians don't always check your levels each year.

Should you get the test? If your blood sugar is normal, a test every few years is fine, but it still might be a good idea to get annual testing. "Some people are 'silent' diabetics who don't have symptoms, and you wouldn't pick this up unless you ordered the test," Dr. Salamon says. People at high risk for diabetes, such as those who are overweight or have diabetes in their family, may need more frequent tests.

A normal fasting blood sugar measurement is less than 100 milligrams per deciliter (mg/dL) of blood; 126 or more can indicate diabetes. "But normal levels change with age and can be slightly higher. Your doctor must interpret the results," Dr. Salamon says.

Should you worry about prediabetes?

You may be at an increased risk for heart attack and stroke.

An estimated 37 million Americans—just over one in 10—have type 2 diabetes. However, approximately 96 million—more than one in three—have prediabetes, a condition in which the average amount of sugar (glucose) in the blood is high, but not high enough to be diagnosed as diabetes. More than 84% of people with prediabetes don't know they have it.

Older adults tend to ignore the seriousness of prediabetes because, on average, they are less likely to get full-blown diabetes compared with younger people. Still, prediabetes can greatly raise their risk for heart attack and stroke.

"Older adults need to understand the potential danger of elevated blood sugar levels even if they are not worrisome yet, so they can address the problem before it worsens," says Dr. Jorge Plutzky, director of preventive cardiology at Harvard-affiliated Brigham and Women's Hospital.

The sticky issue of glucose

How does prediabetes (and diabetes) occur? When you eat, your body breaks down carbohydrates from food into a simple sugar called glucose. At the same time, your pancreas produces a hormone called insulin that signals the body's cells to absorb glucose from the bloodstream.

Type 2 diabetes, the most common type, happens when the body has trouble using glucose for energy because cells become resistant to the action of insulin. So your pancreas makes more insulin to try to get cells to respond. Eventually, the pancreas can't keep up, and blood sugar builds up in the bloodstream.

The difference between diabetes and prediabetes is how high blood sugar levels get. Diabetes is known to increase a person's risk of heart attack and stroke. But prediabetes also can be dangerous. "Even mildly elevated glucose levels can trigger inflammation that damages blood vessels, cause them to narrow, and lead to blockages," says Dr. Plutzky. That's why it's so important for people with prediabetes to lower other cardiovascular risk factors by controlling blood pressure and cholesterol levels.

Prediabetes usually has no symptoms, which is why many people are unaware they have it. The common risk factors are the same as those for full-blown type 2 diabetes, such as excess weight, poor diet, and a family history of diabetes. Less often, some people with prediabetes notice dark patches on the skin around their armpits, elbows, knees, knuckles, or neck.

The big three

Older adults should get their blood sugar levels checked even if they are in good health overall.

"Those are often the people who need to be the most mindful," says Dr. Plutzky. (See "Blood check.")

The best way to treat prediabetes is also the best way to prevent it. You need to focus on the big three: weight, exercise, and diet.

Weight. If you are overweight, even a small amount of weight loss—5% to 7%—can lower your risk of prediabetes and protect against diabetes. "Focus on smaller amounts at first, like five

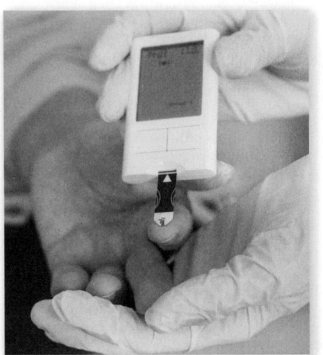

© AndreyPopov | Getty Images

Blood check

As with diabetes, prediabetes is diagnosed from blood sugar tests. Your doctor will probably suggest one of these:

▶ A hemoglobin A1c test reflects your average blood sugar for the past two to three months.

▶ A fasting plasma glucose test measures your blood sugar after you've avoided eating or drinking for at least eight hours.

▶ An oral glucose tolerance test checks how well the body processes sugar after drinking a sweet drink.

According to the American Diabetes Association, prediabetes is suspected with an A1c from 5.7% to 6.4%, a fasting blood sugar level of 100 to 125 milligrams per deciliter (mg/dl), or a blood sugar level of 140 to 199 mg/dl during an oral glucose tolerance test.

pounds, and when you reach that, aim for another five pounds," says Dr. Plutzky.

Exercise. Staying active even when you carry a higher-than-ideal weight is associated with a lower risk of prediabetes. Dr. Plutzky suggests looking beyond traditional workouts, and adopting sports and physical activities you like, such as golf, dancing, or yoga. "If you enjoy it, you'll do it more often, and consistency is what's important," he says.

Diet. Reduce your intake of simple carbs, such as bread, pasta, rice, potatoes, and high-sugar beverages like fruit juice and soda. These carbs are quickly digested and can cause blood sugar levels to quickly rise and fall. Simple carbs also can trigger cravings that may lead to overeating and weight gain. In turn, replace simple carbs with complex ones, such as those in whole grains, beans, and lentils. Also, eat more fiber-rich foods. Fiber slows the absorption of sugar and helps balance blood sugar levels.

If you are diagnosed with prediabetes, Dr. Plutzky suggests getting another blood test in two to three months after adopting these changes. "The results will determine if you need to make any adjustments," he says. "If your numbers have improved, seeing the change can inspire you to keep going."

What's new in diabetes drugs

Two classes of drugs have gotten much attention lately.

Watch TV lately, and you may have noticed a slew of advertisements for two classes of diabetes drugs—GLP-1 receptor agonists and SGLT-2 inhibitors. Why are these medications being marketed so heavily?

Sure, these new drugs add significant revenue to pharmaceutical companies. But they also offer health benefits beyond just keeping blood sugar levels controlled.

Growing problem

Type 2 diabetes (by far the most common type) remains a serious health risk for many Americans, especially older adults. About 37 million adults have type 2 diabetes, according to the CDC. Based on current trends, the CDC predicts that one in five American adults will have diabetes by 2025, and the number could reach one in three by 2050.

Oral metformin remains the first go-to drug in the treatment of type 2 diabetes. It's available as a generic, so it's very affordable. Also, metformin does not cause hypoglycemia (low blood sugar) when used alone. The most common side effects are abdominal discomfort and irregular bowel habits.

According to new guidelines from the American Diabetes Association (ADA), doctors should consider adding either a GLP-1 receptor agonist or SGLT-2 inhibitor if blood sugar levels are still too high despite metformin or a person has an increased

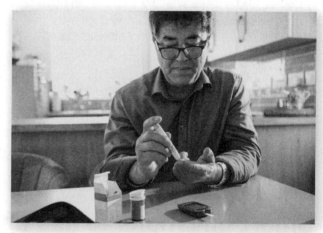
Current trends suggest more older adults will be diagnosed with diabetes in the coming years.

risk of cardiovascular or kidney disease. The ADA recognizes that many patients won't be able to afford these drugs today.

Tale of two drugs

The two drug classes work to manage glucose (sugar) levels but in different ways. You can take one or the other, or in some cases, both. Here is a look at how each works.

GLP-1 receptor agonists. These mimic the hormone glucagon-like peptide 1 (GLP-1). People with diabetes don't make enough. GLP-1 is released from

The extra advantages

The real excitement about GLP-1 receptor agonists and SGLT-2 inhibitors relates to their additional health benefits for those with and without diabetes. For example:

Weight loss. Both can help a person with diabetes shed pounds. But the GLP-1 receptor agonists are more effective for weight reduction compared with the SGLT-2 inhibitors. In fact, two of the GLP-1 receptor agonists, liraglutide (Saxenda) and semaglutide (Wegovy), are FDA approved for long-term weight management in people with obesity who don't have diabetes.

Heart disease. Drugs from both classes lower the risk of heart attack and stroke in people with diabetes. For people with heart failure and diabetes, SGLT-2 inhibitors have been shown to decrease hospitalizations and improve survival. Because of these benefits, doctors are beginning to use SGLT-2 inhibitors even in nondiabetic heart failure patients.

Chronic kidney disease. SGLT-2 inhibitors can slow down the progression of diabetic kidney disease and may help prevent kidney failure related to other conditions.

the intestines when you eat. It signals the pancreas to produce extra insulin and tells the liver to stop making glucose, both of which balance blood sugar levels. The hormone also signals the brain that you have eaten, which helps you avoid overeating.

Most GLP-1 receptor agonists are injected. There are two types: short-acting formulas taken once or twice daily, and long-acting formulas taken once a week.

Short-acting GLP-1 receptor agonists include exenatide (Byetta), lixisenatide (Adlyxin), liraglutide (Victoza), and semaglutide (Rybelsus, available in tablet form). Long-acting versions are dulaglutide (Trulicity), exenatide extended release (Bydureon BCise), and semaglutide (Ozempic). Side effects may include nausea and other gastrointestinal problems like vomiting and diarrhea, but these are usually short-lived.

SGLT-2 inhibitors. These daily oral drugs block the kidneys from reabsorbing glucose. Instead, excess sugar passes out of the body in urine, thereby lowering blood sugar levels. This way, the body doesn't have to work harder to manage glucose, says Dr. Susan Herzlinger-Botein, a clinical researcher at Harvard-affiliated Joslin Diabetes Center. The ones currently available are canagliflozin (Invokana), dapagliflozin (Farxiga), empagliflozin (Jardiance), and ertugliflozin (Steglatro).

"The drugs might make a person urinate more at first, but the frequency goes away over time," says Dr. Herzlinger-Botein. The drugs also may increase the risk of urinary tract infections, a problem that is more common in women than men.

SGLT-2 inhibitors have a few caveats. The drugs are not for people with type 1 diabetes or those with type 2 diabetes who follow strict low-carb diets, need dialysis, or have had recent surgery. They also can raise the risk of low blood pressure.

Smart questions to ask about a new prescription

Getting answers can help you avoid costly medication mistakes.

When your doctor prescribes a new drug, you might not think of all the questions you should ask about it. Maybe your appointment is rushed, you're focused on a diagnosis, or you just don't feel well.

That's all understandable. But without enough information, you might be vulnerable to the consequences of a medication error (such as taking too much or too little of the drug). Such errors result in 1.3 million emergency department visits each year in the United States. If you don't ask questions when you get a prescription, seek information as soon as possible and write down the answers. Here are ideas to get you started.

Why is this being prescribed?

"You need to be in on your treatment so you understand what your condition is, how a particular medication will help you, and what would happen if you didn't take it. A good example is high blood pressure. Since it often doesn't cause symptoms, some people don't realize that if high blood pressure is not controlled, it can lead to a heart attack or stroke," says Joanne Doyle Petrongolo, a pharmacist at

Harvard-affiliated Massachusetts General Hospital.

What is the name of the drug?

Make sure you get the name of the medication, so you'll be able to recognize it on a pill bottle and know how to refer to it.

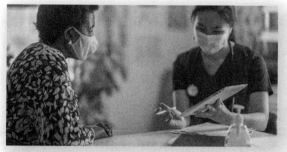

Bring a list of questions to an appointment, in case your doctor prescribes something new.

What are the side effects?

Medications often have the potential to cause side effects such as dizziness, drowsiness, nausea, or headache. Find out what the common side effects are for the drug you're getting, and what to do if you notice them. For example, "some medications for anxiety or depression may cause you to be sleepy, so you may want to take the medication only while you're at home, and avoid driving," Doyle Petrongolo says. "Find out how your body reacts to it so you can plan your day."

What are the drug instructions?

Medication instructions vary widely. Some are simple, like taking a drug with food (to ward off stomach irritation) or without food (to promote better absorption). Others are more complicated. An example is alendronate (Fosamax) to treat osteoporosis. "You need to take it on an empty stomach one hour before meals or two hours afterward, with a large glass of water, and you can't lie down for one hour after taking it because it can irritate the esophagus," Doyle Petrongolo says.

Ask about the best way to fit a new medication into your existing regimen.

How long will I need to take it?

The length of time you need to take a prescription drug also varies, depending on your needs. But not everyone gets that message. "For example, I run into problems with some patients thinking they only have to take a blood pressure medication for a month or until refills run out, although they really need to take it indefinitely," Doyle Petrongolo says. "On the other hand, a drug like a pain reliever might only be intended for the short term."

Ask up front how long your doctor thinks you'll need to take the drug, and how you'll know when to stop.

Will it affect my other medications?

Many pills—including over-the-counter remedies and supplements—have harmful interactions with others, such as amplifying the effect of one or making another too weak. For example, taking calcium can block the effect of levothyroxine (Synthroid, Tirosint) that is taken to treat an underactive thyroid.

Some interactions can be dangerous. "A lot of antibiotics can interact with the blood thinner warfarin [Coumadin], increasing the risk for bleeding." Doyle Petrongolo says. Make sure your doctor knows about everything you're taking at the time a new drug is prescribed.

What if I miss a dose?

In some cases, it might be okay to skip a dose or take the medication when you realize you missed it. In others, it depends on when you make the discovery.

For example, with metformin (Glucophage, Riomet) for diabetes: "If you're supposed to take doses at 8 a.m. and 6 p.m., and you discover at midnight that you forgot your 6 p.m. dose, you might need to skip it and wait until the morning. Otherwise, it could make the morning dose too strong. But you'd need guidance from your doctor or pharmacist," Doyle Petrongolo says.

More questions

Here are other important questions:

- How much does the drug cost?
- Can I get it in a generic form?
- How will we know it's working?
- Is it safe to drive while taking it?
- Can I drink alcohol while taking it?
- How can I get refills?
- How should I store it?
- Are there drug-free alternatives?

"And if more questions occur to you," Doyle Petrongolo says, "don't be embarrassed to ask them."

Is it okay to use proton-pump inhibitors on demand?

It depends on your health and the frequency of symptoms, but it can be done in certain instances.

Proton-pump inhibitors (PPIs) are effective treatments for chronic heartburn caused by gastroesophageal reflux disease (GERD). Several, such as omeprazole (Prilosec, Zegerid), lansoprazole (Prevacid), and esomeprazole (Nexium), are available over the counter as well as by prescription.

But they don't rapidly relieve symptoms like two other classes of heartburn drugs—antacids and H2 blockers. That's important to understand when your doctor says you can take PPIs "on demand."

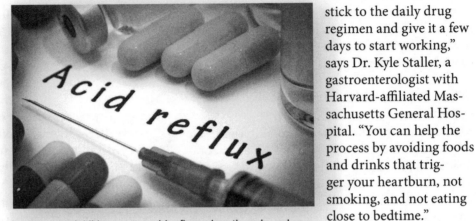

Proton-pump inhibitors tame acid reflux or heartburn by reducing stomach acid levels.

© GreenApple78 | Getty Images

How do PPIs work?

PPIs stifle the production of stomach acid. This is important in GERD, which occurs when stomach acid and digestive enzymes squirt back up (reflux) into the esophagus, the tube that carries food from the mouth to the stomach.

The stomach juices irritate and inflame the esophagus lining, causing heartburn—a burning feeling in the chest—as well as a bitter taste in the mouth, difficulty swallowing, a sore throat, or coughing. Over time, GERD can cause permanent damage to the esophagus and increase the risk of esophageal cancer.

PPIs help by lowering stomach acid levels, which relieves heartburn and reduces the risk for esophageal damage.

Taking PPIs

A usual course of PPIs lasts two to eight weeks, depending on what your doctor prescribes. The drugs are taken once a day on an empty stomach, 30 to 60 minutes before breakfast. Your doctor might also recommend taking a PPI before a big meal.

But don't expect immediate relief. "You have to stick to the daily drug regimen and give it a few days to start working," says Dr. Kyle Staller, a gastroenterologist with Harvard-affiliated Massachusetts General Hospital. "You can help the process by avoiding foods and drinks that trigger your heartburn, not smoking, and not eating close to bedtime."

After PPI therapy

Stopping PPI therapy gets tricky. Going cold turkey can lead to heartburn that's worse than it was before PPI therapy. "It's a rebound phenomenon," Dr. Staller says. "The PPI turns off the acid production, but when you stop the PPI, acid production gets turned back on suddenly, and that leads to symptoms."

To avoid a rebound, Dr. Staller advises a few strategies. "Taper off of PPIs slowly," he says. "If you're on a

Are PPIs safe?

You may have heard that proton-pump inhibitors (PPIs) are associated with dangerous side effects. In the past, small studies suggested that the drugs might reduce levels of vitamin B_{12}, magnesium, and calcium and increase risks for hip fractures, pneumonia, kidney or cardiovascular disease, and dementia. However, large studies published in 2019 and 2020 found no links to such risks.

"The new studies are more reliable and show no evidence of adverse outcomes, at least in a three-year period," says Dr. Kyle Staller, a gastroenterologist with Harvard-affiliated Massachusetts General Hospital.

"But if you don't have any symptoms, and you don't have any damage in your esophagus due to heartburn, there's no reason to continue taking PPIs."

high dose, go to a lower dose for a few days. Then start an overlap period where you alternate a PPI one day and an H2 blocker the next." Examples of H2 blockers include famotidine (Pepcid) and cimetidine (Tagamet).

"After a week of overlap, stop the PPI altogether and take the H2 blocker each day for another week. Then stop the medications and see how you feel," Dr. Staller suggests.

What if symptoms return?

The way to treat recurring symptoms depends on the type of GERD you have. If GERD has damaged the lining of your esophagus, you'll likely need to stay on a long-term PPI regimen to reduce the risk for further damage and cancer. People who don't have such damage from GERD can use PPIs "on demand," according to guidelines from the American College of Gastroenterology, published in January 2022 in the *American Journal of Gastroenterology*.

While you might take H2 blockers to rapidly suppress GERD symptoms, just one or two at a time, that's not the way to use PPIs. "It's usually a two-week course," Dr. Staller says, "You probably won't need to taper off the drugs in this case, but you may need to experiment and see what works for you. If this round of PPIs treats your heartburn, you can go off of them again. If your symptoms persist, you may need to go back to long-term maintenance therapy with PPIs."

Is your medication making you lightheaded?

Many drugs can cause this symptom. Consider strategies to manage the risks.

You're taking a new prescription, and you're feeling a little lightheaded. Are the two connected? It's an important question, since many drugs are known to cause lightheadedness. And lightheadedness comes with a dangerous risk: falling.

"Just being older increases your risk for falls. If you add three or four medications—or even just one with a known side effect of lightheadedness—it increases risk even more," notes Joanne Doyle Petrongolo, a pharmacist at Harvard-affiliated Massachusetts General Hospital.

Recognize the symptom

Lightheadedness can mean many things. You may think of it as feeling faint or about to pass out, off-balance, nauseated, confused, or weak. All of those symptoms fall under the umbrella term of "lightheadedness."

But lightheadedness is not a sensation of the world moving or spinning around you. Such a sensation is vertigo, which occurs when the body's sensory inputs (such as vision or sense of touch) send confusing messages to the brain. Vertigo is often associated with inner ear disorders.

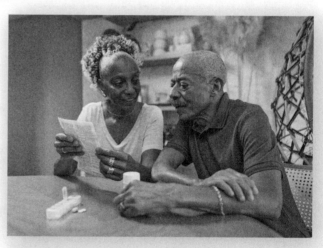

Check the list of a drug's possible side effects, and be on alert if lightheadedness is a risk.

Why do some drugs cause lightheadedness?

There are many reasons why medications cause lightheadedness. Sometimes they simply work too well. In the case of diabetes drugs, your blood sugar may fall too low, which can cause lightheadedness. "And with some blood pressure medications, you may urinate a lot of fluid and become dehydrated, which lowers your blood pressure too much. Or the blood pressure drugs might drop your pressure when you stand up suddenly, causing you to feel temporarily lightheaded. Or the medicines may keep your blood pressure below normal all the time, not just when you stand up, which also can make you lightheaded," Doyle Petrongolo says.

What you can do

Learn about the potential side effects of all your medications, and be on high alert if lightheadedness is a possibility. Jot down the day and time you take a pill and the side effects you experience: your record of those details can help your doctor determine if you need a change in your regimen.

"With blood pressure medications, antidepressants, antipsychotics, and antiseizeure medications, lightheadedness should subside after about a week or two," Doyle Petrongolo says. "If it doesn't, report it to your doctor. You may need a lower dose or a different medication."

If a drug has a high likelihood of causing lightheadedness, Doyle Petrongolo says you may

Lightheadedness culprits

Many medications commonly cause lightheadedness. Common offenders include

- antidepressants, such as fluoxetine (Prozac), sertraline (Zoloft), paroxetine (Paxil), and amitriptyline (Elavil)

- antipsychotics, such as quetiapine (Seroquel) and olanzapine (Zyprexa)

- antiseizure drugs, such as gabapentin (Neurontin), which is often given to treat neuropathy or shingles pain

- blood pressure drugs, including diuretics such as hydrochlorothiazide (Hydrodiuril), ACE inhibitors such as lisinopril (Zestril), calcium-channel blockers such as diltiazem (Cardizem), and beta blockers such as metoprolol (Lopressor)

- diabetes drugs, such as glipizide (Glucotrol) and glyburide (Diabeta)

- pain medications, such as oxycodone (Oxycontin)

- sedatives, such as lorazepam (Ativan) and diazepam (Valium)

- sleep medications, such as zolpidem (Ambien)

- urological medications that work by relaxing bladder muscles, such as tamsulosin (Flomax), which is prescribed to help urine flow more easily, and oxybutynin (Ditropan), which is used to treat overactive bladder.

Take melatonin supplements for sleep? Check your dosage

Melatonin supplement use to improve sleep has jumped 425% in the past two decades, with the number of people taking large amounts (more than 5 milligrams per day) at an all-time high, according to a study published Feb. 1, 2022, in *JAMA*. These findings highlight potential safety concerns.

Like other supplements, melatonin products are not subject to the same regulations and quality standards as prescription drugs. The authors pointed out that the actual amount of melatonin in a given pill can be significantly higher than what the label shows. This can cause people to take too much, especially since many use melatonin regularly.

While melatonin is generally considered safe in low doses taken in the short term, high amounts for long periods can cause side effects, such as nausea, dizziness, headaches, and anxiety. Melatonin, the so-called sleep hormone, keeps your circadian rhythm (your 24-hour internal clock) in sync. Evidence suggests melatonin supplements may help some people fall asleep faster, but it has minimal effect on sleeping throughout the night.

want to take it at night—so you don't experience the symptom during the day. "And if you know a medication makes you lightheaded, don't get up abruptly from a chair or bed. Give yourself a chance to get your bearings."

Other tips include staying hydrated throughout the day and checking your blood pressure regularly with a home monitor. "If your blood pressure is normal, but on the low side of normal, or if it's unusually low for you, give that information to your doctor," Doyle Petrongolo says. "You may need a medication adjustment."

Tips to manage tinnitus

Treating underlying causes, practicing mindfulness, and living a healthy lifestyle may help reduce the volume and distress.

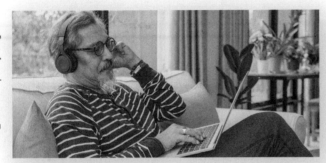

Playing music helps distract your brain, so you pay less attention to your tinnitus.

The distant peal of bells from a town square or church can be a lovely and even comforting sound. The ringing of tinnitus in your ears is quite the opposite. The internal high-pitched ringing, whooshing, or hissing noise can cause great distress.

"Having tinnitus can make it hard to concentrate, reduce sleep quality, and cause irritability, nervousness, anxiety, depression, or feelings of hopelessness. This, in turn, can lead to mental, physical, and social repercussions, causing people to withdraw from the company of others," says Emma Alscher, an audiologist at Harvard-affiliated Massachusetts Eye and Ear.

While it's not always possible to eliminate tinnitus, the following strategies may help ease symptoms.

Check for underlying conditions. Tinnitus is often seen in people with hearing loss. It also can be a side effect of some medicines. In rare cases, it's caused by a tumor involving the nerve responsible for hearing. See an ear, nose, and throat specialist who can diagnose the cause of your tinnitus and perhaps help you reverse or alleviate it.

Learn your triggers. Write down the circumstances when tinnitus symptoms bother you. "It helps you to anticipate, prevent, and change situations that may make tinnitus worse," Alscher points out. For example, some people feel their tinnitus worsens after drinking alcohol or caffeinated drinks, although there's little evidence that alcohol or caffeine causes tinnitus very often.

Get hearing aids. "If you have hearing loss, there's a good chance that hearing aids will both provide some relief for your tinnitus and help you hear better," Alscher says.

Try a masking device. This device looks like a hearing aid and produces sounds (such as nature sounds) that make tinnitus seem quieter. "The sound distracts the brain, and tinnitus symptoms become easier to tolerate. If you have hearing loss as well as tinnitus, the masking device and hearing aid may operate together as one instrument," Alscher says. "Many such combination instruments also have Bluetooth streaming capabilities, so you can find a unique sound you prefer and stream the sound directly to your hearing instrument."

Exercise. "Regular physical activity can reduce the frequency and intensity of tinnitus, and the distress it causes, in some people," Alscher says. "And higher levels of physical activity can improve overall health and the quality of your sleep, both of which can help you cope with tinnitus."

Try mindfulness. "A program called Mindfulness Based Tinnitus Stress Reduction builds skills in deep breathing, yoga, relaxation, and meditation to help a person to deal with tinnitus," Alscher says. "Mindfulness programs have been shown to reduce depression and anxiety while improving social

© Six_Characters | Getty Images

functioning and overall mental health in people with tinnitus."

Try cognitive behavioral therapy (CBT). CBT helps you identify negative thoughts about tinnitus and reframe the way you think about and react to tinnitus. CBT is often used in conjunction with mindfulness.

Join an online tinnitus support group. "These groups can promote feelings of hope and control. Members often share strategies they have found successful in dealing with their tinnitus," Alscher says. You can find these groups on Facebook (search for "tinnitus support") or at the American Tinnitus Association (www.ata.org; click on "Support").

Consider giving tinnitus retraining therapy a try. This therapy uses counseling and sound masking to help the brain relearn hearing patterns so tinnitus is less noticeable.

Reduce stress. Being stressed out may increase your perception of tinnitus and increase your reaction to it. To reduce stress, try such strategies as relaxation exercises and mindfulness breaks.

Stay socially active. Sometimes tinnitus can become so unbearable that it leads to isolation, loneliness, and a focus on tinnitus symptoms. Make it a point to spend time with people whose company you enjoy, even if it's just a text or phone call. The exchange will take the focus away from tinnitus and improve your feelings of well-being, hope, and happiness.

Do-it-yourself sound masking

You don't always need a fancy ear device to mask tinnitus sounds. Playing music or "white noise" helps distract your brain, so you pay less attention to the tinnitus.

It's especially helpful at night, when it's quiet and tinnitus can interfere with sleep. "Using a bedside sound generator or a fan can help people with tinnitus fall asleep easier and reduce tinnitus distress. You can also use the sound machine during the day," says Emma Alscher, an audiologist at Harvard-affiliated Massachusetts Eye and Ear.

Earbuds or headphones will also do the job. "It's just individual preference," Alscher says. "But we don't recommend noise-canceling headphones or earbuds, as they cancel out ambient and background noise, both of which can be helpful for tinnitus."

Reduce your fear of falling

Improving your balance, strength, flexibility, and gait will give you the confidence to stay active.

Falling poses a major risk for injury as we get older, and it's no wonder that many of us have a real fear of it. Unfortunately, fear of falling often winds up increasing the chance of a devastating spill. To protect your mobility and independence, it's important to address this fear.

Fear factors

Fear of falling often develops for two reasons. One is an awareness of age-related changes. Body systems that keep you steady—your muscles, joints, cognition, vision, hearing, nerves, and reaction time—all start to decline. You wind up being weaker and less flexible. You might have chronic aches and pains. That leads to heightened caution.

"Our natural instinct is to slow down so we don't fall. We shuffle our feet and take shorter strides; our feet don't clear the ground as high as they used to; walking speed slows. As that happens, we become apprehensive about taking a step," explains Michael Clem, a physical therapist with Spaulding Rehabilitation Hospital. "I have two patients with this problem right now. They tend to reach out for things and not move their feet. But trying to grab on to a piece of furniture that's a little out of reach can make you lose your balance and fall."

A history of falls is another contributor to fear; if you've already fallen, you know how quickly it happens and how easy it would be to fall again. "And when fear increases, for any reason, people don't want to be as active as they were. That makes physical decline happen faster," Clem points out.

Regaining your confidence

To reduce your fear of falling, you'll need to address underlying conditions, such as poor eyesight or joint problems.

It will also help to work with a physical therapist to improve your balance and gait (walking pattern). The therapist will evaluate your physical strengths and weaknesses and try to understand your specific

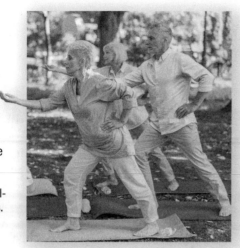

Practicing tai chi can improve balance by boosting leg strength, flexibility, and reflexes.

The final piece

When you're feeling stronger and more confident about performing activities without fear, you'll focus on improving your gait.

"We use metronomes to increase walking speed. We start off with 80 beats—and thus, steps—per minute, which is on the low end, and work up to 100," Clem says. "Then we work on walking with your gaze ahead of you, so you don't look down. People start shuffling less, walking faster, and becoming more confident."

Eventually, you'll tackle walking short distances as your physical therapist coaches you. "The goal is to get you back to being able to walk in and out of your house, through a grocery store, or into a doctor's office," Clem says. At that point, the course of physical therapy will end. But, of course, the real work will begin. You'll need to continue doing strength, stretching, and balance exercises on your own.

"If you don't, your fear may return and your fall risk will increase," Clem says. "To counter it, we'll want you to exercise and stay active for as long as possible."

concerns about falling. "I'll want to know what someone is afraid of," Clem says. "Is it stepping off a curb or a set of stairs in the backyard? We can build exercises to address that one specific issue as well as any other weaknesses."

Starting slowly

You won't be thrown into a rigorous exercise program. "We stay in a person's comfort zone with a program that challenges them while they still feel safe," Clem says. "I select exercises they'll succeed at."

For balance exercises, that could mean standing with your arms at your sides and your feet together, with a railing or walker nearby for support. "I might have the person look left or right, and then reach for a target. This can be challenging, and they may sway, but they won't fall. I'm right there behind them, and they can grab on to something if they need to," Clem says.

From there, you might work on standing with one foot in front of the other (see "Tandem standing"), or standing on one leg at a time. Then you might try taking steps forward, backward, or to the side.

As you learn to improve balance, you'll also work on boosting muscle strength, flexibility, and range of motion. Expect a focus on the muscles in your buttocks, hips, thighs, and calves.

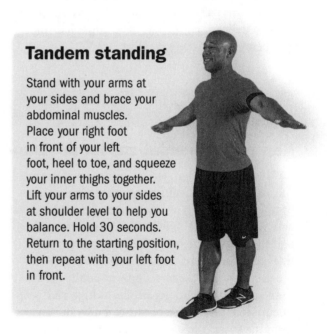

Tandem standing

Stand with your arms at your sides and brace your abdominal muscles. Place your right foot in front of your left foot, heel to toe, and squeeze your inner thighs together. Lift your arms to your sides at shoulder level to help you balance. Hold 30 seconds. Return to the starting position, then repeat with your left foot in front.

When medication deliveries hit a snag

Whether by mail carrier or local courier, deliveries have some risks. Here's what to do if there's a problem.

Getting prescription medications delivered to your home is an important service, and many millions of Americans rely on it. But it comes with snafus, especially as the United States faces challenges with its work force, supply chain, and postal service.

One national survey conducted in August 2020, for example, suggested that one in four mail-order prescription users had experienced a problem with medication delivery the week before. That was particularly true early in the pandemic, and delivery issues may have improved since then, depending on where you live.

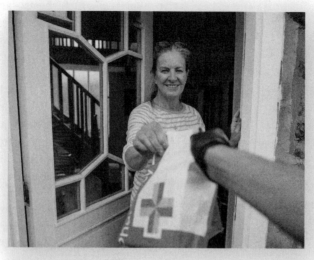

What can go wrong?

Prescription deliveries have the potential for several problems, says Joanne Doyle Petrongolo, a pharmacist at Harvard-affiliated Massachusetts General Hospital. For example, they might be delayed, damaged, delivered to the wrong address, lost, or stolen.

You can miss a delivery if it requires a signature and you're not home—or you can't get to the door before the delivery person leaves.

Or the package may be left in an unusual spot. "I have one patient whose medication was left

---

IN THE JOURNALS

New recommendations for pneumococcal vaccination

The CDC has changed its guidelines for vaccinating adults against pneumococcal disease by approving two new pneumococcal conjugate vaccines (PCVs): PCV15 (Vaxneuvance) and PCV20 (Prevnar 20). The updated guidelines, published Jan. 28, 2022, in *Morbidity and Mortality Weekly Report*, apply to adults older than age 65 and younger people at high risk for pneumococcal disease because of a weakened immune system or a chronic medical condition. People can get either vaccine, as the CDC does not endorse one over the other.

Pneumococcal disease refers to infections caused by *Streptococcus pneumoniae* bacteria. Examples include pneumonia, bloodstream infections, ear and sinus infections, and meningitis (swelling of the membranes covering the brain and spinal cord). Previous guidelines recommended two other vaccines: PCV13 and PPSV23. A person who hasn't received one of these earlier vaccines should have a single dose of the new PCV20 or PCV15, followed a year or more later with a "chaser" of PPSV23. (This period can be shortened to eight weeks for people at high risk.)

People who've had one of the earlier vaccines should follow these guidelines: PPSV23 recipients should have one of the new PCVs at least a year after their PPSV23 vaccination. PCV13 recipients don't need one of the new PCVs at this time, but, if not already received, they should get a PPSV23 vaccination six to 12 months later.

on the back porch instead of the front porch. He didn't find it until two days later," Doyle Petrongolo says. "Perhaps the delivery person thought the package was less likely to be stolen from the back porch."

What you can do

Take action when medications don't arrive. First, see if the package was left in a spot you hadn't anticipated (such as a mailbox or back porch). If you live in an apartment or a condo, check the mailroom.

Avoiding delivery problems

The following steps may help you avoid medication delivery problems, or at least give you the tools to act if something goes wrong.

▶ Consider ordering as much medicine at a time as your insurance allows, such as a three-month supply. That means fewer deliveries, and thus fewer opportunities for a delivery failure.

▶ Once medication is ordered, confirm which service is delivering it.

▶ Provide specific delivery instructions.

▶ Ask for a signature to be required upon receipt (if you'll be able to answer the door promptly and sign for the package). This may require an additional fee.

▶ Keep the delivery company's customer service phone number handy.

▶ Ask about the delivery company's lost package policy.

▶ Ask your insurance company what would happen in the event of a medication delivery problem.

▶ Ask your pharmacy to alert you when your medication goes out.

▶ Get tracking information as soon as it's available, and follow your package's delivery progress online.

▶ Find out when the package will be delivered, and try to be home then.

▶ For apartment or condo dwellers, notify your front desk that you're expecting an important package and you'll need it as soon as it arrives.

▶ Be on the lookout for your package and take action if it doesn't arrive.

IN THE JOURNALS

Vaccination still recommended after a shingles infection

The CDC recommends people ages 50 and older get the Shingrix vaccine to protect against shingles. But suppose you haven't been vaccinated and you get shingles for the first time. In that case, you should still receive the shot to reduce your risk of future attacks, says a study published Sept. 1, 2021, in the *Journal of the American Academy of Dermatology*.

Shingles causes a painful, burning rash that usually develops on one side of the body, often the face or torso. The rash consists of blisters that typically scab over in a week to 10 days and clears up within two to four weeks. For some people, the pain from shingles lasts for months or even years after the rash goes away. The researchers looked

at the recurrence rate among 17,413 people who had a first-time shingles attack. They found that approximately 4% had another outbreak later. Those ages 45 to 54 had a recurrence after two years on average, while people ages 55 and older had one three years later on average. People with weaker immune systems were at a higher risk for a second shingles attack.

Given the recurrence rates, the researchers said that people who'd already had shingles would still benefit from getting the vaccine. Shingrix is administered in two doses, two to six months apart. The vaccine should not be given during a shingles outbreak or when someone is taking antiviral medications.

Next, contact the delivery service, whether it's a local courier (such as Shipt or Instacart) or a mail service (such as the USPS or FedEx). Having a tracking number will help in locating your medication.

If you don't know which service is delivering your medications and you don't have a tracking number, Doyle Petrongolo says the pharmacy should be able to give you that information and tell you when the package left the pharmacy. "They may even be able to contact the delivery service," she notes.

Lost, stolen, or damaged drugs

Do call your pharmacy if you believe your medication has been lost, stolen, or damaged. But brace yourself: getting a replacement may be complicated. "In order to legally send out another prescription, we need a prescription that allows for refills, or we need a new prescription from the doctor," Doyle Petrongolo says.

Who'll pay for a replacement? It might be you, since the insurance company paid for the first prescription that went out.

"But there may be policies for the pharmacy to get a 'lost prescription override' so the insurance will pay for it again," Doyle Petrongolo explains. "It depends on the insurance."

Is home delivery worth the risk?

Most deliveries go smoothly, but there's no guarantee. If you're concerned about the delivery of extremely urgent, expensive, or temperature-sensitive medications, consider another way to get your prescriptions.

"If you're homebound or in a rural area, there may not be another option," Doyle Petrongolo says. "Just be as knowledgeable about the delivery as possible, so you'll be better equipped to act if things go awry. We want you to feel empowered."

Are you too embarrassed to go to the doctor?

Here are some tips for those times when you feel uncomfortable, shy, or even ashamed at the physician's office.

Doctors are charged with caring for every aspect of our health, right down to our birthday suits and our most private mental and physical issues. It's just part of the job for the experts, who deal with intimate details all day, every day.

However, you may feel embarrassed being up-front or vulnerable with professionals you see only a few times a year—or have just met. That may keep you from being honest during a doctor visit; some research suggests up to 81% of patients withhold details about their health habits from doctors because they don't want to be judged or lectured. Or you may avoid making an

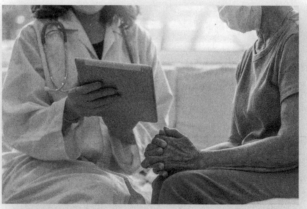

You may be more comfortable talking to your doctor privately, without other staff present.

appointment in the first place. And that hesitation may have health consequences.

Common concerns

There are many reasons why you might feel reluctant to talk with a doctor. For example:

You didn't follow the doctor's advice. Maybe you didn't take medications, exercise, cut back on alcohol, lose weight, or stop smoking, as your doctor recommended. "I think a lot of patients are afraid they'll be punished in some way. They may even lie about their self-care," says Dr. Suzanne Salamon, associate chief of gerontology at Harvard-affiliated Beth Israel Deaconess Medical Center.

You feel the stigma of a condition or disease. It may be difficult to talk about sensitive health issues—such as sexual dysfunction, sexually transmitted disease, diarrhea, gas, or mental illness. "Some people feel embarrassed or ashamed about having a particular condition. They don't want people to know about it," Dr. Salamon says.

You're overweight. It can be embarrassing to step on a scale, especially in a public area like the hallway of the doctor's office.

You don't want to disrobe. "Some people don't want to undress because they're shy or they're unhappy with their body image," Dr. Salamon says.

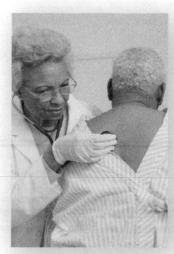

It's okay to ask about staying partly covered during an exam.

Health consequences

Avoiding doctor appointments for any reason—including embarrassment—may mean that your health will suffer.

"I know people who keep postponing going to a doctor because they're overweight. But being overweight can lead to high blood pressure or cholesterol, which are risk factors for heart disease—just like obesity," Dr. Salamon says. "We have good treatments for high blood pressure and cholesterol, but if a patient is too embarrassed to seek our help, we'll be unable to diagnose and treat these conditions."

Skipping medical care can be particularly dangerous if you have a family history of disease or if you ignore recommended health screenings, such as skin checks or a colonoscopy.

Tips to cope

It's common to feel embarrassed about something when you're seeing your doctor. "These feelings appear to be even more common among people who had to put off routine care during the pandemic," says Dr. Jennifer Gatchel, a geriatric psychiatrist with Harvard-affiliated Massachusetts General Hospital. "The key is to accept that your feelings are normal and address them head-on." Here are some ways to do that.

Do a reality check. Question whether your concerns or fears are realistic. "For example, if you're worried your doctor will be mad at you about something, and lecture you, ask yourself if that's ever happened before," Dr. Gatchel says. If so, perhaps you should seek a new doctor. If not, consider that you might be overlooking alternative outcomes, such as your doctor expressing understanding and working with you to get back on track.

Talk to a trusted friend. "Getting another perspective can help," Dr. Gatchel says. "For example, if you aren't on track with your medications, and you're worried a doctor will berate you, talk to a friend. The friend may be able to help you evaluate your expectations about this and provide a more neutral perspective—perhaps asking how many doses you've missed, and noting that they've also missed doses and that it's common."

Practice relaxation strategies before the appointment. People who get very nervous about seeing the doctor can benefit from using various relaxation techniques before the visit, including meditation, guided imagery, or even light stretching or yoga.

Advocating for yourself

Speak up at the doctor's office when you're feeling embarrassed. Here are ways to troubleshoot in the moment.

If you're embarrassed because you didn't heed advice. "It's your body, and you can choose to follow or not follow the advice you're given," Dr. Salamon says. "Be up-front and explain why you haven't done something." Perhaps you haven't had enough time (or enough money) to do exactly as your doctor has advised. "Maybe you're taking too many medications and adding another is too confusing. The doctor often can help you simplify your treatments," she says.

If you're embarrassed about your weight. "Tell your doctor you're sensitive about it, you've been struggling with it, and ask for ways to work with those feelings. For example, maybe you can have your weight measured in a private room, where no one but the medical assistant taking your weight can see the result," Dr. Gatchel says.

If you're uncomfortable with others in the room. "These days it's common for another health professional to be in the room with you and your doctor. If that makes you uncomfortable, it's okay to ask to speak with the doctor alone," Dr. Gatchel suggests.

If you're sensitive about a particular condition. "If you have a condition that is stigmatized, like HIV, consider going to a clinic that deals only with that condition. Your condition won't be unique there, it will be the norm, and that may make you may feel more comfortable," Dr. Salamon says.

If you're shy about undressing. "Ask if you can keep your clothes on for an exam, or at least keep some of your clothes on," Dr. Salamon says. "Or get a doctor of the same sex, which might make it easier for you."

What else can help

Try not to beat yourself up if you feel embarrassed at the doctor's office. Many people feel the same. You live in the real world; doctors don't expect perfection; they have plenty of patients who have been unable to follow medical advice or to achieve a medical goal, like losing weight. Above all, don't avoid medical care because you fear a negative interaction with your doctor. You should be able to express your concerns, and your doctor should respond with empathy. If that doesn't happen, it's probably time to look for a new doctor.

Difficulty seeing at night? Try these tips to cope

Slight changes at home and on the road may make a difference.

Cats, owls, raccoons, and deer—they're among the animals with exceptional night vision. We humans aren't on the list. Our eyes have just a fraction of the same visual machinery needed to see well in the dark, and our limited ability deteriorates with age (see "How our night vision changes" on the next page). The resulting poor night vision sets us up for difficulty driving at night or stumbling in a darkened room, which can lead to accidents and injuries.

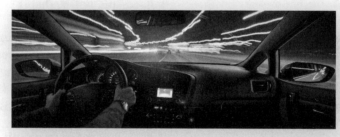

Dim your dashboard when driving at night. It reduces some glare so you can see better.

How can you stay safe? There's no one medical treatment to restore night vision, but the following approaches can help.

Get regular eye exams. You need a comprehensive eye exam every year or two, depending on your vision. This will identify early signs of eye disease and keep your eyeglasses prescription current. "Uncorrected vision is one of the most common causes of difficulty seeing at night. Often, an updated eyeglasses prescription reduces glare when driving at night," says Dr. Haley Italia, an optometrist at Harvard-affiliated Massachusetts Eye and Ear.

Treat underlying conditions. Dry eyes and cataracts (clouding of the lens inside the eye) make it harder to see at night. Treating them should improve night vision.

Keep a flashlight handy. Get a flashlight app on your smartphone or carry a pocket-sized flashlight in case you need help to see where you're walking.

Turn on the lights. "Consider adding more lamps to brighten your home, and install night lights throughout the house. For reading, I recommend gooseneck lamps, which can be adjusted easily," Dr. Italia says. Also: keep window shades or blinds open during the day.

Maintain your eyeglasses. Wash lenses regularly, and take them to an optician to buff out small scratches or add antireflective coatings that reduce headlight glare.

Keep your windshield and headlights clean. Even a little dirt or dust can make it harder to see the road at night. Get your car washed, and keep windshield washer fluid levels high.

Adapt your night driving. Dim your dashboard lights, which cause glare. Look at right lane markings

© Ru_Foto | Getty Images

when oncoming traffic headlights are bothering you. Use the night setting on your rearview mirror. "And use familiar roads and well-lighted streets, which will be easiest to navigate at night," Dr. Italia suggests.

What if these strategies don't work? "It could be that you'll need to limit driving to daytime only," Dr. Italia says. "It's inconvenient, but it's better to be safe."

How our night vision changes

We need at least a little bit of light (like moonlight) to see in the dark. We also need the ability to make use of that light: the eye collects and focuses the light and sends signals to the brain, which translates the light into images. Age-related changes can affect this process. Here are some examples:

We lose certain light-sensitive eye cells (photoreceptors). Very sensitive photoreceptors called rods are essential for night vision. The number of rods in our eyes diminishes with age.

Our pupils get smaller. The pupils—small openings that look like black dots—allow light to enter the eyes. The size of the pupil (and amount of light that enters) is controlled by muscles in the iris (the colorful part of the eye). "These muscles weaken with age, making the pupils smaller and allowing less light into the eyes. For this reason, you need more light to see comfortably," explains Dr. Haley Italia, an optometrist at Harvard-affiliated Massachusetts Eye and Ear.

Our eyes react more slowly to changes in light. At any age, the photoreceptors need time to adjust after we look into

bright headlights or when we walk into a dark room from a bright room. In older people, this process takes longer.

Our eye lenses get cloudy. "The lens inside each eye goes through microscopic changes over time that ultimately lead to a clouded lens called a cataract. Even the early changes, before there is a cataract, cause light to scatter as it enters the eye, reducing the quality of vision or causing glare around headlights or streetlights," Dr. Italia notes.

Our eyes get drier. We make fewer tears when we're older, which can irritate the outer surface of the eye (the cornea) and scatter incoming light. "Dry eyes are especially noticeable at the end of the day and can cause glare or blurry vision at night," Dr. Italia says.

Our vision worsens. The quality of vision decreases with age, which can make it harder to see at night. "Even if you're lucky and still have 20/20 vision when you're 70, it probably won't be as crisp as it was 50 years ago. Your remaining photoreceptors are less densely packed and less able to discern fine detail," Dr. Italia notes.

Watch out for these balance busters

Health problems, medications, and environmental hazards can throw off balance and increase your fall risk.

Our balance wanes as we age, putting us in jeopardy. The problem reflects a mix of issues that set us up for falls, which are a major cause of hip fractures, head injuries, and disability.

The good news is that you can fight back by recognizing and addressing potential balance busters. "Everything we do to maintain our health, alertness, fitness, and mobility will slow the trajectory of our declining balance," explains Dr. Steven Rauch, medical director of the Balance and Vestibular Center at Harvard-affiliated Massachusetts Eye and Ear.

What is balance?

Your balance is controlled by a miraculous system—one that involves your whole body.

"Your eyes tell you where you are in space. Balance organs in your ears read your head movements. Nerves send information about the position of your body. All these signals from your eyes, ears, and nerves are processed by your brain, which then sends messages back to your sensory nerves, muscles, and joints that help you keep your balance. As a result, you can walk, keep your gaze stable while you move,

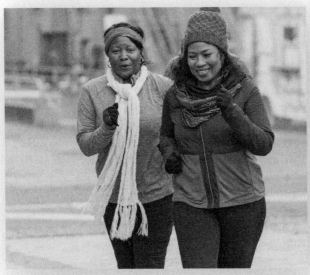

Watch out for icy sidewalks and uneven pavement on your walk.

or catch yourself after tripping," Dr. Rauch explains.

These different parts of our balance system decline as we age. "Vision and hearing don't work as well as they used to, messages in the nerves can get garbled, muscles shrink and get weaker, joints wear out, and our brain may not be as quick to make adjustments to maintain balance," Dr. Rauch says.

Health-related balance risks

Many health conditions can hurt balance. Here are some common culprits.

Vision problems. Eye diseases can reduce the ability to relay your location to the brain. Three conditions in particular become more common with age: cataracts (cloudy eye lenses), glaucoma (which causes loss of side vision), and macular degeneration (which destroys central vision).

Inner ear conditions. Some disorders can impair balance organs and trigger a sense of spinning (vertigo). Three common conditions are benign paroxysmal positional vertigo (caused by loose ear crystals), inner ear infections, and Ménière's disease (in which fluid buildup leads to pressure and damage).

Neuropathy. This type of nerve damage, often caused by diabetes or compressed nerves in the spine, causes tingling, numbness, or pain in the limbs and limits your brain's ability to sense your legs and feet.

Foot conditions. Anything that affects the way you walk threatens your balance, whether it's a heel problem or fallen (painful) arches.

Orthostatic hypotension. This means your blood pressure dips too low when you stand up, which can make you feel dizzy and fall. It becomes more common with age and can be a side effect of medicines.

Mild cognitive impairment. This slight but noticeable change in memory and thinking skills is sometimes a precursor to dementia. The condition can affect your attention, reaction time, and ability to sense where you are in space.

Medication-related balance risks

Many medications can make you woozy and cause you to lose your balance. These include

- some antidepressants
- drugs to treat anxiety, such as benzodiazepines
- antihistamines
- blood pressure drugs, such as ACE inhibitors, angiotensin-receptor blockers (ARBs), and beta blockers
- diabetes drugs, such as insulin, glipizide (Glucotrol), and glyburide (DiaBeta, Glynase)
- drugs to treat irregular heartbeat
- prescription pain medications, such as opioids
- sleep medications, such as sedatives and hypnotics.

Environmental balance risks

Hazards in your environment threaten your balance and can make you trip and fall. Watch out for the following:

Outdoor hazards, such as icy walkways, uneven pavement, poorly lighted walkways or parking lots, paths blocked by shrubs or large tree roots.

Indoor hazards, such as floor clutter, throw rugs, poorly lighted hallways or stairways, furniture that blocks your path, extension cords, loose carpeting, loose handrails, slippery bathroom floors, broken steps, and tile floors.

Pets that can get underfoot, such as cats and small dogs.

Ill-fitting shoes that keep you from sensing the ground properly, such as shoes that are too loose or squishy.

What you can do

There's plenty you can do to improve your balance and reduce your fall risk. Start at home: get rid of hazards and add anti-slip equipment. "Install grab

Try this balance exercise

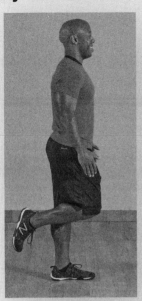

Stand upstraight with your feet together and arms at your sides. Bend your right knee, lifting that foot several inches off the floor, and balance on your left leg. Hold, then lower to starting position. Now try the exercise with your left leg. Repeat both exercises 10 times.

bars by the tub and toilet, nonslip treads in places that get wet, night lights so you don't bump around in the dark, and handrails that can support your body weight," Dr. Rauch advises.

Ask your doctor if any of your health problems or medications could be increasing your fall risk. Ask if you might benefit from physical therapy, and if an assistive walking device (like a cane or rollator) might improve your balance.

Wear supportive shoes with laces to keep them snug on your feet.

And hone your balance skills by challenging your balance safely. "Stand on one foot when you brush your teeth in the morning, then stand on the other when you brush at night—holding the sink counter for balance. Use the stairs instead of the elevator. And exercise: walk, cycle, do tai chi or yoga or dance," Dr. Rauch urges. "Use your balance, because there's no question that good balance is a use-it-or-lose-it proposition."

IN THE JOURNALS

Beware of possible rise in blood clot risk when binge-watching television

Watching television for four or more hours a day is linked to a higher risk of developing dangerous blood clots, recent research suggests. The study included more than 131,000 people, all ages 40 and older without venous thromboembolism (VTE). VTE includes two serious conditions: pulmonary embolism (clots in the lungs) and deep-vein thrombosis (clots in deep veins, usually in the legs). Participants who reported watching television at least four hours a day were categorized as prolonged viewers, while those who watched less than 2.5 hours per day were deemed never-viewers or

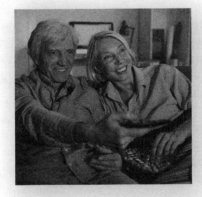

seldom-viewers. During the follow-up (which ranged from just over five years to nearly 20 years), prolonged television viewers were 1.35 times more likely to develop VTE compared with never- or seldom-viewers. While the findings don't prove cause and effect, the connection makes sense because sitting for long periods causes blood to pool in the legs, which can raise blood clot risk, according to the authors, who published their findings Jan. 20, 2022, in the *European Journal of Preventive Cardiology.*

When imaging tests reveal unexpected findings

Finding an "incidentaloma" presents challenges for doctors and patients alike.

Thanks to advances in medical imaging, cardiologists can now visualize the heart in more detail than ever before. The information can help determine if you need medications or a procedure to reduce your risk of a heart attack or stroke. Sometimes high-tech heart scans enable people to avoid more invasive procedures (see "Heart scanning techniques").

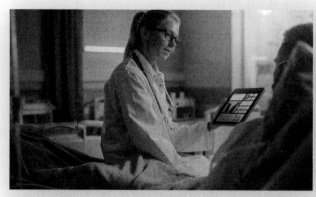

Imaging tests can reveal unexpected "spots" that usually turn out to be harmless.

© gorodenkoff | Getty Images

may show subtle changes in one of the heart's valves. It might be an infection or a less-concerning buildup of calcium caused by normal aging. For these and other incidentalomas, it's often tricky to know whether more tests are warranted—or a waste of time. Clear communication with your doctor can help, however.

But the use of more advanced cardiac imaging means doctors are also seeing more potentially worrisome abnormalities both within and near the heart. "Sometimes a scan detects an unexpected finding that's unrelated to the original reason for the test," says cardiologist Dr. Jason H. Wasfy, director of cardiology outcomes research at Harvard-affiliated Massachusetts General Hospital and associate professor at Harvard Medical School.

Incidentalomas: Troublesome or helpful?

Known as an "incidentaloma," these findings might be a nodule or tumor (abnormal growths that may be benign or malignant) or more subtle but unusual changes in the heart, lungs, or other nearby areas of the body.

When doctors image the heart, they often see things in the lungs. Detecting a suspicious lung growth often leads to additional imaging tests and possibly biopsies. For patients, this often translates to considerable inconvenience, stress, expense, and risks (such as from radiation exposure and contrast dye that can harm the kidneys). More often than not, the suspicious growth turns out to be harmless. But in rare cases, it ends up being an early cancer, says Dr. Wasfy.

An echocardiogram may also reveal unanticipated findings. For example, using this test to assess heart function in someone with shortness of breath

Heart scanning techniques

In a matter of minutes, cardiac CT angiography (CCTA) can capture a detailed, three-dimensional image of the blood vessels and other structures of the heart. Although this test requires an arm injection of contrast dye to "light up" the blood vessels, it's far less invasive than traditional coronary angiography, which delivers contrast dye to the heart through a thin tube (catheter) that's snaked through a blood vessel in the upper leg or wrist. For people who are unlikely to have narrowed arteries, CCTA can rule out that problem without resorting to invasive angiography.

Here are some other methods for heart imaging

Coronary artery calcium scanning uses a special CT scanner that detects and measures the amount of calcium in the walls of the heart's arteries. It involves small amounts of radiation but no contrast dye.

Cardiac MRI uses magnets, radio waves, and a computer to create images of the heart and nearby blood vessels. It may require a contrast injection but involves no radiation exposure.

Echocardiography uses sound waves to create moving pictures that show the size and shape of the heart as well as the function of the heart's chambers and valves. It typically involves no dye and no radiation.

Two things you can do

First, ask your physician to explain the rationale for any imaging tests he or she recommends. Be sure you understand how the results may change your treatment, which may involve stopping or starting medications or undergoing a procedure. Sometimes, doctors order tests without confirming that the patient would agree to the potential intervention, says Dr. Wasfy. "For example, it doesn't make sense to look for a narrowing of the coronary arteries if a person doesn't want to get a stent," he says. Stents—tiny mesh tubes used to prop open narrowed arteries—can be lifesaving if you're having a heart attack.

But if you are not, growing evidence suggests that medications (such as those to lower cholesterol and blood pressure) are just as effective as stents in preventing heart attacks and premature death from cardiovascular disease.

Second, if you're found to have an incidentaloma on an imaging test, consider getting a second opinion from a cardiologist or radiologist with extensive experience interpreting scans of the organ or area in question. "Getting a specialist's opinion can give you more confidence that a concerning finding is treated appropriately," Dr. Wasfy says.

IN THE JOURNALS

Treating low vitamin D levels may help people live longer

It's well established that having a low level of vitamin D can lead to bone disease, like rickets in children and osteoporosis in adults. But it may also increase the risks for heart attack and premature death. The Endocrine Society defines vitamin D deficiency as a blood level of less than 20 nanograms per milliliter (ng/mL), while vitamin D insufficiency is 21 to 29 ng/mL. Optimal levels are 30 to 100 ng/mL. In a study published in October 2021 in *The Journal of the Endocrine Society*, researchers identified 19,092 people who showed vitamin D deficiency on at least two tests and who'd never had a heart attack. Everyone was divided into three groups. People in group A were not treated, and their blood levels remained below 20 ng/mL. Those in group B received vitamin D supplements that raised their levels into the range of 21 to 29 ng/mL. Those in group C took enough supplements to raise their levels to 30 ng/mL or higher.

The researchers found the risk of heart attack was lower in group C than in both of the other groups. However, people in groups B and C (who all took supplements) had a lower risk of death from any cause than those in group A, who remained deficient in vitamin D. The connection? Other evidence has linked low blood levels of vitamin D to cardiovascular risk factors, such as high blood pressure, diabetes, obesity, and chronic kidney disease.

Index

ABCD2 score, 94
abdominal aortic aneurysm (AAA), 89–90, 246
ACE inhibitors, 52, 79, 308, 318
acetaminophen (Tylenol), 54, 128, 152
  high blood pressure and, 54
Achilles tendinitis, 138, 182
acid reflux, 223, 306
acne, 4
acute inflammation, 13
acute pain, 134–35
acyclovir (Zovirax), 151
adalimumab (Humira), 6, 11, 14
adenomyosis, 235
adipocytes, 240
adjuvant radiation therapy, 174
adrenal glands, 56, 175
aducanumab (Aduhelm), 33, 34, 36
Advil. See ibuprofen
aerobic exercise, 54, 59, 61, 128, 129, 178, 198, 207, 291
aging skin, 228–30
alcohol use, 266
  amount, 82, 163, 215, 265
  atrial fibrillation and, 21
  bone health and, 122
  brain health and, 32
  cancer risk from, 160, 164, 214
  heart disease and, 213–15
  incontinence and, 234
  urinary problems and, 247
  women and, 213–15
aldosterone, 53, 56
alendronate (Fosamax), 305
Aleve. See naproxen
alfuzosin (Uroxatral), 248
alirocumab (Praluent), 60
allergies, 4
almond milk, 155, 224
almonds, 9
5-alpha-reductase inhibitors (5 ARIs), 248–50
alpha blockers, 248–50
alprostadil, 252
ALS (amyotrophic lateral sclerosis), 36
alternate nostril breathing, 270
Alternative Healthy Eating Index, 8
Alzheimer's disease, 4, 23, 24, 27, 46, 278
  diagnosing, 34
  family history and, 155
  gum disease and, 33
  medications for, 33–36, 256
  noise pollution and, 41
  statins and, 63
  symptoms of, 36
Ambien, 42, 308
amitriptyline (Elavil, Endep), 42, 308
Amulet, 92

AMX035, 36
amyloid beta protein, 33–36, 46
anal cancer, 166
anaplastic large-cell lymphoma (ALCL), 227
anastrozole (Armidex), 169
androgen suppression therapy (ADT), 174, 176
androgens, 174–76
anemia, 99, 236, 264, 300
aneurysms, 89–90, 214
angina, 84, 88
angioplasty, 83–84
angiotensin II receptor blockers (ARBs), 52, 79, 318
angle push-ups, 202
ankle injuries, 182, 198
ankle osteoarthritis, 138
ankylosing spondylitis, 136
antacids, 300, 306
anthocyanins, 8, 9
anti-anginal drugs, 84
anti-clotting medications, 87, 91, 92, 194, 292
anti-inflammatory diet, 7–9, 105
antibiotics, 231–33, 254, 305
anticholinergics, 42, 234
anticoagulants, 92, 175
antidepressants, 42, 53, 136, 236, 257, 308, 318
  side effects from, 163, 308
antidiuretic hormones, 250
antihistamines, 42, 247, 248, 318
antimicrobial peptides, 102
antimuscarinics, 250
antioxidants, 105, 115, 161, 171
antipsychotics, 308
antiseizure drugs, 308
anxiety, 32, 224, 264
aortic aneurysm, 89–90, 213, 214
appetite
  aging and, 122
  leptin and, 240
aquablation, 249
arm raises, 190
aromatase inhibitors, 169
arterial plaque, 9, 65, 69, 176, 215–17. See also atherosclerosis
arteries
  peripheral artery disease (PAD), 141
  radial, 83–84
  renal, 56
  retinal, 73
arthritis, 4–6
  exercise. See Exercise(s)
  inflammatory, 5–6
  psoriatic, 4, 6, 10
  rheumatoid (RA), 4, 5, 10, 11, 13

sex life and, 259
  tooth brushing and, 279
  treatment for, 6, 137
arthrodesis, 147
arthroplasty, 147
artificial intelligence, 297
aspirin, 4, 5, 84, 87
  diverticulosis and, 260
  with heart disease, 68–71, 77
  for ischemic stroke prevention, 68
assistive walking devices, 319
asthma, 4
asymptomatic bacteriuria, 232
atherosclerosis, 4, 19, 50, 87, 169, 180, 200
  See also arterial plaque
Ativan, 308
atorvastatin (Lipitor), 64
atrial fibrillation (afib), 87
  alcohol use and, 213, 214
  exercise and, 200, 296
  heart rate and, 292, 295
  ministrokes and, 92–94
  screening for, 292–94, 296, 298
  silent stroke and, 292
  sleep apnea and, 293
  stroke risk from, 50, 91, 92
  transradial angioplasty and, 83
atypical hyperplasia, 168
autism, 23
autoimmune diseases, 4, 225
autoimmune systemic inflammatory diseases, 10
avanafil (Stendra), 257
avascular necrosis, 128
avocados, 118
axial spondyloarthritis, 136

back pain, 126, 134–37, 196
bacon, 110
bacteria, 15–17, 19, 20, 23, 33, 102, 231–32, 312
balance, 179, 184, 185, 198, 317–19
  exercises, 61, 143, 187, 194, 311, 319
  falls and, 163, 187, 310, 311
beans, 164
beauty product safety, 166
bedtime, depression and, 32
bempedoic acid (Nexletol), 60, 62, 66
benign paroxysmal positional vertigo (BPPV), 318
benign prostatic hyperplasia (BPH), 247–51
benzodiazepines, 318
berries, 8, 9, 106
beta blockers, 17, 59, 78, 79, 84, 264, 292, 308, 318
beta carotene, 106, 161
bilateral adrenal hyperplasia, 56

bioidentical hormones, 222
biologic drugs, 10, 11, 14, 15, 18
biopsy, in prostate cancer screening, 244
birth control pills, 15, 220, 236
birth weight, 237
bisphenol A, 166
blackberries, 9
bladder, 174, 175, 231–32, 234, 247, 248
   cancer, 156
   infections. See urinary tract infections
      (UTIs)
   sling surgery, 234
   stones, 247
bleeding
   aspirin therapy and, 68–70
   from blood thinners, 92
   gums, 70, 87
   perimenopausal, 235–36
   transradial angioplasty and, 83–84
blisters, 197
blood brain barrier, 42, 52
blood clots
   aspirin therapy and, 68–70
   atrial fibrillation and, 50
   diet and, 111
   edema and, 237
   heart attacks from, 65
   strokes from, 9, 73, 75, 91
   television watching and, 319
blood glucose test, 246
blood pressure. See also high blood
      pressure; low blood pressure
   breath training and, 57
   categories of, 51
   cortisol and, 261
   diastolic, 51, 54, 57–58, 116, 246
   diet and food choices, 114, 170, 266
   exercise, 180, 200, 202, 203
   guidelines, 48, 49, 51
   home monitoring of, 54, 55, 246, 292,
      309
   measuring, 246
   medical appointments and, 162
   POTS (postural orthostatic
      tachycardia syndrome), 80–81
   salt and, 52, 53, 57, 58, 62, 82, 114–16
   seasonal changes and, 52
   systolic, 48–51, 54, 57–58, 116, 246
   weight gain, 163
blood pressure medications, 236, 250,
   307–8
   balance risk and, 318
   exercise and, 264
   for heart failure, 79
   heart rate and, 292
   for older adults, 87
blood pressure monitors, 54, 55
blood sugar
   exercise and, 202–3
   hormone therapy and, 176
   measurement of, 301
   prediabetes and, 301–2

tracking, 293–94, 296, 298
blood tests, 300–303
blood thinners. See anticoagulants
blood vessels, 232
   exercise and, 180, 201
blueberries, 9, 161
body fat facts, 240
body mass index (BMI), 75, 241–42, 245,
   260, 265, 289
bone density scan, 163
bone health, 121–22, 217, 224, 300
botulinum (Botox) injections, 234
boundaries, establishing in relationships,
   218–19
bowel cancer, 15
bowel movements, rectocele and, 227
brachytherapy, 175
bradycardia, 295
brain cancer, 167
brain-derived neurotrophic factor
      (BDNF), 24
brain fog, 41–42, 219–21, 292
brain health
   amount of sleep and, 46
   dehydration and, 231–32, 268
   diet and, 32
   electronic programs and, 31–33
   exercise and, 24–25, 90
   gut, connection to, 23
   high blood pressure and, 50–51
   lifestyle for, 44–45
   music and, 32
   oral hygiene and, 33
   social interactions and, 32, 44–45
   social media and, 37–38
   statins and, 63
   vertigo and, 307
   worst habits for, 44–46
breads, healthy, 118
breakfast, 117–18, 155, 256
breast cancer
   alcohol use and, 213
   exercise and, 156
   family history and, 220
   hormone therapy and, 169–70, 220
   incidence and death rates of, 167
   mammogram screening for, 163–65,
      167, 168, 220
   proliferative lesions and, 167
   ultrasound screening and, 168
   weight and, 165
breast implants, 226–28
breath training, blood pressure and, 57
breathing techniques, 60, 269–70, 281
breathlessness, 71, 79, 84
bridges, 194
bruising, aspirin therapy and, 70
bunions, 149
burgers, 110–11
bursitis, 128
butter, 120–21
C-reactive protein, 8, 9, 266

testing, 11–13
caffeine, 30, 55, 221, 234, 247, 248, 256,
   268
calcifications, arterial, 76
calcium, 76–77, 121–22, 143, 154, 223–25,
   300, 320
calcium channel blockers, 78, 79, 84,
   292, 308
calories, 108, 109
   fiber and, 260
   on nutrition labels, 109
   in plant oils, 82
   recommended intake, 112
   weight gain and, 81, 240–41, 266
cancer
   coffee and, 171
   diagnosis of women and, 167
   diet and food choices and, 160–62,
      164
   exercise and, 156, 165
   family history and, 155–56, 164
   preventing, 105, 106, 108, 110, 160–62,
      164–66
   risk factors for
      alcohol consumption, 160, 164,
         214
      environmental hazards, 166
      heart disease. See heart disease
      nails, 164
      radiation exposure, 173–75, 216,
         320
      vitamin D deficiency, 154
      weight and obesity, 165, 242
   screening tests for, 158–60
   sleep quality and, 166
   support groups, 173
   types of
      anal, 166
      anaplastic large cell lymphoma,
         227
      bladder, 156
      brain, 167
      breast. See breast cancer
      cervical, 163, 165, 166, 236
      colon (colorectal), 154, 156, 158–61,
         164, 165, 245
      endometrial, 165
      esophageal, 156, 161, 214, 306
      head and neck, 166
      kidney, 165
      liver, 156, 165–67, 214
      lung, 4, 161, 166, 167
      ovarian, 165
      pancreatic, 4, 161, 167, 246
      penile, 166
      prostate. See prostate cancer
      skin, 4, 122, 154, 170, 243
      stomach, 156
      testicular, 246
      thyroid, 165, 246
      uterine, 156, 167, 236
      vaginal, 165, 166

vulvar, 166
vitamin D deficiency and, 66, 134, 154–55, 300
candesartan, 52
canned foods, 81, 100
canola oil, 82, 101, 113
capsaicin, 115, 142, 152
carbohydrates, 20, 35, 102, 123–24, 240, 241
cardiac CT angiography (CCTA), 320
cardiac arrest, 69–71, 78
Cardiac Lifestyle Program, 88, 89
cardiac rehabilitation (rehab), 88–89, 200, 203
cardiac stress test, 237
cardio rheumatology, 10
cardiometabolic disease, 258
cardiomyopathy, 213
cardiorespiratory fitness (CRF), 179–81, 202
cardiovascular disease. *See also* coronary artery disease; heart attacks; heart disease; strokes
  inflammation and, 8
  risk factors for
    atherosclerosis, 4, 19, 50, 87, 169, 180, 200
    diabetes. See diabetes
    dietary, 102, 110, 114, 123
    gum disease, 19
    high cholesterol. See cholesterol
    high systolic blood pressure, 57–58
    hormone therapy, 169–70
    obesity, 75
    prediabetes, 302
    in pregnancy, 237
    sitting, 189, 200, 201
    stress, 217–19
  risk reduction methods
    dietary, 9, 77, 81–82, 111
    drug therapy, 11, 64
    exercise, 24–25, 171, 180, 195, 198–201, 270
cardioversion, 78
carotenoids, 171
carotid arteries, 214
cataract removal, dementia risk and, 26
cataracts, 316–18
catecholamines, 18
catheter ablation, 78
CCTA, 320
celiac disease, 141, 223, 246
cereal, 117, 118, 155, 224
cervical cancer, 163, 165, 166, 236
chair squats, 202
chair stand, 196
chair twists, 190
chair yoga, 187
chemicals, 166
chest pain, 88
  causes of, 71, 84–86
  gender and, 211

symptoms of, 212
chia seeds, 9
chickenpox, 150, 151
chiropractic, 137
cholesterol, 8, 10, 216, 300
  cortisol and, 261
  diet and food choices and, 105, 112, 118, 120, 160, 170, 172, 256, 266
  exercise and, 200
  health risks from LDL, 48, 71
  hormone therapy and, 176
  medications and, 48, 59–63, 66, 73, 76, 120, 216, 321
  methods lowering LDL, 60–62, 66, 73, 120
  testing, 72, 73
chondroitin supplements, 233
chronic degenerative meniscal tears, 131–32
chronic inflammation, 4–9, 13–15
chronic kidney disease, 4
chronic obstructive pulmonary disease (COPD), 105, 246
chronic pain, 126, 136, 144, 149, 288
chronotype, 32
Cialis, 248, 250, 257
cimetidine (Tagamet), 307
circadian rhythm, 274, 283, 308
cirrhosis of liver, 246
citalopram (Celexa), 257
clamshells, 194
coenzyme Q10, 66
coffee, 45, 171, 268
cognitive behavioral therapy (CBT), 126–27, 135, 221, 290, 310
cognitive behavioral therapy for insomnia (CBT I), 36, 283–84
cognitive decline, inflammation and, 8, 9
collagen supplements, 228–30
Cologuard, 159, 245
colon, diverticulosis and, 259–60
colon (colorectal) cancer, 154, 156, 158–61, 164, 165, 245
colonoscopy, 158–60, 163, 165, 245, 260
colorectal cancer, 154, 158–61, 164, 165
compression stockings, 238
computer games, 31
concentration, 29–30, 309
congenital long QT syndrome, 71
constipation, 227, 259–61, 268
contact sports, 197
continuous glucose monitors, 293–94, 296, 298
contrast dye, 320
cooling systems, for sleep, 284
COPD, 105, 246
core strength, 87, 136, 191, 192, 194–97, 207
corn oil, 113
coronary angiography, 320
coronary artery calcium (CAC) scan, 65, 69, 76–77, 215–17, 320

coronary artery disease, 65, 87, 213, 214
coronary bypass surgery, 68, 84, 88, 114
coronary calcium tests, 65, 69, 76–77, 215–17
corticosteroids, 13, 15, 53, 143, 147, 260
cortisol, 56, 184, 217, 261
Coumadin, 92
COVID-19 pandemic, 80, 126, 127, 158, 162, 163, 194, 217, 261, 312, 315
COVID-19 vaccine, 151, 163
CPPD (calcium pyrophosphate deposition disease), 6
cranberry, 233
creatinine, 163
Crohn's disease, 4, 15
cruciferous vegetables, 161, 170
crunches, 196
CT (computed tomography) scans
  colonography, 245, 260
  coronary artery calcium (CAC) scan, 65, 69, 76–77, 215–17
  fat measurement and, 242
  for lung cancer screening, 246
Cushing's syndrome, 56
cycling, 129, 179, 194–95, 197, 199, 272
cystic fibrosis, 223
cytokines, 18

D-mannose, 233
dabigatran (Pradexa), 92
dairy products, 121, 122, 160, 224
dancing, 303, 319
  for brain health, 32
DASH diet, 8, 11, 160, 161, 164, 170, 256
deadlifts, 263
decision making, improving, 272
decongestants, 53, 247, 248
deep vein thrombosis (DVT), 319
defribrillator, 294
dehydration, 140, 198, 268–69, 308
dementia, 318
  cataract removal and, 26
  diet and, 35, 105
  exercise and, 25–26, 156
  hearing loss and, 27–28
  high blood pressure and, 52
  job type and, 40
  noise pollution and, 41
  oral hygiene and, 33
  statins and, 63
  tea and coffee consumption and, 45
  testing for, 34
dental care, 277–79
dental cleanings, 162, 278
depression
  antidepressants, 42, 53, 136, 236, 257, 308, 318
  bedtime and wake time and, 32
  in caregivers, 217, 218
  exercise and, 264
  menopausal, 219, 221, 224
  music and, 32

pain and, 290
pandemic and, 163
prolonged grief disorder and, 262
sleep and, 36, 46
social media and, 37
tinnitus and, 309, 310
diabetes
aspirin therapy and, 68
blood sugar testing, 301
exercise and, 156, 180, 195, 200
family history and, 155
health checks for, 245–46
heart disease and, 212, 216
inflammation and, 8, 10
medications for, 303–5, 307, 308
neuropathy with, 140
prediabetes and, 246, 301–3
in pregnancy, 237
risk factors for
blood sugar spikes, 163, 293–94, 296
dietary, 102
insulin resistance, 102, 123, 165
silent heart attacks and, 75
visceral fat, 240
weight gain and obesity, 163, 242, 245
risk reduction methods
checking blood sugar, 293–94, 296, 298
dietary, 82, 119
exercise, 202, 303
medications, 76, 303–5
type 1, 4
diabetic retinopathy, 73
diaphragmatic (belly) breathing, 270
diastolic heart failure, 211
diazepam (Valium), 308
diet and food choices
blood sugar and, 296, 303
brain health and, 32
breakfast, 117–18, 155, 256
for cancer prevention, 160–62, 164, 173
carbohydrates, 20, 35, 102, 123–24, 240, 241
collagen in, 230
DASH diet, 8, 11, 160, 161, 164, 170, 256
effect on calorie intake, 81
exercise and, 264
fiber. See fiber
food shortcuts, 99–101
food staples, 98
frozen foods, 81, 82, 98, 100, 101
glycemic index (GI), 102, 123
grocery store list, 97–98
gum disease and, 20
heart healthy, 81–82, 88, 96–97, 108–24, 143, 255–56, 265–66
high blood pressure and, 53
high-glycemic diet, 102

inflammation and, 7–9, 11, 16
magnesium in foods, 9, 121
meat, 96, 99, 110–11, 160, 170, 173, 224
Mediterranean diet, 7–8, 16, 32, 105, 160, 162, 164, 170, 173, 240
nutrition labels, 98, 100, 108, 109
olive oil, 82, 105, 113, 170, 278
plant-based diets, 110–11, 170, 172, 223, 224, 255
prediabetes and, 303
processed foods, 14, 82, 96, 100, 108, 110, 111, 121, 160, 173
prostate cancer and, 170–71, 255
serving sizes, 82, 161
16/8 method, 266
snacking, 117, 119–20, 261, 266
soups, 103–4
spices, 115–16
urinary problems and, 247
vitamin B12 and, 300
vitamin D and, 154–55, 223, 300
Dietary Approaches to Stop
Hypertension diet. See DASH diet
Dietary Guidelines for Americans, 154
digestive health, 4, 223
digital rectal examination (DRE), 244, 248
dihydrotestosterone (DIT), 175
diphenhydramine, 42
direct oral anticoagulants (DOACs), 92
diuretics, 53, 59, 79, 223
diverticulitis, 260
diverticulosis, 259–60
dizziness
fraility and, 194
heart rate and, 78, 292
hydration and, 198
iron levels and, 99
from low blood pressure, 58, 140
from medications, 305, 307–9
vertigo, 307, 318
DMARDs, 6
DNA testing kit, 157
DOACs, 92
dopamine, 188
dry eyes, 316, 317
dry mouth, 279
dual energy x-ray absorptiometry (DEXA), 242
duloxetine (Cymbalta), 142
dutasteride (Avodart), 248, 249
dynamic exercises, 61
dysbiosis, 16

ear infections, 312
earbuds, 310
for sleep, 283
early coronary artery disease, 69–71
echocardiogram, 75, 77, 94, 320
eczema, 4
edema (swelling), 236–38

egg muffins, 118
eggs, 118
ejection fraction (EF), 77–78
Elavil, Endep, 42, 308
electrocardiogram (ECG), 65, 75, 76, 246, 292, 293, 295
electrolytes, 163, 264
elliptical trainers, 129–30, 187
empagliflozin (Jardiance), 79, 304
empowered relief, 135
Endep, 42, 308
endometrial cancer, 165
endometrium, 236
endothelial dysfunction, 58
endoxaban (Savaysa), 92
Entresto, 79
environmental hazards, 166
epithelial proliferation (EP), 220
epithelial proliferation with atypia (EPA), 220
erectile dysfunction (ED), 172, 248, 249, 252–53, 255, 257, 275
erectile function (IIEF) questionnaire, 253
escitalopram (Lexapro), 257
esomeprazole (Nexium), 306
esophageal cancer, 156, 161, 214, 306
estradiol, 232
estrogen, 165, 169, 221, 224
estrogen therapy
etanercept (Enbrel), 11, 14
evolocumab (Repatha), 60
exemestane (Aromasin), 169
exercise-induced ischemia, 86
exercise stress test, 85, 203
exercise(s). See also stretching; tai chi; walking; yoga
aerobic, 54, 59, 61, 128, 129, 178, 198, 207, 291
balance, 61, 143, 187, 194, 311, 319
benefits of, 29–30
afib prevention, 200, 296
cancer prevention, 156, 165
diabetes prevention or control, 202, 303
edema, 238
energy levels, 186
eye-hand coordination, 188–89
functional fitness, 189–90
hand pain, 147
heart health, 24–25, 54, 88, 198–201
incontinence prevention, 234
inflammation, 18
knee, 131
longevity, 269
menopause, 221, 224
pain relief, 129–31, 143
posture improvement, 136
POTS and, 81
sleep, 186
bone health and, 122
breathing, 269–70

cardiovascular, 24–25
for core strength, 87, 136, 195–97
easing into, 311
effort levels and, 264
for fall prevention, 163, 311
fatigue and, 264
fitness buddies, 178, 185, 187, 209
fitness trackers and, 126, 179, 201, 286–87, 289
hearing or vision impairment and, 186–87
heart rate and, 59, 291–92
high-intensity interval training (HIIT),171, 201–4, 254–55
home equipment for, 129–30
home workouts, 208–9
injuries, 196–97
for lifting and carrying ability, 144
muscle strengthening, 191, 262–63
for older adults, 86–87, 193–94
personal trainer for, 263
pickleball, 188, 189
prostate cancer and, 171, 173
pushing and pulling, 191–92
rowing and paddling, 206–8
sense of purpose and, 180
shoulder, 143
SMART (Specific, Measurable, Achievable, Relevant, and Time Based) exercise strategy, 178–79
stair climbing, 204–6
strength training, 61, 128, 198, 201
tinnitus and, 309
video workouts, 208–9
walk and carry, 196–97
for weight loss, 200, 241
external beam radiation, 174–75
external memory aids, 284–85
eye exams, 162
eye (ocular) strokes, 73
eyeglasses, 187
eyes and vision
balance risk and, 318
exercise and, 186–87, 205
heart disease and, 72–74
night vision, 316–17
ezetimibe (Zetia), 60, 62, 66

FACES of heart failure, 79
fainting, 58, 71, 78, 140, 194
fallen arches, 149, 318
falls, 70, 87, 91, 130, 144, 163, 187, 194, 198, 307, 310–11, 317–19
famiciclovir (Famvir), 151
familial hypercholesterolemia, 61, 71–73
family history, 155–57, 220, 265
famotidine (Pepcid), 307
farmer's carry, 196–97
fasting, intermittent, 266
fatigue, chest pain and, 211, 212
fats, dietary, 240, 241. See also omega-3 fatty acids; saturated fats;

unsaturated fats
fecal transplantation, 16
feet, 149–50, 318
femory artery, in angioplasty, 83–84
Fermara (letrozole), 169
fetal immunochemical test (FIT), 159, 245
fiber
amount of, 260–61
breakfast, 117
carbohydrates, 123–24
diverticulosis and, 260
on nutrition labels, 109
fibroadenomas, 168, 220
fibrocystic breast changes, 167, 220
fibroids, uterine, 235
fibromuscular dysplasia, 56
fibromyalgia, 126
fight-or-flight response, 86, 269
finasteride (Proscar), 248, 249
fingernails, melanoma and, 164
fingers, 146–48
fish, 100, 122, 224
good fats in, 9
health benefits of, 82, 139, 170
migraines and, 139
vitamin D in, 154
fish oil supplements, 225
FIT DNA test, 159
fitness trackers, 126, 179, 201, 286–87, 289
flaxseeds, 9
flexibility, 178, 179, 198, 310
flexible sigmoidoscopy, 245
floor dips, 202
flossing, 279
flu shots, 163
fluciclovine F 18 (Axumin), 244
fluoxetine (Prozac), 257, 308
fluvastatin (Lescol), 64
folic acid, 223
food staples, 98
foot pain, 149–50, 182, 197–98
forgiveness, 276–77
fractures, 143
fraility, 193–94
free radicals, 8
frozen foods, 81, 82, 98, 100, 101
fructose, 109
fruit juices, 121–22, 155
fruits, 8, 117, 164. See also specific fruits
climateric and non climateric, 98
diverticulosis and, 260
fiber in, 106
in heart healthy diet, 81, 96, 104–7, 121–23, 160, 255, 261
servings of, 106–7
stone, 107
functional fitness, 189–90
fungi, 15
gabapentin (Neurontin), 42, 142, 308
gallium-68 PSMA-11 test, 244

gamma secretase inhibitors, 35
gantenerumab, 35
gardening, 129, 272
gastric bypass surgery, 223
gastroesophageal reflux disease (GERD), 306–7
gastrointestinal bleeding, 69, 70
gene therapy, 265
genetics
diet and food choices and, 170
family history and, 155–57
inflammatory bowel disease (IBD) and, 15
longevity and, 265
osteoarthritis and, 128
small-fiber neuropathy and, 141
GERD, 306–7
gingivitis, 19–20, 278
glaucoma, 162, 186, 318
Gleason score, 172–75
glipizide (Glucotrol), 308, 318
GLP-1 receptor agonists, 76, 303–4
glucagon-like peptide 1 (GLP-1), 303–4
glucose, 82, 109, 123, 165, 186, 202, 301, 302
glucosinolates, 161
glyburide (DiaBeta, Glynase), 308, 318
glycemic index (GI), 102, 123
glycemic load, 123
glycemic variability, 296
golf, 195, 198, 303
golfer's elbow, 198
gout, 6–8, 14, 128
granola, 118
grief and grieving, 39–40, 261–62
grocery store list, 97–98
guaiac-based fecal occult blood test (gFOBT), 159, 245
guided imagery, 290
gum disease, 19–20, 87, 278
gut health, 15
guttate psoriasis, 18

H2 blockers, 306, 307
HALT acronym, 218
hammertoes, 149
hamstring stretch, 133
hand pain, 128, 145–48
happiness, 271–72
HDL (good) cholesterol. See cholesterol
head and neck cancers, 166
head trauma, 70
headaches, 140, 305
hearing aids, 187, 298, 309
hearing impairment, exercise and, 186–87
hearing loss, 27–28, 163, 246, 298, 309
heart attacks. See also heart disease
angina and, 84
cardiac arrest and, 69–71
inflammation and, 10
premature, 69–71

prevention methods
  cardiac rehab programs, 88–89
  CCTA, 320
  dietary, 82
  drug therapy, 68–69, 321
risk factors for
  alcohol use, 214
  blood clots, 9
  coronary artery disease, 65
  diabetes, 302
  diet, 111
  exercise, 198, 200
  gum disease, 19
  high cholesterol, 75
  hormone therapy, 169
  low diastolic blood pressure, 58
  overweight, 75
  salt consumption and, 82, 114
  sex and, 204, 258
  stress, 85–86
  symptoms of, 74, 211
  in women, 85
silent, 74–76, 292
  heart disease, 4, 96. *See also*
     cardiovascular disease;
     coronary artery disease; heart
     attacks
angina and, 84, 88
aspirin therapy and, 68–69
assessing risk for, 48
cancer risk and, 161
coffee and, 45
exercising with. See exercise(s)
family history and, 155
frailty and, 193–94
gender and, 211–12
risk factors for
  alcohol use, 213–15
  diabetes, 212, 216
  eyes, 72–74
  family history, 69–72, 200
  high homocysteine, 300
  solo dining, 212
  stress, 85–86, 217–19
  visceral fat, 75, 240
  weight and obesity, 242
risk reduction methods
  bedtime and wake time and, 32,
     45, 274
  coronary artery calcium (CAC)
     scan, 65, 69, 76–77, 215–17
  dietary, 77, 81–82, 105, 116, 119,
     123, 160, 170
    exercise, 77, 156, 179, 198–201,
     203, 254–55, 280–81
sex life and, 258–59
heart failure, 77–79, 88, 169, 199, 200
heart failure with preserved ejection
     fraction (HFpEF), 78–79, 199, 211
heart failure with reduced ejection
     fraction, 211
heart rate

and exercise, 59, 287, 291–92
  monitors, 199, 287, 291–92
  POTS (postural orthostatic tachycar-
    dia syndrome), 80–81
  resting, 291, 292, 295
  slow, 292, 295
  tachycardia, 78
heart scanning techniques, 320
heart stents, 84, 88, 114, 321
heart surgery, 92, 295
heart transplant, 88
heart valve infections, 295
heart valve replacement, 87
heartburn, 223, 300, 306–7
heel problems, 318
hemarthrosis, 128
hemoglobin A1c, 296, 302
hemp seeds, 9
hepatitis, 4
hepatitis B, 166, 246
hepatitis C, 165, 246, 301
herbs, 115, 233
high blood pressure. *See also* blood
     pressure
  aneurysm and, 90
  contributors to
    alcohol use, 213, 214
    eye strokes, 73
    hormone therapy, 169
  DASH diet for, 256
  diagnosing, 58
  family history and, 155
  inflammation and, 10
  magnesium and, 62
  medications, 48, 50–53, 79
  migraines and, 231
  pre-eclampsia and, 170
  in pregnancy, 237
  resistant hypertension, 53–54, 57
  secondary hypertension, 56–57
  strength training and, 61
  yoga and, 60
high cholesterol. *See* cholesterol
high-glycemic diet, 102
high glycemic load, 123
high-intensity interval training (HIIT),
     171, 201–4, 254–55
high-resistance inspiratory muscle
     strength training (IMST), 57, 270
high-sensitivity C-reactive protein
     (hsCRP) test, 11
hiking, 184–85
hip pain, 128–30
HIV (human immunodeficiency) virus,
     246, 301, 316
holmium laser enucleation of prostate
     (HoLEP), 248
homocysteine, 300
honey, sugar in, 82
hormone therapy, 169–70, 174, 220, 221
  for prostate cancer, 175–76
hormones

decrease in menopause, 221
  levels of, 165
hot flashes, 176, 220, 221, 224
HPV (human papillomavirus) vaccine,
     165, 166
hyaluronic acid, 233
hydration, 268–69, 309
hydrochlorothiazide, 59
hydrophilic statins, 64
hyperaldosteronism, 56
hypermobile Ehlers Danlos syndrome,
     80
hyperplasia, 168, 236
hypertension. *See* high blood pressure
hypertrophic cardiomyopathy, 71
hypofractionated radiation therapy, 175
hypoglycemia (low blood sugar), 303
hypotension, orthostatic, 80, 140, 318.
     See also low blood pressure
hypothyroidism, 141, 295

ibuprofen, 5, 6, 13, 54, 135, 146, 152, 260
iliotibial band syndrome, 198
imaging tests, 320–21
immunosupressants, 13–14
implantable cardioverter defribillator
     (ICD), 294
incidentalomas, 320
inclisiran (Leqvio), 60, 62
incontinence, urinary, 233–34
indigestion, 223
Indocin (indomethacin), 5
infections. *See specific infections*
infertility, 212
inflammation, 111, 225
  acute, 13
  chronic, 4–6
  Crohn's disease, 15
  diet preventing, 7–9, 11, 16, 105, 171,
     266
  diseases linked to, 4–5
  exercise and, 201
  history of, 4–5
  medication and, 13–14, 63
  microbiome and, 16–17
  weight and, 165
inflammatory arthritis, 5–6
inflammatory bowel disease (IBD), 4, 13
  causes of, 15
  management of, 15
  types and symptoms of, 14–15
inflixima (Remicade), 11, 14
injuries
  exercise related, 197–98
  from falls, 70
inner ear conditions, 307, 318
insomnia, 36, 221, 284
insulin, 123, 124, 165, 200, 294, 296, 302,
     304, 318
insulin resistance, 102, 123, 165
intensity-modulated radiation therapy
     (IMRT), 174

intermittent fasting, 266
interval training, 171, 184, 199–200, 201–4
interval walking, 181
intraductal papillomas, 168
intrinsic factor, 300
inverse psoriasis, 18
inversions, 60
irisin, 24
iron, 99, 223–25
irritable bowel syndrome, 259
isolated systolic hypertension, 58
isometric exercises, 61
itching, 140, 152

Jalyn, 249, 250
Jardiance, 79, 304
Janus kinase (JAK) inhibitors, 6
jogging, 179, 194
joint fusion, 147
joint pain, 5–6, 30
joint replacement, 147

kidney cancer, 165
kidney disease, 4, 180, 264
kidney function, 300
kidney stones, 268
kidneys
    creatinine levels, 163
    renal artery stenosis and, 56
    water consumption and, 268
knee lift, 192
knee pain or injury, 128–34, 138

lansoprazole (Prevacid), 306
lateral epicondylitis (tennis elbow), 138, 198
laughter, 272
laundry basket carry, 196
laxatives, 261
LDL (bad) cholesterol. See cholesterol
leafy green vegetables, 9, 106, 116, 121, 122, 224
leaky gut, 15
leaky heart valve, 72, 73
lecanemab, 34
left atrial appendage (LLAA), 91
left-sided heart failure, 77–79
left ventricular hypertrophy, 199
leg pain
legumes, 8, 82, 121–23, 160, 170
leptin, 240
Levitra, 257
levothyroxine (Synthroid, Tirosint), 305
lidocaine, 152, 257
life expectancy, 173, 265–66
lifestyle choices, 5, 13–15, 18, 53–54, 58, 86, 122, 141, 152, 164–66, 170, 173, 200, 216, 234, 247–48, 256, 266
lifting and carrying ability, 61, 144
light therapy, 145

lightheadedness. See dizziness
linoleic acid, 139
lipid test (lipid profile), 73
lipids, 240
lipophilic statins, 64
lipoprotein(a), 72
lisinopril, 52
listening, 218
liver, fat in, 202, 240
liver cancer, 156, 165–67, 214
liver disease, 165, 166, 214, 246, 264
liver function, 300, 304
loaded carries, for core strength, 196–97
longevity, 87, 265–66, 269, 273
Lopressor, 59, 308
lorazepam (Ativan), 308
Lou Gehrig's disease, 36
lovastatin (Altoprev), 64
low blood pressure, 49, 58, 140
low-carb diets, 241, 304
low glycemic load, 123
low-impact exercises, 130
Lp(a), 72
lung cancer, 4, 161, 166, 167
lung cancer screening, 163
lung function, 320
lung transplant, 88
lunges, 202, 263
lupus, 4, 10
lycopene, 171
Lyme disease, 292

macular degeneration, 4, 186, 318
magnesium, 62, 106, 121, 223
mammogram, 163–65, 167, 168, 220
maple syrup, sugar in, 82
masking devices, 309, 310
meat, 96, 99, 110–11, 160, 170, 173, 224
medial epicondylitis, 198
medical appointments, 162–63, 314–16
medical errors, 304–5
medications. See also specific medications
    for Alzheimer's disease, 33–36, 256
    anti-clotting, 87, 91, 92, 194, 292
    balance risk and, 318
    benign prostatic hyperplasia (BPH), 248, 250
    blood pressure. See blood pressure medications
    cardiac rehab and, 88
    for chest pain, 84
    cholesterol, 48, 59–63, 66, 73, 76, 120, 216, 321
    for diabetes, 303–5
    diverticulosis and, 260
    drug interactions, 162, 305
    edema and, 236–37
    effect on concentration, 30
    for erectile dysfunction (ED), 172, 248, 249, 252–53, 256, 257
    errors with, 304–5

heart rate and, 292
home delivery of, 312–14
incontinence and, 234
instructions for taking, 305
memory loss and, 41–42
missing doses, 314, 315
for older adults, 87
for pain relief, 135, 136, 142, 146–47
for premature ejaculation, 257
prostate cancer and, 249, 250
reminders for taking, 285
sexual enhancement products and, 243
for shingles, 152
side effects, 163, 176, 223, 234, 236–37, 252, 254, 279, 305–9
statins. See statins
for urinary problems, 247–50, 254, 308
meditation, 60, 127, 173, 247, 281, 290
Mediterranean diet, 7–8, 16, 32, 105, 160, 162, 164, 170, 173, 240
medium glycemic load, 123
melanoma, 164, 167
melatonin, 308
memory
    brain fog, 41–42, 219–21, 292
    cardiovascular exercise and, 24
    maximizing, 30
    vitamin B12 deficiency and, 224
memory enhancers, 284–86
memory lapses, 43
memory loss. See also Alzheimer's disease; dementia
    common memory situations, 43–44
    medications and, 41–42
    stroke and, 51, 163
    vitamin B12 and, 300
Ménière's disease, 318
meninges, 140
meningitis, 15, 312
menopause, 212
    brain fog and, 219–21
    depression in, 219, 221, 224
    exercise and, 221, 224
    hormone therapy and, 170, 220–22, 236
    migraines and, 231
    perimenopausal bleeding, 235–36
    sleep disruptors in, 221, 224
    strokes and early, 232
    symptoms of, 176, 220, 221, 224
    vaginal laser therapy in, 226
menstruation, 223, 235–36
mental health. See anxiety; depression; stress
mental stress ischemia, 85–86
metformin (Glucophage, Riomet), 303, 305
methotrexate (Rheumatrex, Trexall), 6, 11, 14
microbiome, 16–17, 102

microvascular disease, 85
migraines, 40, 126, 139, 231
milk, 155
mind body awareness, 280–81
MIND diet, 173
mindfulness, 30, 127, 181–82, 256, 290,
    309–10, 332–33
mindset, 22–23
ministrokes, 92–94
mirabegron (Myrbetriq), 234
mitochondria, 186
monk fruit sweetener, 108–9
monoclonal antibodies, 34–35
mononucleosis, 80
monounsaturated fats, 105, 113, 118, 240
Motrin. See ibuprofen
mouth, cancer of, 214, 246
MRI (magnetic resonance imaging) scan
    for breast implant screening, 228
    for fat measurement, 242
    for heart, 320
    for prostate screening, 173, 244, 248
multiple sclerosis, 4
multitargeted stool DNA (mt-sDNA)
    test, 159
multivitamins, 155, 223
muscle aches, from statins, 66
muscle strengthening, 191, 262–63. See
    also strength training
MUSE (medicated urethral system for
    erection) therapy, 252
music, 173
    brain health and, 32
    tinnitus management and, 309, 310
musical instrument, playing for brain
    health, 32
myofascial release, 133

nails, melanoma and, 164
names, remembering, 43
napping, 46
naproxen, 5, 54, 135, 146, 260
nausea
    chest pain and, 211, 212
    from medications, 305
nephritis, 4
neurogenesis, 24
neuroinflammation, 36
Neurontin, 42, 142, 308
neuropathy, 139, 318
neuroticisn, 258
night sweats, 224
night vision, 316–17
nitrates, 108, 110, 116, 259
nitric oxide, 57, 116
nitrites, 108, 110
nocebo effect, 66
noise pollution, 41
nonalcoholic fatty liver disease, 75
noncontact boxing, 188
Nordic walking, 181
norepinephrine, 80

nortriptyline (Aventyl, Pamelor), 42
NSAIDs. See also aspirin; ibuprofen;
    naproxen
    for arthritis pain, 6, 128, 146
    for back pain, 135
    development of, 4–5
    diverticulosis and, 260
    health risks from, 15, 53, 54
    for inflammation, 11, 13–14
nutrition labels, 98, 100, 108, 109
nuts, 8, 9, 82, 105, 113, 119, 121–23, 164,
    170, 261

oat milk, 155
oatmeal, 118, 261
obesity and overweight, 96
    body mass index (BMI) and, 75,
        241–42
    diabetes and prediabetes and, 302–3
    diverticulosis and, 260
    fitness trackers and, 289
    health risks from, 75, 211, 220, 240,
        301, 302
    incontinence and, 233
    medical appointments, 315
    processed foods and, 82
    surgery for, 223
olive oil, 82, 105, 113, 170, 278
omega-3 fatty acids, 9, 139, 171, 225
omega-6 fatty acids, 139
omeprazole (Prilosec, Zegeride), 70, 306
open heart surgery, 92
opiates, 260
opioids, 42, 288, 318
optimism, 22–23
organic produce, 98
Ornish Reversal Program, 88
orthostatic hypotension, 80, 140, 318
orthotics, 149, 198
osteoarthritis, 6–8, 126–29, 132, 145–47
osteoclasts, 121
osteopenia, 122
osteoporosis, 122, 163, 246, 305
ovarian cancer, 165
ovaries, removal of, 232
overactive bladder, 308
overweight. See obesity and overweight
oxybutrin (Ditropan), 234
oxygen, 180, 186
oxytocin, 23

P-tau levels, 34
pacemakers, 294
pain
    acute, 134–35
    at-home management of, 126–27
    back, 126, 134–37, 196
    bursitis, 128
    chronic, 126, 136
    foot and ankle, 149–50, 182, 197
    gout, 6–8, 14, 128
    hand, 128, 145–48

headache, 140
hip, 128–30
joint, 128–31
knee, 128–34, 138
leg, 141
muscle, from statins, 66
osteoarthritis, 126–29
shingles, 150–52, 163, 313
shoulder, 142–44
small-fiber neuropathy, 139–42
pain relief devices, 144–45, 288–90
painkillers, 308
    acetaminophen (Tylenol), 54, 128, 152
    memory loss and, 42
    NSAIDs. See NSAIDs
    opioid, 42, 288, 318
    OTC, 128, 152
    topical, 142, 146
palm oil, 82, 112
pancreas, 4, 161, 302, 304
pancreatic cancer, 4, 161, 167, 246
Pap test, 163, 165
parasites, 15
parathyroid gland, 121
Parkinson's disease, 4, 23, 223
paroxetine (Paxil), 257, 308
passwords, 44
patellofemoral pain, 131
Paxil, 257, 308
PCSK9 inhibitors, 60, 62
peanut oil, 113
pelvic floor exercises, 234
pelvic floor physical therapy, 227
penile band (ED ring), 252
penile cancer, 166
pericarditis, 72
peridontal disease, 19–20
perimenopausal bleeding, 235–36
peripheral artery disease (PAD), 141, 300
personal trainers, 263
pessary, 227, 234
PET (positron emission tomography)
    scan, 244
phenols, 105
phenylephrine, 53
phosphorus, 121, 122
phototherapy (light therapy), 17–18
phthalates, 166
physical activity. See exercise(s)
phytochemicals, 8, 161
pickleball, 188, 189
pistachios, 9
pitavastatin (Livalo), 64
pizza crust, 109–10
placebo, 66, 225, 230
placental abruption, 237
plank (exercise), 196, 202
plant-based diets, 110–11, 170, 172, 223,
    224, 255
plant stanols, 120–21
plantar fasciitis, 150, 182
plaque. See arterial plaque

plaque psoriasis, 18
plastics, 166
platelet rich plasma (PRP) injections, 137–38
platelets, in blood clots, 69, 70
pneumococcal conjugate vaccines (PCVs), 312
pneumonia, 163, 312
polypharmacy, 42, 87
polyphenols, 45
polyps
    colon, 159, 165, 245
    uterine, 235, 236
polyunsaturated fats, 113, 118, 240
positive attitude, 33
postbiotics, 102
posterior vaginal prolapse, 227
postherpetic neuralgia, 150
posture, 136
potassium, 56, 58, 106, 107, 121, 163, 223
potatoes, 101, 124
POTS (postural orthostatic tachycardia syndrome), 80–81
pravastatin (Pravachol), 64
pre-eclampsia, 170
prebiotics, 16–17, 102, 104
prediabetes, 246, 301–3
prednisone, 13
pregabalin (Lyrica), 142
pregnancy
    adverse outcomes, 237
    iron in, 223
Premarin, 222
premature ejaculation, 257
premature heart contractions, 69–71
Prempro, 222
prescription delivery, 312–14
preterm birth, 237
pretzel stretch, 130
Prevacid, 306
priapism, 252
Prilosec, 70, 306
primary care doctors, 162
probiotics, 16, 102
processed foods, 14, 82, 96, 100, 108, 110, 111, 121, 160, 173. See also ultra-processed foods
proliferative lesions, 167
prolonged grief disorder, 261–62
prostaglandins, 5, 6, 13
prostate artery embolization (PAE), 249
prostate cancer
    diet and food choices, 170–71, 255
    erectile dysfunction and, 172, 176
    exercise and, 171, 173
    monitoring, 172–73, 175
    predicting risk of, 172–73
    PSA levels and, 172, 173, 176, 243–44, 250
    screening for, 163, 243–44
    sexual function and, 176
    treatments for, 173–76, 249

prostate enlargement, 244, 247–50
prostate specific membrane antigen (PSMA), 244
prostatectomy, 173, 175, 176
prostatic urethral lift, 249
proteins, 8, 35, 82, 108, 117, 122, 143, 240, 241, 263
    structure of, 297
proton beam therapy, 174–75
proton pump inhibitors (PPIs), 70, 223, 306–7
Prozac, 257, 308
PSA (prostate specific antigen) testing, 163, 173, 174, 176, 243–44, 246
pseudogout, 6
psoriasis, 4, 10, 17–18, 225
psoriatic arthritis, 4, 6, 10
psychomotor speed, 63
pulmonary embolism, 319
pulsating pupil, 72, 73
pumpkin seeds, 9
pupils, 317
purpose, sense of, 180, 273

quadriceps stretch, 130, 133

radial artery, 83–84
radial scars, 168
radiation exposure, from imaging tests, 216, 320
radiation therapy, for prostate cancer, 173–75
radiofrequency (RF), 145
radon, 166
raloxifene (Evista), 169
racquet sports, 188
raspberries, 9
reading glasses, 187
rectocele, 227
rectum, 174, 175
red blood cells, 99, 223, 224, 300
red wine, 213, 214
relationship stress, 217–19
relaxation techniques, 86, 135, 219, 270, 281, 315
renal artery stenosis, 56
repetitive strain injuries, 198, 207
resistance training, 240, 241
resistant hypertension, 53–54, 57
resistant starches, 124
respiratory health, 105
restaurant eating, 101
resting heart rate, 291, 292, 295
restless legs syndrome, 30
retina, 727–73
retinal degeneration, 4
retrograde ejaculation, 248, 249
Rezum, 249
rheumatic disease, 128
rheumatoid arthritis (RA), 4, 5, 10–11, 13, 225
rilonscept (Arcalyst), 72

rivoxaban (Xarelto), 92
rosuvastatin (Crestor), 64
rotator cuff injuries, 142–44
rowing and paddling, 206–8
rowing machines, 130
running, 197, 198
running shoes, 183, 197

sacubitril, 79
safflower oil, 82, 113
salt, 11, 110
    blood pressure and, 52, 53, 57, 58, 62, 82, 114–16
    in canned and frozen foods, 81, 100
    edema and, 238
    low-salt diet, 114
    on nutrition labels, 109
    POTS (postural orthostatic tachycardia syndrome) and, 80, 81
    weight gain and, 79
saturated fat, 82, 105, 108–10, 117, 118, 121, 172
    limiting, 112–13
    list in selected foods, 113
sausage, 108
sclerosing adenosis, 168
sedatives, 308, 318
sedentary lifestyle. See sittiing
seeds, 8, 9, 121, 122, 261
seizures, 71
selective estrogen receptor modulators (SERMs), 169
selective serotonin reuptake inhibitors. See SSRIs
self-care, 219
self-forgiveness, 276–77
seltzer, 109
sensitivity, teeth, 279
sertraline (Zoloft), 257, 308
serving sizes, 82, 161
sexual enhancement products, 243
sexual function
    exercise and, 264
    heart disease and, 258–59
    new ways of thinking about, 275–76
sexual problems, 219, 221, 257, 258
    erectile dysfunction (ED), 172, 248, 249, 252–53, 255, 257, 275
SGLT-2 inhibitors, 76, 79, 303–4
shingles, 150–52, 163, 313
Shingrix vaccine, 151–52, 313
shoes
    choosing, 197–98, 319
    ill fitting, 318
    walking, 130, 181–83
short-chain fatty acids, 102
shortness of breath, chest pain and, 211, 212
shoulders, 142–43
side-leg raise, 132
sildenafil (Viagra, Revatio), 256, 257
silent stroke, 51, 74–76, 90, 292

silodosin (Rapaflo), 248
simvastatin (Zocor), 64
single-leg lift, 132
sinus problems and infections, 312
sit-to-stand exercise, 190
sitting, health risks from, 44, 180, 200, 201
16/8 method, 266
skin cancer, 4, 122, 154, 170, 243
skin care
    collagen supplement and, 228-30
    edema and, 238
sleep
    amount needed, 46, 166, 219
    bedtime and wake time and, 32, 45, 274
    brain health and, 46
    for concentration, 29-30
    exercise and, 264
    for heart health, 88, 256
    improving quality of, 283-84
    medications, 42, 308, 318
    naps, 46
sleep apnea, 30, 53, 56, 246, 256, 295
sleep education therapy (SET), 36
slow heart rate, 292, 295
small-fiber neuropathy, 139-42
SMART (Specific, Measurable, Achievable, Relevant, and Time Based) exercise strategy, 178-79
smart watches, 294-96
smartphone apps, 31, 286, 288
    for sleep, 283-84
smiling, 272
smoking, health risks from, 79, 89, 90, 122, 163, 166, 260, 265, 266
snacking, 117, 119-20, 261, 266
social interactions
    brain health and, 32, 44-45
    happiness and, 271
    older adults and, 87, 163
    tinnitus and, 310
    volunteering and, 273
social media
    brain health and, 37-38
    stressful relationships and, 218
socks, 183
soda, consumption of, 96, 109, 111, 123, 160, 234
sodium. See salt
solanezumab, 34
sound machines, 283
soups, 103-4
soy milk, 155, 224
soybean oil, 113
spices, 115-16
spirituality, 40
splinting, 146
squats, 263
SSRIs, 257
stair climbing, 204-6, 258-59
standing side leg lift, 196, 197

starches, 124
statins, 77
    for chest pain, 84
    for cholesterol reduction, 48, 59-63, 73, 216
    nonadherence and, 65
    side effects of, 62-66
stationary bikes, 130, 187, 194-95, 255
Stendra, 257
stents. See heart stents
step-up exercises, 204-6
stereotactic body radiation therapy (SBRT), 175
steroid drugs, 56, 236
stomach acid, 306
stomach cancer, 156
stomach ulcers, 69
stone fruits, 107
stool softeners, 261
stool tests, for colon cancer screening, 158, 159, 245
strawberries, 9
strength training, 61, 128, 198, 201, 262-63
stress
    breathing exercises and, 269-70
    caregiving and, 217, 218
    heart disease risk and, 85-86
    psoriasis and, 17
    relationships and, 217-19
    stroke and, 91
    tinnitus and, 310
Stress Management and Resilience Training (SMART) program, 86
stress reduction
    for brain health, 45-46
    for heart health, 256
    for pain relief, 290
    techniques, 207
stress tests, 85, 203, 237
stretching, 61
    exercises for, 130, 133, 143
    for muscle aches, 66, 131
    for shoulders, 143, 144
strokes
    cancer risk and, 161
    hemorrhagic, 232
    ischemic, 68, 91, 232
    risk factors for
        alcohol use, 213, 214
        atrial fibrillation, 91, 92, 292
        blood clots, 9, 73, 75, 91
        blood pressure, 68
        diabetes, 302
        early menopause, 232
        eye (ocular) strokes, 73
        gum disease, 19
        high blood pressure, 50-51, 74
        high cholesterol, 74
        high homocysteine, 300
        hormone therapy, 169
        ministrokes, 92-94

overweight, 75
    silent heart attacks and, 74-76, 292
    stress, 91
    risk reduction methods
        dietary, 82, 105, 114
        exercise, 156, 200
        tea and coffee consumption, 45
    silent, 51, 74-76, 90, 292
    symptoms of, 90, 93
subcutaneous fat, 75, 240, 242
sugar
    carbohydrates, 123
    limiting, 82
    monk fruit sweetener vs., 108-9
    names for, 82
    on nutrition labels, 109
sugar cycle, 119
sugary drinks, 82, 96, 109, 111, 160, 173
suicide, 262
suitcase carry, 197
sun protection, 122, 154, 208
sunflower oil, 101
sunflower seeds, 9
sunrise alarm, 283
support groups
    fitness, 178
    online, 127
supraventricular tachycardia (SVT), 78
swimming, 129, 130, 137, 188, 195, 197, 198, 199
sympathomimetics, 234
synuclein, 23
systemic lupus erythematosus, 10

tachycardia, 78
tadalafil (Cialis), 248, 250, 257
tai chi, 128, 130, 143, 188, 192, 311, 319
tamoxifen (Novaldex), 169
tamsulosin (Flomax), 248-50
tandem standing, 311
target heart rate, 204
tau tangles, 35-36
tea, 45, 268
tear production, 205
tendinitis, 128, 147, 198, 207
tennis, 188, 195, 198
tennis elbow, 198
testicular cancer, 246
testosterone
    low, 262
    prostate cancer and, 175
tetanus, 163
thirst, 268
three-dimensional conformal radiation therapy (3D-CRT), 174
throat cancer, 214
thyroid cancer, 165, 246
thyroid disorders, 56, 225, 264, 292, 295, 305
thyroiditix, 4

tinnitus, 28
tips for managing, 309–10
TNF-alfa inhibitors, 11
toenails
ingrown, 149–50
melanoma and, 164
tofacitinib (Xeljanz), 6, 14
tomatoes, 170–72
tooth loss, 33, 278
toremifene (Fareston), 169
tracking devices, 285–86
transcatheter aortic valve replacement (TAVR), 87
transcutaneous electrical nerve stimulation (TENS), 145
transient ischemic attacks (TIAs), 92–94
transradial angioplasty, 83–84
transurethral resection of prostate (TURP), 248, 249
triglycerides, 73, 176
trimethylamine N-oxide (TMAO), 111
Tylenol, 54, 128, 152

ulcerative colitis, 4, 15, 223
ulnar artery, 84
ultra-processed foods, 82, 240–41.
See also processed foods
ultrasound, 69, 73, 228, 236, 246, 248
under-desk cycling machines, 195
unsaturated fats, 82, 113, 117, 118, 164
urethra, 231, 233, 234, 247–49, 252
urethral bulking agents, 234
uric acid, 6, 7, 14
urinary dribbling, 234, 247
urinary incontinence, 172, 233–34, 247
urinary symptom score, 251
urinary tract infections (UTIs)
causes of, 231–32
dehydration and, 231–32, 268
medications and, 304
prevention of, 232–33
symptoms and treatment of, 232, 254, 308
urinary urgency and frequency, 232, 234
urine, hydration and, 268
UroLift, 249
urological medications, 308
uterine cancer, 156, 167, 236
uterine fibroids, 235, 236
uterus, 235
uveitis, 4

vaccines, 151–52, 163, 232, 312, 313
vacuum pump, 253
vaginal cancer, 165, 166
vaginal dryness, 224, 226, 275
vaginal laser therapy, 226
vagus nerve, 270
valacyclovir (Valtrex), 151
Valium, 308
valsartan, 79
vaporization, BPH and, 248

vardenafil (Levitra), 257
Vazalore, 71
vegan diet, 160, 224
vegetables, 8, 9, 117, 164
cruciferous, 161, 170
diverticulosis and, 260
fiber in, 106
in heart healthy diet, 81, 96–97, 104–7, 121–23, 160, 255, 261
in Mediterranean diet, 160
servings of, 106–7
in soups, 103–4
stir fry, 101
storage of, 98
vegetarian foods, 99, 100, 110, 160, 224
venous insufficiency, 236, 238
venous thromboembolism (VTE), 319
ventricular fibrillation (v fib), 78
ventricular tachycardia (VT), 78
vertigo, 307, 318
Viagra, 256, 257
vinegars, 116
virtual reality (VR), 288–90
visceral fat, 75, 240, 242
VITAL study, 154
vitamin A, 18, 107
vitamin B12
testing and, 300
vitamin B6 deficiency, 141
vitamin B12 deficiency, 141, 223–25, 300
vitamin C, 106-7, 117
vitamin D, 121, 122, 143
deficiency, 66, 134, 154–55, 223–25, 246, 300, 321
testing and, 300–301
vitamin E, 161
volunteering, 271, 273–74
vulvar cancer, 166

waist size, 241, 242
wake time, depression and, 32
walk-and-carry exercise, 196–97
walking, 179, 272, 300, 319
gait, 310, 311
health benefits of, 87, 122, 126, 129, 130, 156, 190, 197–201
hiking, 184–85
intensities of, 180, 201
interval, 181
leg pain and, 141
mindful, 181–82
Nordic, 181
shoes for, 130, 182–83
speed and aging and, 310, 311
timing and, 130, 178, 190, 201
walnuts, 9
warfarin (Coumadin), 92
Watchman, 91–92
water consumption, 80, 81, 109, 198, 227, 231, 232, 268–69, 309
water vapor thermal therapy, 249
weight gain

cancer and, 165
high-glycemic diet and, 102
osteoarthritis and, 128
pandemic and, 163
prostate cancer and, 173
psoriasis and, 17
seasonal, 52
weight lifting, 61
weight loss, exercise and, 200, 241
weight training, 122, 129, 241, 262–63
weighted blankets, 283
white blood cells, 9, 300
white-coat syndrome, 246
white matter, 51
whole foods, 119
whole grains, 8, 82, 96, 101, 103–5, 117, 122, 123, 160, 161, 164, 170, 261
wine, 213, 214
wooziness. *See* dizziness
wrists, 148

xanthelasmas, 73–74
Xarelto, 92

yoga, 60, 126, 128, 143, 179, 187, 198, 261, 280–81, 303, 319
yogurt, 224

Zoloft, 257, 308
zolpidem (Ambien), 42, 308
Zostavax, 151–52
Zostrix, 152